STUDY GUIDE TO ACCOMPANY
BRUNNER AND SUDDARTH'S TEXTBOOK OF

Medical-Surgical
Nursing EIGHTH EDITION

STUDY GUIDE TO ACCOMPANY
BRUNNER AND SUDDARTH'S TEXTBOOK OF

Medical-Surgical Nursing EIGHTH EDITION

Mary Jo Boyer, R.N., D.N.Sc.
Associate Dean
Allied Health and Nursing
Delaware County Community College
Media, Pennsylvania

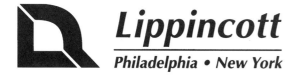

Lippincott
Philadelphia • New York

Acquisitions Editor: Lisa Stead
Assistant Editor: Brian MacDonald
Project Editor: Tom Gibbons
Production Manager: Helen Ewan
Production Coordinator: Kathryn Rule
Design Coordinator: Melissa Olson

8th Edition

ISBN: 0-397-55230-0

The material contained in this volume was submitted as previously unpublished material, except in the instances in which credit has been given to the source from which some of the illustrative material was derived.

Any procedure or practice described in this book should be applied by the health-care practitioner under appropriate supervision in accordance with professional standards of care used with regard to the unique circumstances that apply in each practice situation. Care has been taken to confirm the accuracy of information presented and to describe generally accepted practices. However, the authors, editors, and publisher cannot accept any responsibility for errors or omissions or for any consequences from application of the information in this book and make no warranty, express or implied, with respect to the contents of the book.

The authors and publisher has exerted every effort to ensure that drug selection and dosage set forth in this text are in accordance with current recommendations and practice at the time of publication. However, in view of ongoing research, changes in government regulations, and the constant flow of information relating to drug therapy and drug reactions, the reader is urged to check the package insert for each drug for any change in indications and dosage and for added warnings and precautions. This is particularly important when the recommended agent is a new or infrequently employed drug.

Materials appearing in this book prepared by individuals as part of their official duties as U.S. Government employees are not covered by the above-mentioned copyright.

9 8 7 6 5 4 3 2 1

This book is dedicated to my family, Bill, Brian, and Susan

Preface

The *Study Guide to Brunner and Suddarth's Textbook of Medical-Surgical Nursing, Eighth Edition,* was developed as a learning tool to help you, a nursing student, focus on content areas considered essential for understanding the concepts, techniques, and disease processes presented in the textbook. A Critical Thinking approach was used to present facts from a knowledge-based level (using multiple-choice, matching, fill-in and crossword puzzles) to the highest levels of analysis and synthesis (using comparison analysis, pattern identification, contradiction recognition, supportive argumentation, and clinical problem solving). The application of theory to practice is tested by having you complete nursing care plans, outline detailed patient teaching guides, and complete decision-making trees and critical clinical pathways. Case studies are offered at the end of most sections.

The answer to every question is presented in the Answer Key at the end of the book and referenced to a page number in the textbook so you can clarify or reinforce information as necessary. Critical thinking, the nursing process, and a community-based focus to nursing care are incorporated throughout; information is tested from the viewpoint of nursing intervention. Pathophysiologic processes are included only if relevant to specific nursing actions.

It was my intent to present information in a manner that will stimulate critical thinking and promote learning. It is my hope that knowledge gained and reinforced will be used to provide competent nursing care to those in need.

Mary Jo Boyer, R.N., D.N.Sc.

Acknowledgments   Special thanks to Kathy Campitelli who carefully typed every page and to the staff of Lippincott-Raven Publishers who pulled everything together.

Contents

UNIT 1
Health Maintenance and Health Needs

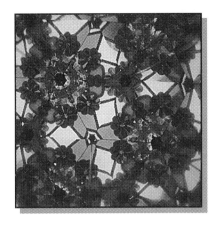

1

Health Care Delivery and Nursing Practice

Chapter Overview

Nursing is a caring-oriented, scientific health profession that helps people to maintain and promote health as well as to prevent illness. Various conceptual models serve as a framework for nursing practice. Basic to all models is the belief that a person is a holistic organism entitled to, and responsible for, an optimum state of health. The modalities of nursing intervention differ slightly among the various conceptual models, but all recognize the science of nursing, its role in research and theory development, and its goal of illness prevention and wellness promotion.

I. Knowledge-Based Questions

Deduction and Interpretation

Read each question carefully. Circle your answer.

1. Several definitions of nursing are currently being accepted. The main theme among all is that registered nurses can and should:
   a. diagnose health alterations and prescribe specific nursing interventions.
   b. promote optimum levels of wellness and prevent illness.
   c. maintain health and assist patients with the dying process.
   d. do all of the above.

2. The appropriate focus for any definition of nursing is the registered nurse's responsibility to:
   a. appraise and enhance an individual's health-seeking perspective.
   b. coordinate a patient's total health management with all disciplines.
   c. diagnose acute pathology.
   d. treat acute clinical reactions to chronic illness.

3. To view a person holistically means to think of him or her conceptually as a:
   a. physical being who experiences pathophysiologic changes.
   b. social being who needs the dynamics of group interaction.
   c. psychological being whose mind influences his or her health status.
   d. biopsychosocial being who is in constant interaction with his or her environment.

4. A Jewish patient who adheres to the dietary laws of his faith is in traction and confined to bed. He needs assistance with his evening meal of chicken, rice, beans, a roll, and a carton of milk. Choose the nursing approach that is most representative of the concept of holism.

 Mary Jo Boyer: Study Guide to Accompany Brunner & Suddarth's Textbook of Medical-Surgical Nursing, 8th ed. © 1996 Lippincott-Raven Publishers

a. Nurse "A" removes items from the overbed table to make room for the dinner tray.

b. Nurse "B" pushes the overbed table toward the bed so that it will be within the patient's reach when the dinner tray arrives.

c. Nurse "C" asks a family member to assist the patient with the tray and the overbed table while she straightens the area in an attempt to provide a pleasant atmosphere for eating.

d. Nurse "D" prepares the environment and the overbed table and inspects the contents of the dinner tray. She asks the patient if he would like to make any substitutions in the foods and fluids he has received.

5. Using the concept of the wellness–illness continuum, a nursing care plan for a chronically ill patient would outline steps to:

a. educate the patient about every possible complication associated with the specific illness.

b. encourage positive health characteristics within the limits of the specific illness.

c. limit all activities because of the progressive deterioration associated with all chronic illnesses.

d. recommend activity beyond the scope of tolerance to prevent early deterioration.

6. A nurse who assesses a patient's psychosocial reaction to illness as being below his or her developmental level would be referencing information to the theories propounded by:

a. E. Erikson.

b. R. Havighurst.

c. J. Piaget.

d. H. Selye

7. Choose the infectious disease that is *not* currently increasing in frequency.

a. AIDS

b. Chickenpox

c. Sexually transmitted diseases

d. Tuberculosis

8. The diagnosis-related groups (DRGs) legislation enacted in 1983 provides for:

a. a fixed rate of Medicare payment, per diagnosis, for hospital services.

b. a retrospective method of reimbursement based on a patient's length of stay.

c. all hospital and extended-care costs (nursing homes, home care) per diagnosis if the hospital participates with a peer review organization (PRO).

d. total reimbursement per diagnosis for as long as the patient requires hospitalization (as long as the patient is eligible for Medicare benefits).

9. To be responsive to the changing health care needs of our society, registered nurses will need to:

a. focus their care on the traditional disease-oriented approach to patient care because hospitalized patients today are more acutely ill than they were 10 years ago.

b. learn how to delegate discharge planning to ancillary personnel so that RNs can spend their time managing the "high-tech" equipment needed for patient care.

c. place increasing emphasis on wellness, health promotion, and self-care, since the majority of Americans today suffer from chronic debilitative illness.

d. stress the curative aspects of illness, especially the acute, infectious disease processes.

10. Certification for registered nursing practice is:

a. mandatory for nurses working in specialty areas.

b. offered by the state boards of nursing at the time a graduate writes for licensure.

c. required in all states after a nurse has been practicing for 5 years.

d. suggested by the ANA as a way of validating expertise in clinical practice.

11. The primary focus of the nurse advocacy role in managing a clinical pathway is:

a. continuity of care.

b. cost-containment practices.

c. effective utilization of services.

d. patient's progress toward desired outcomes.

12. Nursing practice in the home and community requires competence and experience in the techniques of:
   a. decision making.
   b. health teaching.
   c. physical assessment.
   d. all of the above.

Read each statement carefully. Write your response in the space provided.

1. It is expected that most nursing practice in the next 5 years will be in community and long-term care settings. This movement reflects legislature and sociologic changes consistent with:

_____   _____

_____   _____

2. According to the Social Policy Statement of the American Nurses' Association (ANA), nursing practice involves the *diagnosis and treatment of human responses to actual or potential health problems.* Choose three health problems and write a human response to each that would require nursing intervention.

Problem	*Human Response Needing Nursing Health Intervention*
a. Fractured right arm	Self-care limitations
b. _____	_____
c. _____	_____
d. _____	_____

3. You are currently a student in a nursing program. You have many demands on your time and you are coping with multiple stressors. List three activities that you can do now to promote positive behaviors directed toward your health and well-being:

a. _____   b. _____

c. _____

4. Managed health care of the 1990s has resulted in:

a. _____   c. _____

b. _____   d. _____

5. Explain the expanded role of the independent nurse practitioner.

_____

_____

6. State the major purpose of the nurse practice acts.

_____

7. List Maslow's hierarchy of needs and give an example for each need.

Need   *Example*

8. List the purpose and goals of case management.

_____

_____

9. Define the term _clinical pathway_ as it relates to the concept of managed care.

_____

_____

_____

II. Critical Analysis Questions

Supporting Arguments

Read the paragraph below. Fill in the space provided with the best response.

Compare the purpose, focus, and characteristics of a job versus a career/profession. Choose four values that you believe represent the profession of nursing. List an activity that you can do now as a student nurse that will reflect each of those values.
(reference readings pp. 8–9)

Values Essential to Nursing Profession	_An Activity that Reflects the Value_
1. Honesty (example)	Document objectively and accurately
2.	
3.	
4.	
5.	

Read the paragraph below. Fill in the space provided with the best response.

Four factors significantly impact on nursing care delivery and nursing education: (a) the aging population, (b) the changing pattern of diseases, (c) the rising cost of health care, and (d) federally legislated health care reform. Choose one factor that you believe has the _most impact_ on changing nursing care and support your argument with data.
(reference readings pp. 9–12)

Most important factor is: _____

Supporting arguments

1. _____

2. _____

3. _____

Recognizing Contradictions

Rewrite each statement correctly. Underline the key concepts.

1. A person with a chronic illness can never attain a high level of wellness because part of his health potential will never be reached.

2. The majority of health problems in the United States today are of an infectious and acute nature.

3. It is predicted that by the year 2000, the elderly in the United States will constitute about 10% of the total population.

4. According to the American Hospital Association (AHA) Patient's Bill of Rights, a patient may not refuse medical and nursing care if the lack of care may endanger health and safety.

5. It is predicted that health care costs will be 11% of the gross national product (GNP) by 2000.

Generating Solutions: Clinical Problem Solving

Complete the following flow charts.

1. Hoffman (1972) states, " . . . the single most important factor in health is lifestyle." Complete this clinical map to illustrate how one lifestyle habit (smoking) can result in illness.

Smoking   **Illnesses**

          ↓ciliary action   ⎫   _____

Respiratory   ↑_____   =   ⎬   _____

Changes   ↑_____   ⎭   _____

           Cardiovascular ⎫   ↑CO levels

           Change   ⎬   ↑_____

                         ⎭   ↑_____

2. Continuous quality improvement (CQI) mandates the standardization of processes that are implemented and improved on a continuous basis. Complete the blank lines on the flow chart for the process of radial pulse assessment.

Radial Pulse Assessment

1.0	2.0	3.0	4.0	5.0
Patient ID	Explain Procedure	Identify Site	Palpate Pulse	Document Results

1.1 ID Patient

1.2 _____

_____

1.3 _____

2.1 Give instruction at level of patient's learning.

3.1 Extend forearm

3.2 _____

_____

4.1 Place pads of index and middle finger over radial artery.

4.2 _____

_____

4.3 _____

_____

_____

4.4 _____

_____

_____

5.1 Note rate and character.

5.2 _____

_____

_____

5.3 _____

_____

_____

_____

2

Community-Based Nursing Practice

Chapter Overview

Since 1984, with the advent of Diagnosis-Related Groups (DRGs), the United States has been moving slowly toward a cost containment model of health care delivery. The response from private and corporate providers of care has been slow and resistive. However, since 1992, managed care providers have rapidly and significantly changed health care delivery in America by reimbursing for treatment for only specific time periods, and, in many cases, only for specific physicians.

This rapidly changing health care finance reform movement has caused an eruption in community-based practice and an exodus of patients, nurses, and physicians from hospital-based practice. Nursing needs to respond to these challenges by becoming expert clinicians, who can independently assess, refer, and manage a variety of patient care situations.

I. Knowledge-Based Questions

Deduction and Interpretation

Read each question carefully. Circle your answer.

1. The shift in health care delivery from acute care to community-based care is primarily the result of:
   a. alternate health care delivery systems.
   b. changes in federal legislation.
   c. tighter insurance regulations.
   d. the interfacing of all three conditions.

2. Choose an alternative health care delivery system that has dramatically reduced patient care days in acute care settings.
   a. Health Maintenance Organizations
   b. Managed Health Care Systems
   c. Preferred Provider Organizations
   d. Each of the three is equally significant.

3. The most frequent users of home health services are:
   a. children with chronic, debilitating disorders.
   b. newborns who are sent home with apnea monitors.
   c. the frail and elderly who need skilled care.
   d. young adults on prolonged IV therapy.

4. The majority of home care expenditures are funded by:
   a. direct patient payments.
   b. Medicaid.
   c. Medicare.
   d. private insurance companies.

5. Discharge planning for home care begins when the:
   a. family is ready to care for the patient.
   b. patient is admitted.
   c. physician writes an official medical diagnosis.
   d. social worker drafts a discharge plan.

6. Home care visits are made by nurses who work for:
   a. hospital-based home care.
   b. public health agencies.
   c. visiting nurse associations.
   d. all of the above type of agencies.

Read each statement carefully. Write your response in the space provided.

1. List specific skills a nurse will need to function in community-based care:

_____

_____

2. The first step in preparing for a home visit is for the nurse to: _____

_____

3. Explain the purpose of the initial home visit: _____

_____

4. List some examples of ambulatory health care settings: _____

_____

5. Name several subspecialities for nurse practitioners: _____

_____

3

Critical Thinking and the Nursing Process

Chapter Overview

The nursing process is a systematic way of providing care that is goal-directed, organized, and capable of being evaluated. The process evolved out of society's demand for a structured approach to the delivery of health care. Its format is correlated with the steps of the scientific method of problem solving. The components of the process—assessment, diagnosis (nursing diagnosis and collaborative problems), planning, implementation, and evaluation—serve as an outline for nursing activity. Nurses are encouraged to use these components to identify basic needs and problems, diagnose, formulate a course of action, perform suggested activities, and evaluate outcome behaviors. The process provides a framework for the justification and validation of nursing care.

I. Knowledge-Based Questions

Deduction and Interpretation

Read each question carefully. Circle your answer.

1. Assessment begins with initial patient contact. Nursing activities during this component of the nursing process include:
   a. interviewing and obtaining a nursing history.
   b. observing for altered symptomatology.
   c. collecting and analyzing data.
   d. all of the above.

2. The end result of data analysis is:
   a. actualization of the plan of care.
   b. determination of the patient's responses to care.
   c. collecting and analyzing data.
   d. identification of actual or potential health problems.

3. A therapeutic communication technique that validates what the nurse believes to be the main idea of an interaction is known as:
   a. acknowledgment.
   b. focusing.
   c. restating.
   d. summarizing.

4. An example of a medical diagnosis, in contrast to a nursing diagnosis, is:
   a. fever of unknown origin.
   b. fluid volume excess.
   c. ineffective-breathing patterns.
   d. sleep pattern disturbances.

5. Choose the nursing action that illustrates planned nursing care prioritized according to Maslow's hierarchy of needs. A nurse would:

a. administer pain medication to an orthopedic patient 30 minutes before transportation to physical therapy for crutch-walking exercises.

b. discourage a terminally ill patient from participating in a plan of care, to minimize fears about death.

c. help a patient walk to the shower while the breakfast tray waits on the overbed table because the shower area is vacant at this time.

d. interrupt a family's visit with a depressed patient to assess blood pressure measurement because it is the scheduled time to take vital signs.

6. Consider the following nursing diagnosis: "Altered nutrition, less than body requirements, related to inability to feed self." An example of an immediate nursing goal is that the patient will:

a. acquire competence in managing cookware designed for handicapped people.

b. assume independent responsibility for meeting self-nutrition needs.

c. learn about food products that require minimal preparation yet meet individual needs for a balanced diet.

d. master the use of special eating utensils to feed self.

7. Nurses are expected to write "outcomes" for all nursing interventions. Outcomes must meet all of the following criteria *except* that they are:

a. measurable.

b. met within the critical time period of 24 to 48 hours.

c. realistic.

d. written in terms of the patient's behavior.

8. Teaching a patient how to self-administer insulin is an example of that component of the nursing process known as:

a. assessment.

b. planning.

c. implementation.

d. evaluation.

9. Registered nurses are responsible for delegating patient care responsibilities to licensed practical nurses (LPNs) and ancillary personnel. The most appropriate task to delegate to a nurse aide is:

a. assessing the degree of lower leg edema in a bed rest patient.

b. making the bed of an ambulatory patient.

c. measuring the circumference of a patient's calf for edema.

d. recording the size and appearance of a bedsore.

10. The basis or framework used to evaluate the patient's response to nursing intervention can be found in the nursing:

a. care plan.

b. diagnosis.

c. goals.

d. interventions.

Read each statement carefully. Write your response in the space provided.

1. Discuss four functions of the nurse's role during the patient interview, a significant component of the nursing process.

_____

_____

_____

_____

2. Suggest an opening statement that a nurse can use during the interview process.

_____

_____

3. Explain the purpose of a complete health assessment.

_____

_____

_____

4. Discuss how formulation of a nursing diagnosis and identification of collaborative problems differs from a medical diagnosis.

_____

_____

_____

5. Write the official definition of *nursing diagnosis* as adopted by NANDA in 1990.

_____

_____

_____

6. Discuss the significance of using outcome criteria during the evaluation phase of the nursing process.

_____

_____

_____

II. Critical Analysis Questions

Generating Solutions: Clinical Problem Solving

Read each nursing diagnosis. Write a specific outcome.

The Planning Phase of the nursing process incorporates documented expected patient outcomes for specific nursing diagnoses (ND). Write one outcome that indicates an improvement for each diagnosis.

1. ND: Activity intolerance, related to dyspnea.

*Outcome:*_____

2. ND: Impaired physical mobility, related to total hip replacement.

*Outcome:*_____

3. ND: Fluid volume excess, related to compromised cardiac output.

*Outcome:*_____

4. ND: Altered nutrition, less than body requirements, related to anorexia.

*Outcome:*_____

5. ND: Sleep pattern disturbance, related to pain.

*Outcome:*_____

Read each statement below. Put an "N" in front of every nursing diagnosis and a "C" in front of every collaborative problem.

1. _____ Anxiety related to impending surgery.

2. _____ Constipation related to altered nutrition.

3. _____ Potential complication: paralytic ileus secondary to postoperative inactivity.

4. _____ Potential complication: sacral decubiti secondary to bedrest.

5. _____ Potential Impairment of Skin Integrity related to prolonged bedrest.

6. _____ Ineffective Breastfeeding related to fear of discomfort.

7. _____ Potential complication: hypoglycemia related to inadequate food intake.

8. _____ Potential complication: phlebitis related to intravenous therapy.

9. _____ Post-Trauma Response related to accident.

10. _____ Potential complication: oral lesions related to chemotherapy.

4

Health Education and Health Promotion

Chapter Overview

People have a right to be aware of all aspects of their health and its care. Nursing, as a health-oriented profession, has an obligation to participate in patient health teaching whenever possible. Statistics from nursing research show that structured health-teaching programs have resulted in modified patient behavior and improved health status. Patient education is so vital that many state nurse practice acts have included health teaching as a nursing responsibility. Therefore, it is up to every nurse to identify opportunities for patient education and to modify each program to meet individual needs and goals.

I. Knowledge-Based Questions

Deduction and Interpretation

Read each question carefully. Circle your answer.

1. Patient health education is:
   a. a primary nursing responsibility.
   b. an essential component of nursing care.
   c. an independent nursing function.
   d. consistent with all of the above.

2. Nursing responsibilities associated with patient teaching include:
   a. determining individual needs for teaching.
   b. motivating each person to learn.
   c. presenting information at the level of the learner.
   d. all of the above.

3. Nursing actions that can be used to motivate a patient to learn include all of the following *except:*
   a. feedback in the form of constructive encouragement when a person has been unsuccessful in the learning process.
   b. negative criticism when the patient is unsuccessful, so that inappropriate behavior patterns will not be learned.
   c. the creation of a positive atmosphere in which the patient is encouraged to express anxiety.
   d. the establishment of realistic learning goals based on individual needs.

4. A nurse assesses that a patient is emotionally ready to learn when the patient:
   a. has accepted the therapeutic regimen.
   b. is motivated.
   c. recognizes the need to learn.
   d. demonstrates all of the above.

5. Normal aging affects changes in cognition. Therefore, when teaching an elderly patient how to administer insulin, the nurse should:

   a. repeat the information frequently for reinforcement.
   b. present all the information at one time so that the patient is not confused by pieces of information.
   c. speed up the demonstration because the patient will tire easily.
   d. do all of the above.

6. The nurse reviews a medication administration calendar with an elderly patient. Being aware of sensory changes associated with aging, the nurse should:

   a. print directions in large, bold type, preferably using black ink.
   b. highlight or shade important dates and times with contrasting colors.
   c. use several different colors to emphasize special dates.
   d. do all of the above.

7. A nursing action(s) that involves modifying a teaching program because a learner is not experientially ready is:

   a. changing the wording in a teaching pamphlet so that a patient with a fourth-grade reading level can understand it.
   b. contacting family members to assist in goal development to help stimulate motivation.
   c. postponing a teaching session with a patient until pain has subsided.
   d. all of the above.

8. A nurse identifies a patient's inability to pour a liquid medication into a measuring spoon. This diagnosis is part of the nursing process known as:

   a. assessment.
   b. planning.
   c. implementation.
   d. evaluation.

9. A nurse develops a program of increased ambulation for a patient with an orthopedic disorder. This goal setting is a component of the nursing process known as:

   a. assessment.
   b. planning.
   c. implementation.
   d. evaluation.

10. Outcome criteria are expressed as expected outcomes of patient behavior resulting from teaching strategies. An example is:

    a. ability to climb a flight of stairs without experiencing difficulty in breathing.
    b. altered lifestyle resulting from inadequate lung expansion.
    c. inadequate ventilation associated with pulmonary congestion.
    d. potential oxygenation deficit related to ventilatory insufficiency.

Read each statement carefully. Write the best response in the space provided.

1. Explain why health education is so essential for those with chronic illness.

   _____

   _____

2. Define the term *adherence* as it relates to a person's therapeutic regimen.

   _____

   _____

3. Name several variables (factors) that influence a person's ability to adhere to a program of care.

   _____

   _____

4. Describe the nature of the teaching–learning process.

_____

_____

5. Discuss how learner readiness affects a learner and the learning situation.

_____

_____

6. Discuss the relation between the nursing process and the teaching–learning process.

_____

_____

II. Critical Analysis Questions

Recognizing Contradictions

Rewrite each statement correctly. Underline the key concepts.

1. Health education is a dependent function of nursing that requires physician approval.

2. The largest groups of people in need of health education today are children and those with infectious diseases.

3. Patients are encouraged to evidence compliance with their therapeutic regimen.

4. Evaluation, the final step in the teaching process, should be summative (done at the end of the teaching process).

5

Ethical Issues in Medical–Surgical Nursing

Chapter Overview

The complexity of contemporary ethical issues in medical–surgical nursing can be correlated with the explosion of scientific discoveries and the development of sophisticated technology, whereby life (and the dying process) can be prolonged, sometimes indefinitely. The rapidly changing health care delivery system directly impacts on the professional nurse, who must expand her practitioner role to include analytical decision-making processes relative to ethical and moral situations. Nurses of today and tomorrow need to learn how to articulate ethical issues and function as change agents in a rapidly expanding health care environment.

I. Knowledge-Based Questions

Deduction and Interpretation

Read each question carefully. Circle your answer.

1. *Morality* is defined as:
   a. adherence to specific codes of conduct.
   b. commitment to an individual value system.
   c. dependence on specified principles of behavior.
   d. understanding of defined rules of behavior.

2. *Descriptive ethics* is an approach to studying ethics that is concerned with:
   a. choosing the morally correct course of behavior.
   b. deciding what one "should do."
   c. identifying various beliefs and behaviors.
   d. understanding what is meant by "good."

3. Choose the situation that *most accurately* represents a *moral problem* in contrast to a *moral dilemma*.
   a. A 3-day postoperative patient requests narcotic pain medication every 3 hours. The nurse administers a placebo that reduces pain.
   b. A 32-year-old father of three with advanced cancer of the lung asks that everything be done to prolong his life, even though his treatments are no longer effective.
   c. A confused 80-year-old needs restraints for protection from injury even though the restraints increase agitation.
   d. A young patient with AIDS has asked not to receive tube feedings to prolong life because of intense pain.

4. When an ethical decision is made based on the reasoning that "good consequences will outweigh bad consequence," the nurse is following the:
   a. deontological theory.
   b. formalist theory.
   c. moral justification theory.
   d. utilitarian theory.

5. Consider the ethical situation in which a nurse moves a confused, disruptive patient to a private room at the end of the hall so that other patients can rest, even though the confused patient becomes more agitated. The nurse's judgment is consistent with reasoning based on:
   a. "consequentialism," by which good consequences for the greatest number are maximized.
   b. "duty of obligation," by which an action, regardless of its results, is justified if the decision making was based on moral principles.
   c. "prima facie" duty, by which an action is justified if it does not conflict with a stronger duty.
   d. the "categorical imperative," by which the results of an action are deemed less important than the means to the end.

6. A hospital board of directors decided to close a pediatric burn treatment center (BTC) that annually admits 50 patients and to open a treatment center for terminally ill AIDS patients (expected annual admission of 200). This decision meant that the nearest BTC for children was 300 miles away. The board's decision was an example of ethical reasoning consistent with:
   a. a formalist approach.
   b. obligation or duty.
   c. "the means justifies the end."
   d. utilitarianism.

7. A terminally ill patient asks the nurse if she is dying. The nurse's response is influenced by the moral obligation to:
   a. communicate the patient's wishes to the family.
   b. consult with the physician.
   c. provide correct information to the patient, to "not lie."
   d. consider all of the above measures before disclosing specific information.

8. A patient with a "Do Not Resuscitate" order requires large doses of a narcotic (which may significantly reduce respiratory function) for excruciating pain. After the patient requested pain medication, the nurse assessed a respiratory rate of 12 breaths per minute. The nurse's ethical decision should be to:
   a. ask the patient to wait 20 minutes and reassess the respiratory rate.
   b. give one-half the prescribed dose.
   c. give the pain medication without fear of respiratory depression.
   d. withhold the pain medication and contact the physician.

Read each statement carefully. Write your response in the space provided.

1. Explain what is meant by a moral dilemma.

   _____

   _____

2. *Ethical pluralism* refers to _____

   _____

   _____

3. Explain the basis for ethical behaviors based on "virtues."

   _____

   _____

4. List two types of "advanced directives," or legal documents that specify a patient's wishes before hospitalization.

   _____   _____

5. Explain the merit of having an "advanced directive."

   _____

Match the definitions of ethical principles listed in Column II with its associated term listed in Column I.

Column I

1. _____ autonomy
2. _____ beneficence
3. _____ justice
4. _____ nonmaleficence
5. _____ paternalism
6. _____ veracity

Column II

a. limiting one's autonomy based on the welfare of another

b. all similar cases should be treated the same

c. the commitment not to deceive

d. freedom of choice

e. the duty to do good and not inflict harm

f. the expectation that harm will not be done

II. Critical Analysis Questions

Analyzing Comparisons

Read each analogy. Fill in the space provided with the best response.

1. Ethics: formal study of beliefs :: Morality: _____

2. Descriptive ethics: understanding behaviors :: Metaethics: _____

3. Applied ethics: morally correct decision-making :: _____

   analyzing a specific course of action.

4. Teleological theory: principle-based behavior ::

   Virtue ethics: _____

Recognizing Contradictions

Rewrite each statement correctly and underline the key concepts.

1. Nursing ethics is considered an applied form of medical ethics because nurses only work under physician direction.

2. A moral dilemma, in contrast to a moral problem, infers no conflict of moral principle.

3. A nurse experiences *moral uncertainty* when he is prevented from doing what he believes is the correct action.

4. A nurse should always honor a terminally ill patient's request to withhold food and hydration if the patient is competent.

5. Living wills, by design, are very prescriptive and are always honored as legally binding documents.

Supporting Arguments

Read each situation. Offer logical supporting arguments for your response.

1. In vitro fertilization, the result of sophisticated technology, has resulted in women in their 50s (and one 62-year-old woman) giving birth. Physicians argue that this is ethically sound if the woman meets the criteria that she is healthy and should live another 25 years. List three rationales to support this argument:

   1. _____

   2. _____

   3. _____

2. You are asked to defend the statement that "life support measures should never be used for anyone with a terminal illness." Develop three supporting arguments.

   1. _____

   2. _____

   3. _____

3. List two rationales to support the argument that age should be used as a criterion for determining the allocation of health care resources.

   1. _____

   2. _____

Generating Solutions: Clinical Problem Solving

Read the following case study. Fill in the blanks below.

CASE STUDY: Ethical Analysis

You are an RN and a board member of the American Red Cross Disaster Relief Services. A cholera epidemic has erupted among thousands of refugees in Rwanda. The board has been asked to decide how to allocate limited resources. The board decided that healthy children, those without symptoms of cholera, would be transported out of the camps and treated at an alternative location. The decision resulted in fewer medical personnel at the camp sites where about 50 children a day were dying; in fact, some orphaned children died crawling up the steps of the clinic to seek help. The framework for decision making followed the *teleological* or *utilitarian approach*. Use the "Steps of an Ethical Analysis," page 59 (Chart 5–3) as a guide, and complete your decision-making process to determine if you agree or disagree with the outcomes.

Assessment

1. List two possible conflicts between ethical principles and professional obligations:

   a. _____

   b. _____

2. People involved in decision making   Those affected by decision

   a. _____   a. _____

   b. _____   b. _____

                                                c. _____

Planning

1. Treatment options   Medical facts

    a. _____   a. _____

    b. _____   b. _____

2. Influencing information

    a. _____

    b. _____

3. Ethical/moral issues   Competing claims

    a. _____   a. _____

    b. _____   b. _____

Implementation

Compare the utilitarian and deantological approach.

Utilitarian   **Deontological**

1. Basis of ethical principles

    a. _____   a. _____

    b. _____   b. _____

2. Predict consequences of actions

    a. _____   a. _____

    b. _____   b. _____

3. Assign a positive or negative value to each consequence.

    a. _____   a. _____

    b. _____   b. _____

4. Choose the consequence, decision, or action that predicts the highest positive value.

    _____

Evaluation

1. The best, morally correct action is to: _____

_____

2. This decision is based on the ethical reasoning that: _____

_____

3. The decision can be defended based on the following arguments.

    a. _____

    b. _____

    c. _____

Learner's Self-Evaluation Tool for End of Unit 1 Review

1. The most important concepts or facts I have learned from this unit are:

   1. _____

   2. _____

   3. _____

2. The most important reference page numbers for test review and clinical concepts are pages:

   _____   _____   _____

   _____   _____   _____

3. The concepts or facts that I do not fully understand are:

   _____

   _____

4. I will get the answer(s) to my questions by _____

   _____

   I will do this on _____ (date and time).

5. I believe my mastery of this unit to be:

   a. 100%   Great job! Good luck!

   b. 90%   2 hours of review recommended.

   c. 80%   4 hours of review recommended.

   d. <80%   Make an appointment with your instructor.

UNIT 2
Health Assessment of the Client/Patient

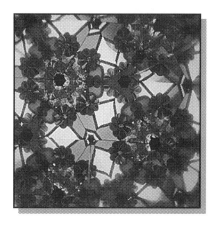

6

Clinical Interviewing: The Health History

Chapter Overview

The clinical interview is a vital part of the assessment component of the nursing process. Nurses obtain data through the interview and the physical examination in order to determine the patient's needs and nursing diagnoses and to develop plans of care based on the nursing diagnoses. Thus, individual needs can be met through systematic delivery of nursing care.

The clinical interview provides an opportunity for establishing a trusting relationship between the nurse and the patient. This trusting relationship lays the foundation for future nursing intervention throughout the patient's cycle of wellness and illness.

I. Knowledge-Based Questions

Deduction and Interpretation

Read each question carefully. Circle your answer.

1. The clinical interview obtained by the nurse should focus on nursing's concern about:
   a. a comprehensive body systems review.
   b. current and past health problems.
   c. family history.
   d. all of the above.

2. A patient has certain rights concerning data collection, such as the right to know:
   a. how information will be used.
   b. that selected information will be held confidential.
   c. why information is sought.
   d. all of the above.

3. Open-ended questions permit persons to express themselves. Choose the sentence that is *not* an open-ended question.
   a. "Describe the pain."
   b. "Tell me more about your feelings."
   c. "How did the accident happen?"
   d. "Is the pain sharp and piercing?"

4. An *inappropriate* interviewer response to the patient statement, "I will not take pain medication when I'm in pain" is:
   a. "Is there another way you have learned to lessen pain when you experience it?"
   b. "Let a nurse know when you're in pain so you can be helped to decrease stimuli that may exaggerate your pain experience."
   c. "Refusing medication can only hurt you by increasing your awareness of the pain experience."
   d. "You have the right to make that decision. How can the nurses help you cope with your pain?"

5. The *single* most important factor in helping the nurse and physician arrive at a diagnosis is the:
  a. family history.
  b. history of the present illness.
  c. past health history.
  d. results of the systems review.

6. Tinnitus and vertigo are assessed during a systems review of the:
  a. ears.
  b. mouth and throat.
  c. nose and sinuses.
  d. skin.

7. Anorexia and hematemesis are symptoms associated with dysfunction of the:
  a. cardiovascular system.
  b. gastrointestinal system.
  c. genitourinary system.
  d. musculoskeletal system.

8. Choose the best question an interviewer would use to obtain educational or occupational information.
  a. "Are you a blue-collar worker?"
  b. "Do you have difficulty meeting your financial commitments?"
  c. "Is your income more than $20,000 per year?"
  d. "What college did you attend?"

9. All of the following are questions that will provide information about a person's lifestyle *except*:
  a. "Do you have any food preferences?"
  b. "Have you always lived in this geographic area?"
  c. "How many hours of sleep do you require each day?"
  d. "What type of exercise do you prefer?"

10. When obtaining a health history from an elderly patient, the nurse must remember to:
  a. ask questions slowly, directly, and in a voice loud enough to be heard by those who are hearing-impaired.
  b. clarify the frequency, severity, and history of signs and symptoms of the present illness.
  c. conduct the interview in a calm, unrushed manner using eye-to-eye contact.
  d. do all of the above.

Read each statement carefully. Write your response in the space provided.

1. Describe how the nursing database differs from the physician's database.

_____

_____

_____

2. Describe the concept of interdependence as it relates to health professionals.

_____

_____

_____

3. Explain how mutual trust and confidence between the interviewer and the patient facilitate the communication process.

_____

_____

4. Differentiate between an inquiring and a therapeutic mode of interviewing.

_____

_____

5. Define the term *chief complaint*.

_____

_____

6. Discuss the focus of information gathering for the patient profile.

_____

_____

II. Critical Analysis Questions

Recognizing Contradictions

Rewrite each statement correctly. Underline the key concepts.

1. According to current health care practices, patient needs and problems are diagnosed only by physicians.

2. During the interview process, verbal communication is more accurate than nonverbal communication.

3. During the interview process, the patient needs to assume a dominant leadership role.

4. It is important during the interview process to document, word for word, information that is necessary for the nursing care plan.

5. The most personal area of assessment on the patient profile is the section on lifestyle.

6. A person's ability to handle stressful situations is influenced by present coping patterns.

7
Physical Assessment and Nutritional Assessment

Chapter Overview

The physical examination is a vital part of nursing assessment. Frequently, inspection, palpation, percussion, and auscultation are necessary to identify symptoms and relate them to pathology. The physical examination provides an atmosphere of intimacy in which the nurse and the patient can exchange information that might not have been shared in a less personal interaction. During the examination, both obvious and hidden needs can be identified, and nursing diagnoses can be developed. This hands-on process is an essential part of nursing assessment that permits validation of stated problems and provides an opportunity to identify new areas of concern that can be met through nursing interventions.

FACT:

- *American Institute for Cancer Research (AICR) toll-free Nutrition Hotline is 1-800-843-8114, Monday through Friday, 9:00 AM to 5:00 PM, Eastern time. Callbacks are guaranteed within 48 hours.*

I. Knowledge-Based Questions

Deduction and Interpretation

Read each question carefully. Circle your answer.

1. On initial impression the nurse assesses a patient's posture, stature, and body movements. This assessment is part of the physical examination process known as:
   a. auscultation.
   b. inspection.
   c. palpation.
   d. percussion.

2. When assessing body temperature variations, it is important to note that most persons achieve their lowest temperature recordings between:
   a. 7:00 AM and 9:00 AM.
   b. 10:00 AM and 12:00 noon.
   c. 1:00 PM and 3:00 PM.
   d. 4:00 PM and 6:00 PM.

3. During a physical examination, the nurse noted hyperresonance over inflated lung tissue in a patient with emphysema. The process used for this assessment was:
   a. auscultation.
   b. inspection.
   c. palpation.
   d. percussion.

4. An examiner needs to determine the upper border of a patient's liver. With the patient in the recumbent position, the examiner would percuss for a:
- a. dull sound.
- b. flat sound.
- c. resonant sound.
- d. tympanic sound.

5. A heart murmur was detected during a physical examination. The process used to obtain this information was:
- a. auscultation.
- b. inspection.
- c. palpation.
- d. percussion.

6. When assessing nutritional intake, the nurse knows that an adult should have a daily intake of:
- a. 1 cup of milk.
- b. 1 ounce of meat.
- c. one serving of fruit.
- d. six servings of bread, rice, or pasta.

7. Peanut butter is a popular food that is classified under the _____ food group.
- a. milk
- b. meat
- c. bread
- d. miscellaneous

8. The triceps skin-fold thickness measurement is a good indicator of protein–calorie malnutrition. The standard female measurement is:
- a. 13.5 mm.
- b. 15.0 mm.
- c. 16.5 mm.
- d. 18.0 mm.

9. A serum albumin level of 2.50 g/dl indicates:
- a. a severe protein deficiency.
- b. low levels of serum protein.
- c. an acceptable amount of protein.
- d. an extremely high measurement of protein.

10. Several factors contribute to the altered nutritional status of the elderly. A *primary nutritional nursing consideration* during physical assessment is:
- a. altered metabolism and nutrient use secondary to an acute or chronic illness.
- b. decreased appetite related to loneliness.
- c. limited financial resources.
- d. the patient's ability to shop for and prepare food.

Match the body area listed in Column II with the descriptive sign of poor nutrition listed in Column I.

Column I	Column II
1. _____ atrophic papillae	**a.** abdomen
2. _____ brittle, dull, depigmented	**b.** eyes
3. _____ cheilosis	**c.** hair
4. _____ flaccid, underdeveloped	**d.** lips
5. _____ fluorosis	**e.** muscles
6. _____ xerophthalmia	**f.** skeleton
	g. teeth
	h. tongue

Read each statement carefully. Write your response in the space provided.

1. Identify two major techniques used to assess the integumentary system.

_____   _____

2. Three health problems related to dietary excess that contribute to the leading causes of illness and death in the United States today are: _____, _____, and _____.

3. The most common anthropometric measurements include height, weight, and the circumference of the
_____, _____, and
_____.

4. Explain the concept of *negative nitrogen balance.*

_____

_____

5. Because the elderly are sensitive to nutritional alterations, the goal of diet therapy is to _____
_____.

Correlate the following statements with the assessment most likely used to obtain the data. Write the word or code on the line provided.

Code:

INS—inspection   PER—percussion
PAL—palpation   AUS—auscultation

1. Asymmetry of movement is associated with a central nervous system disorder. _____

2. Clubbing of the fingers is a diagnostic symptom of chronic pulmonary disorders. _____

3. Tenderness is present in the area of the thyroid isthmus. _____

4. Tactile fremitus is diagnostic of lung consolidation. _____

5. Tympanic or drumlike sounds are produced by pneumothorax. _____

6. The first heart sound is created by the simultaneous closure of the mitral and tricuspid valves. _____

_____

7. A friction rub is present with pericarditis._____

8. Nodules present with gout lie adjacent to the joint capsule. _____

II. Critical Analysis Questions

Generating Solutions: Clinical Problem Solving

Read the following case study. Fill in the blanks below.

CASE STUDY: Mrs. Allred

> Part I: Estimate ideal body weight
> Part II: Calculate a balanced diet using the Food Guide Pyramid as a reference

Mrs. Allred is a 40-year-old, 5′ 5″ tall Hispanic with three children under the age of 5. She weighs 180 lb. She had no known previous history of any physical illness before experiencing fatigue and irritability that she believed was the result of her parenting responsibilities. Mrs. Allred does not exercise regularly, eats snack foods while watching TV with her children, and is too tired to prepare balanced meals for her family. She orders fast food or pizza for dinner at least three times a week:

Part I: Estimating ideal body weight

1. Calculate Mrs. Allred's frame size based on a wrist circumference of 16 cm.
  a. small frame
  b. medium frame
                                              c. large frame

2. Calculate Mrs. Allred's ideal body weight (IBW): _____ lb.
Therefore, she needs to (gain/lose) _____ lb. (approximate).

Part II: Calculate a balanced diet for Mrs. Allred's ideal body weight, as determined in Part I. Use the Food Guide Pyramid (Figure 7–7) and Chart 7–1 as a reference. Use the following guidelines.

1. Convert IBW in pounds to kilograms. _____

2. Determine basal energy needs (1 kcal/kg/hr) _____ calories

3. Increase by 40% (moderate activity) _____ calories

4. Divide calories into:

Carbohydrates   (50%) _____

Fat   (30%) _____

Protein   (20%) _____

5. Estimate grams for each:

Carbohydrates _____   Fats _____   Protein _____

6. Patient teaching guidelines:

_____

_____

_____

Learner's Self-Evaluation Tool for End of Unit 2 Review

1. The most important concepts or facts I have learned from this unit are:

1. _____

2. _____

3. _____

2. The most important reference page numbers for test review and clinical concepts are pages:

_____   _____   _____

_____   _____   _____

3. The concepts or facts that I do not fully understand are:

_____

_____

4. I will get the answer(s) to my questions by _____

_____

I will do this on _____ (date and time).

5. I believe my mastery of this unit to be:
   a.   100%   Great job! Good luck!
   b.   90%   2 hours of review recommended.
   c.   80%   4 hours of review recommended.
   d.   <80%   Make an appointment with your instructor.

UNIT 3
Biophysical and Psychosocial Concepts

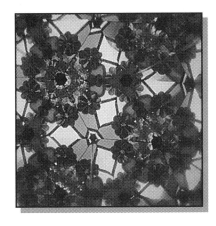

8

Homeostasis and Pathophysiologic Processes

Chapter Overview

Homeostasis is a dynamic state of motion and reaction in which the body attempts to maintain constancy of its internal environment. Negative feedback is one example of the way in which physiologic processes attempt to compensate for deviations. Sometimes the compensatory mechanisms can lead to the death of the organism. When this threat exists, humans intervene with various medical–surgical modalities.

I. Knowledge-Based Questions

Deduction and Interpretation

Read each question carefully. Circle your answer.

1. An example of a functional, yet maladaptive, response of the body to a threat is:
   a. collateral circulation subsequent to diminished tissue perfusion.
   b. decreased cardiac output subsequent to cardiomegaly.
   c. increased pulmonary ventilation subsequent to increased levels of carbon dioxide.
   d. muscle atrophy subsequent to disuse.

2. Health promotion should be initiated before compensatory processes become maladaptive. Preventive nursing measures include all of the following *except*:
   a. demonstrating wound cleansing to a patient who has a necrotic leg ulcer resulting from vascular disease.
   b. showing a patient with a casted extremity how to perform isometric exercises.
   c. suggesting stress-reducing measures for a patient with a diagnosis of angina pectoris.
   d. teaching weight management to a patient who has a family history of obesity and a blood pressure reading of 125/90.

3. Maladaptive compensatory mechanisms result in disease processes in which cells may be:
   a. dead.
   b. diseased.
   c. injured.
   d. affected in all of the above ways.

4. Adaptation to a stressor is positively correlated with:
   a. previous coping mechanisms.
   b. the duration of the stressor.
   c. the severity of the stressor.
   d. all of the above.

5. An example of a negative feedback process is increased:
    a. aldosterone secretion in burn trauma, resulting in excess sodium retention.
    b. cardiac output in hemorrhage, resulting in increased blood loss.
    c. secretion of antidiuretic hormone (ADH) in congestive heart failure, causing increased fluid retention.
    d. secretion of thyroid-stimulating factor (TSF), which stops when circulating thyroxin levels reach normal.

6. A patient experiences lower leg pain associated with lactic acid accumulation (an example of a local response involving a feedback loop). The nurse expects the pain to lessen when:
    a. aerobic metabolism is reinstituted.
    b. anaerobic metabolism becomes the major pathway for energy release.
    c. muscle use and subsequent glucose catabolism increase.
    d. vasoconstriction diminishes blood flow, thereby slowing the removal of waste products.

7. A patient has a diagnosis of hypertrophy of the heart muscle (an example of cellular adaptation to injury). The nurse expects all of the following *except*:
    a. compromised cardiac output.
    b. muscle mass changes evident on radiologic examinations.
    c. cellular alteration compensatory to some stimulus.
    d. decreased cell size, leading to more effective ventricular contractions.

8. Cell injury results when stressors interfere with the body's optimal balance by altering cellular ability to:
    a. grow and reproduce.
    b. synthesize enzymes.
    c. transform energy.
    d. do all of the above.

9. An adult patient's hemoglobin is 7 g/dl. This should alert the nurse to assess for signs and symptoms associated with:
    a. hyperemia.
    b. hypertension.
    c. hypoglycemia.
    d. hypoxia.

10. A diabetic is admitted to the hospital with a blood suger level of 320 mg/dl. The nurse decides to monitor fluid intake and output because:
    a. decreased blood osmolarity causes fluid to shift into the interstitial spaces, resulting in polydipsia.
    b. polydipsia occurs when glucose catabolism is accelerated, thereby increasing the body's need for fluids.
    c. polyuria results from osmotic diuresis, which is compensatory to hyperglycemia.
    d. the blood's hypotonicity will result in tissue fluid retention and weight gain.

11. Nursing care for a patient with a fever is based on all of the following body responses *except* one. Indicate the exception.
    a. Diaphoresis, which is a compensatory mechanism that cools the body.
    b. Increased heart rate, which helps to meet increased metabolic demands.
    c. Increased nutrient catabolism, which will influence the body's caloric needs.
    d. Vasodilation of surface blood vessels, which will prevent excessive heat loss.

12. Anti-infectives are not useful against biologic agents known as:
    a. bacteria.
    b. fungi.
    c. mycoplasmas.
    d. viruses.

13. Viruses are infectious agents that:
    a. burst out of invaded cells to enter other cells.
    b. infect specific cells.
    c. replicate within invaded cells.
    d. do all of the above.

14. Genetic disorders arising from inherited traits include all of the following *except*:
    a. hemophilia.
    b. meningitis.
    c. phenylketonuria.
    d. sickle cell anemia.

15. A nurse who is caring for a patient with a localized response to a bee sting expects symptoms to include all of the following *except*:
    a. blanching due to compensatory vasoconstriction.
    b. hyperemia due to increased blood flow.
    c. pain due to pressure on the nerve endings.
    d. swelling due to increased vascular permeability.

16. While caring for a patient with an infected surgical incision, the nurse observes for signs of a systemic response. These include all of the following *except*:
    a. leukopenia owing to increased white blood cell (WBC) production.
    b. a febrile state caused by the release of pyrogens.
    c. anorexia, malaise, and weakness.
    d. loss of appetite and complaints of aching.

17. A nurse is assigned to care for a patient whose abdominal wound is healing by second intention. The nurse expects to observe:
    a. a clean, dry wound.
    b. approximated edges of the wound.
    c. minimal scar formation.
    d. necrotic material with peripheral granulation tissue.

18. A patient is diagnosed in the emergency department with acute gastritis, and questions the nurse regarding the meaning of the diagnosis. The nurse explains that the diagnosis refers to an inflammation that:
    a. may be present for several weeks to months, depending on the causative organism.
    b. will probably result in permanent epigastric discomfort.
    c. is debilitating and has long-term effects.
    d. will subside with treatment, and normal function will return.

II. Critical Analysis Questions

Analyzing Comparisons

Read each analogy. Fill in the space provided with the best response.

1. Homeostasis: rapid bodily adjustments :: _____ : adjustments over time.

2. Negative feedback: altered action and compensation :: positive feedback: _____

3. Hypertrophy: enlarged muscle mass (e.g., the heart) :: atrophy: _____, (e.g., _____)

4. Acute inflammation: histamine and kinin secretion with increased vascular permeability :: chronic inflammation: _____

Generating Solutions: Clinical Problem Solving

Read the following case study. Fill in the blanks below.

Case Study:

Use the "Representative Pathophysiologic Process: Hypertensive Heart Disease (pp. 103–104) as a guide. Develop a nursing plan of care, using the nursing process as a guide, for each compensatory mechanism. The answers to the first mechanism, decreased renal blood flow, are given in the Answer Key.

- Renin secretion is compensatory to decreased renal blood flow. Renin indirectly leads to sodium and water retention by stimulating the release of aldosterone. This mechanism initially results in increased cardiac output.

Selected Compensatory Mechanisms	Nursing Implications	Rationale
a. Renal blood flow is decreased as a result of hypertensive heart disease.	*Assessment*	
	Nursing Diagnosis/ Collaborative Problem	
	Planning	
	Implementation	
	Evaluation	
b. Arteriole constriction occurs, resulting from renin secretion.		
c. Sodium and water retention occurs subsequent to aldosterone secretion.		
d. Increased cardiac output is due to increased extracellular fluid.		

9

Stress and Adaptation

Chapter Overview

Stress is an essential part of everyday life. Stressors, both physiologic and psychosocial, stimulate us to function within our capabilities and, occasionally, motivate us to achieve beyond our potential. Distress is produced when our bodies cannot adapt to the quantity or the duration of various stressors. With prolonged distress the organism may fail. Nurses need to be able to recognize the influence of stressors and to be aware of interventions that will help people maintain health and adapt to illness. If adaptation is not realistic, the nurse needs to help the patient cope with death.

I. Knowledge-Based Questions

Deduction and Interpretation

Read each question carefully. Circle your answer.

1. Stress is a change state perceived as:
   a. challenging.
   b. damaging.
   c. threatening.
   d. having all of the above characteristics.

2. Elizabeth is newly admitted to the medical unit. She has periodic episodes of shortness of breath and tightness in her throat. She is crying. To evaluate the impact of physiologic and psychological components on her illness, the nurse should:
   a. perform a thorough physical examination and include subjective patient statements as well as objective laboratory data.
   b. focus primary attention on the respiratory system because this is the patient's chief complaint.
   c. determine that the patient is not in acute distress, then perform a complete physical examination and include data about her lifestyle and social relationships.
   d. attempt to discover the reasons behind the patient's anxieties because stress can cause breathing difficulties.

3. During the nursing interview, a patient with shortness of breath reveals that she is in the process of getting a divorce. This information alerts the nurse to *initially*:
   a. try to determine if there is a psychological basis for the physical symptoms.
   b. restrict family members from visiting because their presence may aggravate the patient's symptoms.
   c. teach the patient specific breathing exercises that can be used to manage symptoms.
   d. request that the physician recommend counseling services.

Mary Jo Boyer: Study Guide to Accompany Brunner & Suddarth's Textbook of Medical-Surgical Nursing, 8th ed. © 1996 Lippincott-Raven Publishers

4. An individual's adaptation to stress is influenced by the stressor's:
   a. frequency and duration.
   b. number of occurrences and magnitude.
   c. sequencing (intermittent or enduring).
   d. combined characteristics as listed above.

5. During the initial stress response, *primary appraisal* refers to:
   a. evaluating the effectiveness of several coping mechanisms.
   b. organizing all available resources to deal with the stressor.
   c. identifying support services needed for coping.
   d. weighing the significance of the stressful event.

6. Helen, age 48, is diagnosed with pneumonia. She has been paralyzed from the chest down for 7 years. The nurse realizes that Helen needs additional support to cope with her infection because:
   a. coping measures become less effective with advancing age.
   b. the patient's available coping resources are already being used to manage the problems of immobility.
   c. an acute infectious process requires more adaptive mechanisms than a chronic stressor.
   d. this additional physical stressor places unmanageable demands on the patient's internal and external resources.

7. Helen cooperates, and willingly follows the treatment regimen. The nurse wonders how Helen can project such a positive outlook and cope with additional stress. Helen's ability to cope is probably due to all of the following *except*:
   a. acceptance that "life is not fair" and that people have limited control over their health.
   b. adoption of the problem-focused method of coping.
   c. her ability to draw on past coping behaviors and apply them to new situations.
   d. the support of family and friends who call and visit frequently.

8. A patient is admitted to the emergency department for observation after a minor automobile accident. Based on an understanding of the sympathetic nervous system's response to stress, the nurse would expect to find all of the following during assessment *except*:
   a. a cold, clammy skin.
   b. decreased heart rate.
   c. rapid respirations.
   d. skeletal muscle tension.

9. Physiologically, the sympathoadrenal response results in all of the following *except*:
   a. decreased blood flow to the abdominal viscera.
   b. decreased peripheral vasoconstriction.
   c. increased myocardial contractility.
   d. increased secretion of serum glucose.

10. The hypothalamic–pituitary response is a long-acting physiologic response to stress that involves:
    a. stimulation of the anterior pituitary to produce adrenocorticotropic hormone (ACTH).
    b. the production of cortisol from the adrenal cortex.
    c. protein catabolism and gluconeogenesis.
    d. all of the above mechanisms.

11. A nurse is assigned to care for a patient who is receiving glucocorticoid therapy. The nurse expects all of the following reactions to drug therapy *except*:
    a. glycosuria.
    b. hypernatremia.
    c. hypoglycemia.
    d. lymphopenia.

12. A patient's serum sodium level rises in association with glucocorticoid therapy. The nurse relates this primarily to an increased secretion of:
    a. adrenocorticotropic hormone (ACTH).
    b. antidiuretic hormone (ADH).
    c. thyroxine.
    d. insulin.

13. Prolonged glucocorticoid therapy inhibits the inflammatory response to tissue injury. A laboratory measurement of this is:
    a. increased hemoglobin.
    b. increased lymphocytes.
    c. lowered erythrocyte count.
    d. lowered eosinophil count.

14. Nursing measures to help a person manage some of the factors involved in the stress process include:
    a. eliminating conditions that produce stress.
    b. promoting healthy behavior to avoid stress.
    c. teaching the use of stress-management techniques to control stress.
    d. all of the above.

15. Nursing assessment to determine individual social support systems includes obtaining information about the person's:
    a. belief that he or she belongs to a group that is mutually dependent and communicative.
    b. concept of being cared for and loved.
    c. impression of being esteemed and valued.
    d. perception of all of the above.

16. Mrs. Talbot is scheduled for a breast biopsy in the morning. There is a history of breast malignancy in her family. While caring for her the evening before surgery, your *most appropriate* nursing action would be to:
    a. administer a soothing back massage to promote relaxation and decrease stress.
    b. make sure she eats all of her evening meal because she will be NPO after midnight.
    c. minimize the emotional impact of surgery by encouraging her to socialize with other patients.
    d. sit with her and provide an opportunity for her to talk about her concerns.

Match the primary category of stressors listed in Column II with its associated stressors listed in Column I.

Column I

1. _____ anxieties

2. _____ genetic disorders

3. _____ hypoxia

4. _____ infectious agents

5. _____ life changes

6. _____ nutritional imbalance

7. _____ social relationships

8. _____ trauma

Column II

a. physiologic

b. psychosocial

Read each statement carefully. Write your response in the space provided.

1. The "father of stress" is _____.

2. Define stress according to Hans Selye.

_____

_____

3. Psychosocial stressors are classified as day-to-day occurrences (daily hassles), major events that affect large groups, and those infrequently occurring situations that directly affect a person. List two examples from your personal experiences that could be included under each classification.

    a. Day-to-day occurrences
    a. _____

       _____

    b. Major events that affect large groups of people
    b. _____

       _____

    c. Infrequently occurring major stressors
    c. _____

       _____

4. Discuss the linkage between illness and critical life events.

_____

_____

_____

5. Discuss how internal cognitive processes and external resources are used by an individual to manage stress.

_____

_____

II. Critical Analysis Questions

Generating Solutions: Clinical Problem Solving

Complete the flow chart.

Fill in the physiologic reactions of the body that respond to sympathetic nervous system stimulation and provide the rationale for each reaction.

General body arousal

Rationale

↑Norepinephrine =   ↑_____   _____
                    ↑_____   ↑_____
                    ↑_____   _____
                    ↑_____   ↑_____

↓

Skeletal muscles   _____   ↑_____
Pupils   _____   ↑_____
Ventilation   _____   _____

10
Human Response to Illness

Chapter Overview

Illness is a unique human experience that elicits as many variable responses as there are people. Experiences are influenced by physiologic adaptability, sociocultural exposures, and psychological stability. Responses influence nursing interventions that aim to meet identified needs. Nursing care plans should be specific for each person. Many people can be helped to cope with the illness experience to the best of their potential.

I. Knowledge-Based Questions

Deductions and Interpretation

Read each question carefully. Circle your answer.

1. It took Mr. "A" 3 months to admit that he was sick, in need of medical and nursing care, and to accept his diagnosis of adenocarcinoma of the right kidney. An emotional response you would expect to see associated with this stage of illness is:
   a. shame.
   b. denial.
   c. guilt and shame.
   d. regression.

2. Mr. "B" always attempts to engage the nurses in lengthy conversations. This behavior to establish mutual interest can be a manifestation of the emotional need for:
   a. affection.
   b. control.
   c. inclusion.
   d. safety.

3. An example of a nursing intervention that meets a patient's need for control is:
   a. arranging a set time each day to communicate with the patient for the purpose of mutual need satisfaction.
   b. assigning the patient to a semiprivate room within view of the nursing station.
   c. encouraging the patient to establish a relationship with another patient that is based on mutual liking.
   d. suggesting that the patient assume some responsibility for decision making about his or her plan of care.

4. The groundwork for the formation of body image occurs during the:
   a. formative preschool years.
   b. maturity years of middle adulthood.
   c. sensitive preadolescent years.
   d. volatile adolescent years.

 Mary Jo Boyer: Study Guide to Accompany Brunner & Suddarth's Textbook of Medical-Surgical Nursing, 8th ed. © 1996 Lippincott-Raven Publishers

5. A condition directly related to a person's altered physical perception of self is:
   a. acute gastritis.
   b. anorexia nervosa.
   c. bronchitis.
   d. serious otitis media.

6. The anxiety process model is a valuable tool that nurses can use to help people manage anxiety reactions because it:
   a. correlates emotional reactions to unmet needs.
   b. explores why an expectation did not occur.
   c. identifies effective relief behaviors.
   d. facilitates coping behaviors by using all of the above mechanisms.

7. The nurse suspects that Mr. Cassidy's physiologic changes are related to anxiety about his impending surgery. To confirm the diagnosis, the nurse observes for all of the following *except*:
   a. cold, clammy skin and increased perspiration.
   b. constricted pupils and bradycardia.
   c. thirst associated with a dry mouth.
   d. increased frequency of urination.

8. Mrs. Daily is frustrated and angry with her diagnosis of thrombophlebitis. To ventilate her anger, she is aggressive and argumentative toward her nurses. To develop a care plan, the nurses recognize that Mrs. Daily is evidencing the defense mechanism known as:
   a. displacement.
   b. projection.
   c. regression.
   d. sublimation.

9. A person who experiences pain, anguish, and an acute sense of sadness is most likely in the stage of mourning known as:
   a. awareness.
   b. disbelief.
   c. shock.
   d. restitution.

10. Nursing interventions to help a person deal with denial include:
   a. allowing the patient to use denial when it serves an immediate purpose and is not harmful.
   b. challenging the patient's use of denial as a defense mechanism.
   c. encouraging the use of denial as a satisfactory method of dealing with illness.
   d. supporting the denial behavior, knowing that the patient needs this coping mechanism.

11. A nurse can motivate a patient to participate in self-care by:
   a. providing positive reinforcement through goal attainment.
   b. recalling previous difficulties with self-management so that the patient can learn from his or her failures.
   c. withholding information about illness that might depress the patient.
   d. doing all of the above.

12. A person's perception of illness as a stressor is primarily influenced by:
   a. finances.
   b. intelligence.
   c. occupational status.
   d. previous coping experiences.

13. A nurse decides to assess psychosocial stressors that may be hindering a person's ability to cope with a minor injury. She should assess the:
   a. influence of an associated illness.
   b. patient and his living conditions.
   c. patient's nutritional status.
   d. presence of pain.

14. To examine a patient's mental status, a nurse should:
   a. analyze the way the patient thinks about stress, illness, and adaptive behavior.
   b. observe the patient's present behavior.
   c. obtain a description of the patient's behavior.
   d. do all of the above.

15. When a patient's nonverbal behavior is in conflict with his verbal expressions, there is said to be a breakdown in that segment of the communication network known as:
   a. I, the sender.
   b. the message being communicated.
   c. the situation influencing the content of the communication.
   d. you, the receiver.

16. A communication breakdown will most probably occur if a nurse:

a. anticipates barriers to communication and works out solutions in advance.

b. clarifies facts about an illness with the patient during the patient's denial of that illness.

c. plans a teaching session for a time when the patient is free from pain.

d. presents a teaching program when the patient demonstrates a readiness to learn.

17. Mr. Emory is a difficult patient whose demanding behavior is disruptive to the staff and other patients. The nurse's plan of care should include all of the following *except*:

a. determining unmet patient needs that may be increasing Mr. Emory's anxiety level.

b. examining the nonverbal behavior of other nurses to determine if any staff members are supporting his behavior.

c. identifying the causes that trigger the disturbed feelings.

d. reinforcing present behavior to gain the patient's confidence so that he will listen to suggestions for modifying his actions in the future.

18. A condition that is generally considered to be psychophysiologic is:

a. emphysema.

b. hepatitis.

c. osteoarthritis.

d. peptic ulcer.

19. Mrs. Renton is hospitalized in the final states of metastatic carcinoma. She tells her physician that she will accept her prognosis if he can keep her alive until her grandchild is born in 3 months. Mrs. Renton is in that stage of dying identified by Kubler-Ross as:

a. isolation.

b. anger.

c. bargaining.

d. depression.

II. Critical Analysis Questions

Generating Solutions: Clinical Problem Solving

Read the following case studies. Circle the correct answer.

CASE STUDY: Hodgkin's Disease

Joan, a 29-year-old mother of two, works 20 hours a week as a secretary. She was diagnosed with Hodgkin's disease the week of her 29th birthday.

1. Joan's reaction to the diagnosis was to increase her working time to 40 hours per week and to increase her social activities. Joan's response is characteristic of the:

a. first stage of illness.

b. second stage of illness.

c. third stage of illness.

d. fourth stage of illness.

2. The most prominent emotion you would expect Joan to experience at the time of her diagnosis is:

a. acceptance.

b. denial.

c. depression.

d. guilt.

3. Nursing intervention at the time of the diagnosis *would not include*:

a. answering questions.

b. listening to the patient ventilate.

c. reinforcing reality.

d. supporting denial.

CASE STUDY: Radical Mastectomy

Kathy, a 45-year-old single executive with a major oil company, lives alone in a high-rise city apartment. She is recovering from a right radical mastectomy performed 3 days ago.

1. Kathy is firm about not bathing in the morning because her normal home routine involves a nightly relaxing tub bath. The nurse should:
   a. document in the plan of care that bathing is to take place near bedtime.
   b. explain the clinical routine to Kathy so she will understand the necessity for each patient to comply so that all patients will receive optimum care.
   c. gently remind Kathy that she is not in control in a hospital; the nurses decide when baths will be taken.
   d. give Kathy a choice of morning bath care or evening shower care because staffing on the evening shift is not sufficient to meet her needs.

2. Kathy refuses to acknowledge that her breast was removed. She believes that her breast is intact under the dressings. The nurse should:
   a. call the physician to change the dressings so Kathy can see the incision.
   b. recognize that Kathy is experiencing denial, a normal stage of the grieving process.
   c. reinforce Kathy's belief for several days until her body can adjust to the stress of surgery.
   d. remind Kathy that she needs to accept her diagnosis so that she can begin rehabilitation exercises.

3. Kathy screams at her nurse because the nurse is 10 minutes late administering Kathy's pain medication. The nurse is aware that anger:
   a. is a maladaptive response to a stressful situation.
   b. is an anticipated reaction to a change in body appearance.
   c. should be reinforced to help reality orientation.
   d. should be repressed so that Kathy can gain control of her surroundings.

4. To help Kathy adjust to her altered body image, the nurse should:
   a. offer acceptance.
   b. reinforce Kathy's concept of self-worth.
   c. understand Kathy's emotional responses to her illness and her surgery.
   d. consider all of the above.

11

Transcultural Perspectives in Nursing

Chapter Overview

Our nation and the world are becoming more culturally diverse as the global market expands, as computer technology brings us closer, and as more individuals value the differences among subcultures. Each of us is identified by our customs, beliefs, values, and family traditions. Our challenge in daily living, and in the delivery of nursing care, is to appreciate each other's uniqueness and to learn how to interpret verbal and nonverbal cues so we can all live in harmony.

I. Knowledge-Based Questions

Deduction and Interpretation

Read each question carefully. Circle your answer.

1. Choose the minority group in the United States that *is not* federally recognized as a minority:
   a. African Americans.
   b. Hispanics.
   c. Native Americans.
   d. Islamics.

2. The nursing profession comprises approximately _____ % ethnic or racial minorities:
   a. 5
   b. 9
   c. 13
   d. 20

3. The most common non-English language spoken in the United States is:
   a. German.
   b. French.
   c. Italian.
   d. Spanish.

4. Personal space is a culturally defined phenomenon. In comparing cultures, individuals who require the most personal space between themselves and others would be from:
   a. Japan.
   b. Latin America.
   c. the Middle East.
   d. the United States.

5. Choose the culture that *does not* consider eye contact impolite when speaking with another:
   a. Americans.
   b. Arabs.
   c. Indo-Chinese.
   d. Native Americans.

6. The cultural group that stares at the floor during conversation is the:
   a. Asians.
   b. Appalachians.
   c. Indo-Chinese.
   d. Native Americans.

 Mary Jo Boyer: Study Guide to Accompany Brunner & Suddarth's Textbook of Medical-Surgical Nursing, 8th ed. © 1996 Lippincott-Raven Publishers

7. The cultural group that has a wide frame of reference for attitudes about time is the:
   a. African-Americans.
   b. Arabs.
   c. Native Americans.
   d. Asians.

8. A nurse would expect that a woman from a(n) _____ culture would want only a female physician to examine her.
   a. Arabian.
   b. Asian.
   c. Japanese.
   d. Latin American.

9. Choose the religious group that shuns the use of caffeine-containing beverages:
   a. Hindus.
   b. Jews.
   c. Mormons.
   d. Seventh Day Adventists.

10. The yin/yang theory of harmony and illness is rooted in the _____ paradigm of health and illness.
   a. biomedical.
   b. holistic.
   c. religious.
   d. scientific.

Read each statement carefully. Write your response in the space provided.

1. Describe the four basic characteristics of culture:

   1. _____
   2. _____
   3. _____
   4. _____

2. Give at least five examples of groupings that can be used to identity subcultures.

   1. _____   4. _____
   2. _____   5. _____
   3. _____

3. List four strategies that individuals tend to use when communication has broken down:

   1. _____   3. _____
   2. _____   4. _____

4. Name four religious groups that routinely incorporate fasting into the religious practice:

   1. _____   3. _____
   2. _____   4. _____

5. Explain the concept of yin-yang: _____

   _____

   _____

12
Health Care of the Older Adult

Chapter Overview

Aging is a normal process that begins with birth and continues throughout life. Most stereotypes concerning the elderly are negative. The aged are thought to be slow-thinking, forgetful, confused, and senile. Erikson's sage of ego integrity versus despair implies that the elderly person will either accept the life he or she has lived or be dissatisfied with its outcome. The aged population is increasing rapidly, and health professionals must meet the challenge to make these added years healthy and productive.

I. Knowledge-Based Questions

Deduction and Interpretation

Read each question carefully. Circle your answer.

1. The study of the aging process is referred to as:
   a. ageism.
   b. geriatrics.
   c. gerontonics.
   d. gerontology.

2. Psychological adjustment to aging is believed to be related to successful completion of:
   a. aging.
   b. developmental tasks.
   c. physical adjustment.
   d. societal position.

3. Nursing interventions to help older people deal with psychological aging include:
   a. attentive listening.
   b. discussing their personal plans for the future.
   c. focusing their attention on the present.
   d. all of the above.

4. All of the following are true concerning Erikson's task of ego integrity *except*:
   a. the person accepts his or her lifestyle as it is.
   b. the person feels dissatisfied with life.
   c. one is still in control of one's life.
   d. the person made the best choices for particular situations.

5. Choose the sociological theory that suggests that adjustment to old age depends on the person's ability to continue life patterns throughout his lifetime.
   a. Activity
   b. Continuity
   c. Disengagement

6. The process most sensitive to deterioration with aging seems to be:
   a. creativity.
   b. judgment.
   c. intelligence.
   d. short-term memory.

 Mary Jo Boyer: Study Guide to Accompany Brunner & Suddarth's Textbook of Medical-Surgical Nursing, 8th ed. © 1996 Lippincott-Raven Publishers

7. The cardiac condition most frequently seen among the aged is:
   a. aortic stenosis.
   b. coronary artery disease.
   c. mitral valve prolapse.
   d. ventricular tachycardia.

8. Respiratory changes associated with aging include all of the following *except*:
   a. decreased residual volume.
   b. changes in the anteroposterior diameter of the chest.
   c. loss of elastic tissue surrounding the alveoli.
   d. reduced vital capacity.

9. Choose the *false* statement concerning genitourinary system changes in the older adult.
   a. The renal filtration rate decreases.
   b. The acid–base balance is restored more slowly.
   c. Bladder capacity increases with advanced age.
   d. Urinary frequency, urgency, and incontinence are common problems.

10. Bone changes associated with aging frequently result from a loss of:
   a. calcium.
   b. magnesium.
   c. vitamin A.
   d. vitamin C.

11. Nervous system changes associated with aging include all of the following *except*:
   a. a decrease in brain weight subsequent to the destruction of brain cells.
   b. an increase in blood flow to the brain to compensate for the gradual loss of brain cells.
   c. atrophy of the convolutions of the brain surface.
   d. widening and deepening of the spaces between the convolutions of the brain.

12. Nursing measures to deal with sensory changes in the aged include:
   a. increasing room lighting without increasing glare.
   b. speaking louder than normal.
   c. suggesting appetite stimulants before meals.
   d. all of the above actions.

13. Drug dosages must be reduced in the elderly because:
   a. cardiac output is significantly reduced.
   b. the number of mucosal cells in the gastrointestinal tract is reduced.
   c. drug biotransformation takes longer in older persons.
   d. all of the above are true.

14. The medications that remain in the body longer in the elderly, because of increased body fat are:
   a. anticoagulants.
   b. barbiturates.
   c. digitalis glycosides.
   d. diuretics.

15. The seventh leading cause of death in older persons is:
   a. accidents.
   b. drug toxicity.
   c. elder abuse.
   d. malnutrition.

16. The major source of public funding that provides nursing home care for the poor elderly is:
   a. Medicaid.
   b. Medicare.

II. Critical Analysis Questions

Recognizing Contradictions

Rewrite each statement correctly. Underline the key concepts.

1. Bones are composed of postmiotic cells that diminish and cause bone density.

2. Osteoporosis, accelerated by the loss of estrogen, can be reversed with a high calcium diet.

3. If the symptoms of delirium go untreated, symptoms will eventually decrease and the person will regain his or her previous level of consciousness.

4. Older persons should "take it easy" and avoid vigorous activity.

5. Back pain is usually the result of fatigue in the elderly and should not be taken seriously.

Generating Solutions: Clinical Problem Solving

Read the following case studies. Circle the correct answer.

CASE STUDY: Loneliness

Suzanne is a 75-year-old retired schoolteacher. She was recently widowed and lives alone. She in financially secure but socially isolated because she has outlived most of her friends. Her children are self-sufficient and very busy with their own lives.

1. Psychological threats that Suzanne may experience include:
   a. a deterioration of self-concept.
   b. a loss of self-esteem.
   c. extensive grief over frequently occurring losses.
   d. all of the above.

2. Suzanne is concerned about the dryness of her skin. Suggestions for skin care include:
   a. applying ointment to the skin several times a day.
   b. avoiding overexposure to the sun.
   c. patting the skin dry instead of rubbing it with a towel.
   d. all of the above measures.

3. Suzanne notices that food does not taste the same as before. She needs to be aware that this sensory change is most probably related to:
   a. a decrease in the number of taste buds.
   b. a loss of appetite associated with a decreased sense of smell.
   c. altered enzyme secretions.
   d. diminished gastric secretions.

4. An analysis of Suzanne's diet shows that it does not contain adequate protein. Her daily protein intake, for a body weight of 134 lb, should be about:
   a. 30 g
   b. 40 g
   c. 50 g
   d. 60 g

5. Most accidents among older people involve falls within the home. Preventive nursing measures include advising Suzanne to:
   a. avoid climbing and bending.
   b. keep personal items stored at a level between her hips and her eyes.
   c. make certain that all her shoes fit securely.
   d. do all of the above.

CASE STUDY: Alzheimer's Disease

Thomas, a 75-year-old retired bricklayer, lives at home with Anne, his 65-year-old wife, who is healthy and active. Lately she has noticed that his is negative, hostile, and suspicious of her. He gets lost in his own home, and his conversations have been accompanied by forgetfulness. Recently his physician has indicated a probable diagnosis of Alzheimer's disease.

1. Choose the statement that is *false* concerning Alzheimer's disease.
   a. It is found only in old persons.
   b. The disease process is irreversible.
   c. The probable cause is neuropathologic and biochemical.
   d. The cells that are affected by the disease are the ones that use acetylcholine.

2. The nurse should suggest that Anne deal with Thomas' behavior by:
   a. reasoning with him.
   b. providing reality orientation.
   c. providing a calm and predictable environment.
   d. not structuring activities for him.

3. An important point to communicate to Anne is:
   a. there are no realistic goals appropriate for Thomas.
   b. lists and written instructions will only tend to confuse him.
   c. Thomas should be restrained when agitated.
   d. maintaining personal dignity and autonomy is still an important part of Thomas' life.

4. Caregivers of patients with Alzheimer's disease should be aware that:
   a. Alzheimer's support groups exist.
   b. Alzheimer's disease does not eliminate the need for intimacy.
   c. socializing with old friends may be comforting.
   d. all of the above are appropriate.

CASE STUDY: Dehydration

Vera, an 89-year-old widow, was transferred from a nursing home to a hospital with a diagnosis of dehydration. Vera needs to be in bed because of her generalized weakness. She is occasionally confused and disoriented.

1. From her knowledge of temperature regulation in the elderly, the nurse should:
   a. make sure that the environmental temperature is adequate.
   b. palpate Vera's skin periodically to assess for warmth.
   c. place extra blankets at Vera's bedside in case she becomes cold, especially in the evening.
   d. do all of the above.

2. The nurse initiates a 2-hour turning schedule for Vera, based on the knowledge that the underlying cause of all decubiti is:
   a. altered skin turgor.
   b. nutritional deficiency.
   c. pressure.
   d. vasoconstriction.

3. Vera has been incontinent of urine since admission. Nursing interventions include all of the following *except*:
   a. initiating a bladder training program.
   b. offering fluids frequently to maintain a minimum daily intake of 2 to 3 L.
   c. providing means for limited daily exercises and ambulation.
   d. securing a physician's order for urethral catheterization.

4. The nurse suggests that Vera sit in a rocking chair for 20 minutes, four times a day. This suggestion is based on the knowledge that rocking:
   a. discourages hypostatic pulmonary congestion.
   b. increases pulmonary ventilation.
   c. improves venous return through contraction of the calf muscles.
   d. does all of the above.

Learner's Self-Evaluation Tool for End of Unit 3 Review

1. The most important concepts or facts I have learned from this unit are:

   1. _____

   2. _____

   3. _____

2. The most important reference page numbers for test review and clinical concepts are pages:

   _____   _____   _____

   _____   _____   _____

3. The concepts or facts that I do not fully understand are:

   _____

   _____

4. I will get the answer(s) to my questions by _____

_____

I will do this on _____ (date and time).

5. I believe my mastery of this unit to be:

    a.   100%   Great job! Good luck!

    b.   90%   2 hours of review recommended.

    c.   80%   4 hours of review recommended.

    d.   <80%   Make an appointment with your instructor.

UNIT 4
Concepts and Challenges in Patient Management

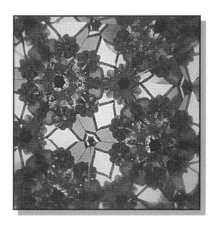

13
Pain Management

Chapter Overview

Pain is a major symptom in many diseases and one of the most common reasons why a person seeks medical attention. Although pain is a common experience, it is a very personal experience and is different for everyone. Care of the person experiencing pain requires an understanding of the physiologic, psychological, and sociocultural aspects of pain, as well as an appreciation of the patient's personal perception of the pain experience.

I. Knowledge-Based Questions

Deduction and Interpretation

Read each question carefully. Circle your answer.

1. Stimuli that result in painful sensations include those classified as:
   a. emotional.
   b. mental.
   c. physical.
   d. all of the above.

2. An individual's perception, tolerance, and management of pain are influenced by the pain and:
   a. age and anxiety.
   b. culture.
   c. gender.
   d. all of the above.

3. The nurse assessing for pain should:
   a. believe a patient when he or she states that pain is present.
   b. doubt that pain exists when no physical origin can be identified.
   c. realize that patients frequently imagine and state that they have pain without actually feeling painful sensations.
   d. do all of the above.

4. Pain in the elderly requires careful assessment because older people:
   a. are expected to experience chronic pain.
   b. have a decreased pain threshold.
   c. experience reduced sensory perception.
   d. have increased sensory perception.

5. Administration of analgesics to the elderly requires careful patient assessment because older people:
   a. metabolize drugs more rapidly.
   b. have increased hepatic, renal, and gastrointestinal function.
   c. are more sensitive to drugs.
   d. have lower ratios of body fat and muscle mass.

6. A nursing measure(s) to manage anxiety during the anticipation of pain should include:
   a. focusing the patient's attention on another problem.
   b. teaching about the nature of the impending pain and associated relief measures.
   c. using an anxiety-reducing technique, such as desensitization.
   d. all of the above.

7. All of the following statements about endorphins are true *except*:
   a. their release inhibits the transmission of painful impulses.
   b. they represent the same mechanism of pain relief as non-narcotic analgesics.
   c. they are endogenous neurotransmitters structurally similar to opioids.
   d. they are found in heavy concentrations in the central nervous system.

8. Acute pain may be described as having the following characteristic. It:
   a. does not usually respond well to treatment.
   b. is associated with a specific injury.
   c. serves no useful purpose.
   d. usually lasts longer than 6 months.

9. Chronic pain may be described as:
   a. attributable to a specific cause.
   b. prolonged in duration.
   c. rapidly occurring and subsiding with treatment.
   d. separate from any central or peripheral pathology.

10. An example of chronic benign pain is:
   a. a migraine headache.
   b. an exacerbation of rheumatoid arthritis.
   c. low back pain.
   d. sickle cell crisis.

11. When a nurse asks a patient to describe the *quality* of his pain, she expects him to use a descriptive term such as:
   a. burning.
   b. chronic.
   c. intermittent.
   d. severe.

12. A physiologic indicator of acute pain is:
   a. diaphoresis.
   b. bradycardia.
   c. hypotension.
   d. lowered respiratory rate.

13. A nursing plan of care for pain management should include:
   a. altering factors that influence the pain sensation.
   b. determining responses to the patient's behavior toward pain.
   c. selecting goals for nursing intervention.
   d. all of the above.

14. The advantage(s) of using intraspinal infusion to deliver analgesics is(are):
   a. reduced side effects of systemic analgesia.
   b. reduced effects on pulse, respirations, and blood pressure.
   c. reduced need for frequent injections.
   d. all of the above.

15. The drug of choice for epidural administration of analgesia is:
   a. codeine.
   b. demerol.
   c. Dilaudid.
   d. morphine.

16. The most worrisome adverse effect of epidural opioids is:
   a. asytole.
   b. hypertension.
   c. bradypnea.
   d. tachycardia.

17. A *preventive approach* to pain relief with nonsteroidal anti-inflammatory drugs (NSAIDs) means that the medication is given:
   a. before the pain becomes severe.
   b. before the pain is experienced.
   c. when pain is at its peak.
   d. when the level of pain tolerance has been exceeded.

18. Cutaneous stimulation is helpful in reducing painful sensations because it:

a. provides distraction from the pain source and decreases awareness.

b. releases endorphins.

c. stimulates large-diameter nerve fibers and reduces the intensity of pain.

d. accomplishes all of the above.

19. The nurse's major area of assessment for a patient receiving patient controlled analgesia (PCA) is assessment of the _____ system.

a. cardiovascular

b. integumentary

c. neurologic

d. respiratory

II. Critical Analysis Questions

Generating Solutions: Clinical Problem Solving

Read the following case study. Circle the correct answer.

CASE STUDY: Pain Experience

Courtney is a young, healthy adult who slipped off the stairs going down to the basement and struck her forehead on the cement flooring. Courtney did not lose consciousness, but did sustain a mild concussion and a hematoma that was 5 cm in width and protruded outward about 6 cm. She experienced immediate acute pain at the site of injury plus a pounding headache.

1. An immediate assessment of the localized pain, based on the patient's description, is that it should be:

a. brief in duration.

b. mild in intensity.

c. persistent after healing has occurred.

d. recurrent for 3 to 4 months.

2. During the assessment process, the nurse attempts to determine Courtney's physiologic and behavioral responses to her pain experience. The nurse is aware that a patient can be in pain yet appear to be "pain free." A behavioral response indicative of acute pain is:

a. an expressionless face.

b. clear verbalization of details.

c. muscle tension.

d. physical inactivity.

3. The nurse uses distraction to help Courtney cope with her pain experience. A suggested activity is:

a. promoting relaxation.

b. playing music or using a videotape.

c. using cutaneous stimulation.

d. any or all of the above.

4. After treatment, Courtney is discharged to home while still in pain. The nurse should:

a. clarify that Courtney knows what type of pain signals a problem.

b. remind Courtney that acute pain may persist for several days.

c. review methods of pain management.

d. do all of the above.

14

Fluids and Electrolytes: Balance and Disturbances

Chapter Overview

Our bodies are constantly striving to maintain physiologic homeostasis, an interdependent process that affects all major body systems. Inherent in each system is a fluid medium that aids in the transport and exchange of various elements, including electrolytes. A deviation in fluid and electrolyte balance can be the cause or result of altered homeostasis. A significant or prolonged deviation can lead to illness and, if untreated, to death. Because of the acuity of symptoms associated with an imbalance, nurses need to familiarize themselves with the principles of fluid and electrolyte balance, recognize parameters of disturbance, make a diagnosis, implement a course of action that will resolve the situation, and evaluate the outcomes on the basis of specific criteria. These nursing activities should follow the nursing process format, which lends itself to problem solving and solution testing.

I. Knowledge-Based Questions

Deduction and Interpretation

Read each question carefully. Circle your answer.

1. A febrile patient's fluid output is in excess of normal because of diaphoresis. The nurse should plan fluid replacement based on the knowledge that insensible losses in an *afebrile* person are normally not greater than:
   a. 300 ml/24 hr.   c. 900 ml/24 hr.
   b. 600 ml/24 hr.   d. 1200 ml/24 hr.

2. A patient's serum sodium is within normal range. The nurse estimates that the serum osmolality should be:
   a. less than 136 mOsm/kg.   c. greater than 408 mOsm/kg.
   b. 280 to 295 mOsm/kg.   d. 350 to 544 mOsm/kg.

3. A nurse is directed to administer a hypotonic intravenous solution. Looking at the following labeled solutions, she should choose:
   a. 0.45% sodium chloride.   c. 5% dextrose in water.
   b. 0.90% sodium chloride.   d. 5% dextrose in normal saline solution.

4. A patient is hemorrhaging from multiple trauma sites. The nurse expects that compensatory mechanisms associated with hypovolemia would cause all of the following symptoms *except*:
   a. hypertension.   c. tachycardia.
   b. oliguria.   d. tachypnea.

5. Nursing intervention for a patient with a diagnosis of *hyponatremia* includes all of the following *except*:
   a. assessing for symptoms of nausea and malaise.
   b. encouraging the intake of low-sodium liquids, such as coffee or tea.
   c. monitoring neurologic status.
   d. restricting tap water intake.

6. A patient with abnormal sodium losses is receiving a house diet. To provide 1600 mg of sodium daily, the nurse could supplement the patient's diet with:
   a. one beef cube and 8 oz. of tomato juice.
   b. four beef cubes and 8 oz. of tomato juice.
   c. one beef cube and 16 oz. of tomato juice.
   d. one beef cube and 12 oz. of tomato juice.

7. To return a patient with *hyponatremia* to normal sodium levels, it is safer to restrict fluid intake than to administer sodium:
   a. in patients who are unconscious.
   b. to prevent fluid overload.
   c. to prevent dehydration.
   d. in patients who show neurologic symptoms.

8. *Hypernatremia* is associated with a:
   a. serum osmolality of 245 mOsm/kg.
   b. serum sodium of 150 mEq/L.
   c. urine specific gravity below 1.003.
   d. combination of all of the above.

9. One of the dangers of treating *hypernatremia* is:
   a. red blood cell crenation.
   b. red blood cell hydrolysis.
   c. cerebral edema.
   d. renal shutdown.

10. Your semiconscious patient presents with restlessness and weakness. He has a dry, swollen tongue. His body temperature is 99.3°F, and his urine specific gravity is 1.020. Choose the most likely serum sodium (Na^+) value for this patient.
    a. 110 mEq/L
    b. 140 mEq/L
    c. 155 mEq/L
    d. 165 mEq/L

11. To supplement a diet with foods high in potassium, the nurse should recommend the addition of:
    a. fruits such as bananas and apricots.
    b. green leafy vegetables.
    c. milk and yogurt.
    d. nuts and legumes.

12. If a patient has severe hyperkalemia, it is possible to administer calcium gluconate intravenously to:
    a. immediately lower the potassium (K^+) level by active transport.
    b. antagonize the action of K^+ on the heart.
    c. prevent transient renal failure (TRF).
    d. accomplish all of the above.

13. A patient is admitted with severe vomiting for 24 hours. She states that she is exhausted and weak. The results of an admitting ECG show flat T waves and ST segment depression. Choose the most likely potassium (K^+) value for this patient.
    a. 4.0 mEq/L
    b. 8.0 mEq/L
    c. 2.0 mEq/L
    d. 2.6 mEq/L

14. A patient complains of tingling in his fingers. He has positive Trousseau's and Chvostek's signs. He says that he feels depressed. Choose the most likely serum calcium (Ca^{2+}) value for this patient.
    a. 11 mg/dl
    b. 9 mg/dl
    c. 7 mg/dl
    d. 5 mg/dl

15. Management of hypercalcemia includes all of the following actions *except* administration of:
    a. fluid to dilute the calcium levels.
    b. the diuretic furosemide (Lasix), without saline, to increase calcium excretion through the kidneys.
    c. inorganic phosphate salts.
    d. intravenous phosphate therapy.

16. A patient is admitted with a diagnosis of renal failure. He also mentions that he has had stomach distress and has ingested numerous antacid tablets over the past 2 days. His blood pressure is 110/70, his face is flushed, and he is experiencing generalized weakness. Choose the most likely magnesium (Mg^{2+}) value.
    a. 11 mEq/L
    b. 5 mEq/L
    c. 2 mEq/L
    d. 1 mEq/L

17. Management of the foregoing patient should include:
    a. a regular diet with extra fruits and green vegetables.
    b. potassium-sparing diuretics.
    c. discontinuance of any oral magnesium salts.
    d. all of the above measures.

18. The most common buffer system in the body is the:
    a. plasma protein buffer system.
    b. hemoglobin buffer system.
    c. phosphate buffer system.
    d. bicarbonate–carbonic acid buffer system.

19. The kidneys regulate acid–base balance by all of the following mechanisms *except*:
    a. excreting hydrogen ions (H^+).
    b. reabsorbing or excreting HCO_3^- into the blood.
    c. reabsorbing carbon dioxide into the blood.
    d. retaining hydrogen ions.

20. The lungs regulate acid–base balance by all of the following mechanisms *except*:
    a. excreting HCO_3^- into the blood.
    b. slowing ventilation.
    c. controlling carbon dioxide levels.
    d. increasing ventilation.

21. Choose the condition that exhibits blood values with a low pH and a low plasma bicarbonate concentration.
    a. Respiratory acidosis
    b. Respiratory alkalosis
    c. Metabolic acidosis
    d. Metabolic alkalosis

22. Nursing assessment for a patient with metabolic alkalosis includes evaluation of laboratory data for all of the following *except*:
    a. hypocalcemia.
    b. hypoglycemia.
    c. hypokalemia.
    d. hypoxemia.

23. Choose the condition that exhibits blood values with a low pH and a high P_{CO_2}.
    a. Respiratory acidosis
    b. Respiratory alkalosis
    c. Metabolic acidosis
    d. Metabolic alkalosis

Read each statement carefully. Write your response in the space provided.

1. The major positively charged ion in intracellular fluid is _____; the major positively charged ion in extracellular fluid is _____.

2. Define *colloidal osmotic pressure*.

    _____

    _____

    _____

3. The major organ that carefully regulates serum potassium balance is the _____.

4. Calcium levels are primarily regulated by _____.

5. The normal blood pH is _____.

6. The upper and lower level blood pH levels that are incompatible with life are _____

    _____

7. Indicate which of the following contribute to hypomagnesemia by writing *low* in the space provided, and which contribute to hypermagnesemia by writing *high* in the space provided.

   a. _____ alcohol abuse

   b. _____ renal failure

   c. _____ diarrhea

   d. _____ gentamicin administration

   e. _____ untreated ketoacidosis

8. Indicate which of the following contribute to hypophosphatemia by writing *low* in the space provided, and which contribute to hyperphosphatemia by writing *high* in the space provided.

   a. _____ hyperparathyroidism

   b. _____ renal failure

   c. _____ major thermal burns

   d. _____ alcohol withdrawal

   e. _____ neoplastic disease chemotherapy

9. Indicate which of the following contribute to hypocalcemia by writing *low* in the space provided, and which contribute to hypercalcemia by writing *high* in the space provided.

   a. _____ hyperparathyroidism

   b. _____ massive administration of citrated blood

   c. _____ malignant tumors

   d. _____ immobilization because of multiple fractures

   e. _____ pancreatitis

   f. _____ thiazide diuretics

   g. _____ renal failure

   h. _____ aminoglycoside administration

10. Indicate which of the following contribute to hypokalemia by writing *low* in the space provided, and which contribute to hyperkalemia by writing *high* in the space provided.

   a. _____ alkalosis

   b. _____ too tight a tourniquet when collecting a blood sample

   c. _____ vomiting

   d. _____ gastric suction

   e. _____ leukocytosis

   f. _____ anorexia nervosa

   g. _____ hyperaldosteronism

   h. _____ furosemide (Lasix) administration

   i. _____ steroid administration

   j. _____ renal failure

   k. _____ penicillin administration

   l. _____ adrenal steroid deficiency

11. Indicate which of the following contribute to hyponatremia by writing *low* in the space provided, and which contribute to hypernatremia by writing *high* in the space provided.

a. _____ vomiting

b. _____ diarrhea

c. _____ watery diarrhea

d. _____ inability to quench thirst

e. _____ burns over large surface area

f. _____ diuretics

g. _____ heat stroke

h. _____ adrenal insufficiency

i. _____ syndrome of inappropriate antidiuretic hormone

j. _____ posttherapeutic abortion

k. _____ diabetes insipidus with water restriction

l. _____ excessive parenteral administration of dextrose and water solution

12. For each of the following indicate the probable cause by writing *m-acid* for metabolic acidosis, *m-alka* for metabolic alkalosis, *r-acid* for respiratory acidosis, or *r-alka* for respiratory alkalosis.

a. _____ sedative overdose

b. _____ lactic acidosis

c. _____ ketoacidosis

d. _____ severe pneumonia

e. _____ hypoxemia

f. _____ acute pulmonary edema

g. _____ diarrhea

h. _____ vomiting

i. _____ hypokalemia

j. _____ gram-negative bacterial infection

13. Explain why the administration of a 3% to 5% sodium chloride solution requires intense monitoring.

_____

_____

14. List several symptoms associated with air embolism, a complication of intravenous therapy.

_____

_____

15. The major complication of intravenous therapy is _____.

II. Critical Analysis Questions

Generating Solutions: Clinical Problem Solving

Read the following case studies. Circle the correct answer.

CASE STUDY: Congestive Heart Failure

George, 88 years old, is suffering from congestive heart failure. He was admitted to the hospital with a diagnosis of extracellular volume excess. He was frightened, slightly confused, and dyspneic on exertion.

1. During the assessment process the nurse expects to identify the following *except*:
   a. a full pulse.
   b. decreased central venous pressure.
   c. edema.
   d. neck vein distention.

2. A manifestation of extracellular volume excess is:
   a. altered serum osmolality.
   b. hyponatremia.
   c. increased hematocrit when volume excess develops quickly.
   d. rapid weight gain.

3. A nursing plan of care for George should include:
   a. auscultating for abnormal breath sounds.
   b. inspecting for leg edema.
   c. weighing the patient daily.
   d. all of the above.

4. Nursing intervention for George should include all of the following *except*:
   a. administering diuretics, as prescribed, to help remove excess fluid.
   b. assisting the patient to a recumbent position to minimize his breathing effort.
   c. inspecting for sacral edema to note the degree of fluid retention.
   d. teaching dietary restriction of sodium to help decrease water retention.

CASE STUDY: Extracellular Volume Deficit

Harriet, 30 years old, has been admitted to the burn treatment center with full-thickness burns over 30% of her upper body. Her diagnosis is consistent with extracellular volume deficit.

1. The major indicator of extracellular volume deficit can be identified by assessing for:
   a. a full and bounding pulse.
   b. a drop in postural blood pressure.
   c. an elevated temperature.
   d. pitting edema of the lower extremities.

2. Manifestations of extracellular volume deficit include all of the following *except*:
   a. collapsed neck veins.
   b. decreased serum albumin.
   c. elevated hematocrit.
   d. weight loss.

3. A nursing plan of care for Harriet should include assessing blood pressure with the patient in the supine and upright positions. A diagnostic reading that should be recorded and reported is:
   a. supine, 140/90; sitting, 120/80; standing, 110/70.
   b. supine, 140/90; sitting, 130/90; standing, 130/90.
   c. supine, 140/90; sitting, 140/85; standing, 135/85.
   d. supine, 140/90; sitting, 140/90; standing, 130/90.

4. Nursing intervention for Harriet includes all of the following *except*:
   a. monitoring urinary output to assess kidney perfusion.
   b. placing the patient in the Trendelenburg position to maximize cerebral blood flow.
   c. positioning the patient flat in bed with legs elevated to maintain adequate circulating volume.
   d. teaching leg exercises to promote venous return and prevent postural hypotension when the patient stands.

CASE STUDY: Diabetes Mellitus

Isaac, 63 years old, was admitted to the hospital with a diagnosis of diabetes mellitus. On admission the nurse observed rapid respirations, confusion, and signs of dehydration.

1. Isaac's arterial blood gas values are pH, 7.27; HCO_3, 20 mEq/L, PaO_2, 33 mmHg. These values are consistent with a diagnosis of compensated:
   a. metabolic acidosis.
   b. metabolic alkalosis.
   c. respiratory acidosis.
   d. respiratory alkalosis.

2. A manifestation *not associated* with altered acid–base balance is:
   a. bradycardia.
   b. hypertension.
   c. lethargy.
   d. hypokalemia.

3. In terms of cellular buffering response, the nurse should expect that the major electrolyte disturbance is:
   a. hyperkalemia.
   b. hypernatremia.
   c. hypocalcemia.
   d. hypokalemia.

4. The nurse should anticipate that the physician will attempt to reverse this acid–base imbalance by prescribing an intravenous administration of:
   a. potassium chloride.
   b. potassium iodide.
   c. sodium bicarbonate.
   d. sodium chloride.

15

Shock and Multisystem Failure

Chapter Overview

The clinical picture of shock can present as a sudden occurrence resulting from bodily insult (hypovolemic shock caused by trauma), or as an insidious progression of cellular deterioration caused by an infectious agent (septic shock caused by gram-negative bacteria). The nurse's role revolves around prevention through health education and accurate and vigilant assessment of patients "at risk." However, once the shock syndrome occurs, the nurse's efforts are directed toward reversing the progression of pathophysiologic responses. Additionally, the nurse works collaboratively with other members of the health care team to manage fluid replacement, nutritional support, and vasoactive drug therapy to prevent the sequence of multiple organ failure (MOF) which has a 25% to 100% mortality rate.

As a student nurse, your efforts need to be directed toward perfecting your physical assessment skills, understanding the underlying physiologic processes involved in the syndrome, and mastering the proficiency of skilled intervention. A multidisciplinary approach to care and cure will help manage the syndrome and decrease its associated morbidity and mortality.

I. Knowledge-Based Questions

Deduction and Interpretation

Read each question carefully. Circle your answer.

1. The primary mechanism of blood pressure regulation results from the initial stimulation of _____ receptors.
   a. chemical
   b. hormonal
   c. neural
   d. pressure

2. Calculate a patient's mean arterial pressure (MAP) when the blood pressure is 110/70.
   a. 65
   b. 73
   c. 83
   d. 91

3. The stage of shock characterized by a normal blood pressure is the _____ stage.
   a. initial
   b. compensated
   c. progressive
   d. irreversible

4. A nurse assesses a patient in shock whose lungs have decompensated. The nurse would *not expect* to find the following symptoms:
   a. a heart rate > 100/min
   b. crackles
   c. lethargy and mental confusion
   d. respirations fewer than 15/min

 Mary Jo Boyer: Study Guide to Accompany Brunner & Suddarth's Textbook of Medical-Surgical Nursing, 8th ed. © 1996 Lippincott-Raven Publishers

5. Oliguria occurs in the progressive stage of shock because the kidneys decompensate. To assess for this condition, the nurse should look for the following signs or symptoms:
   a. congestive heart failure
   b. decreased capillary permeability and localized edema
   c. increased BUN and serum creatinine
   d. systolic BP > 120 mmHg

6. Hematologic system changes in progressive shock would *not* be characterized by:
   a. generalized hypoxemia.
   b. hypertension.
   c. metabolic acidosis.
   d. sluggish blood flow.

7. Depleted ATP stores and multiple organ failure are characteristic of the _____ stage of shock.
   a. initial
   b. compensatory
   c. progressive
   d. irreversible

8. The primary goal in treating cardiogenic shock is to:
   a. improve the heart's pumping mechanism.
   b. limit further myocardial damage.
   c. preserve the healthy myocardium.
   d. treat the oxygenation needs of the heart muscle.

9. The drug of choice for cardiac pain relief is IV:
   a. codeine.
   b. Demerol.
   c. Dilauded.
   d. morphine.

10. Sympathomimetic drugs increase cardiac output by all of the following measures *except* by:
    a. decreasing preload and afterload
    b. increasing myocardial contractility
    c. tachycardia
    d. vasoconstriction

11. The vasoactive effects of dopamine are diminished when high doses are given because vasoconstriction increases cardiac workload. Doses are titrated for therapeutic range. A nontherapeutic drug dose for a 154-lb (70-kg) man would be:
    a. 210 μg/min.
    b. 350 μg/min.
    c. 490 μg/min.
    d. 630 μg/min.

12. The negative effect of intravenous nitroglycerin (Tridil) for shock management is:
    a. reduced preload.
    b. reduced afterload.
    c. increased cardiac output.
    d. increased blood pressure.

13. Intra-aortic balloon counterpulsation (IABC) is a mechanical, assistive device used as a temporary means of improving the heart's pumping ability. IABC is primarily meant to:
    a. decrease cardiac work.
    b. decrease stroke volume.
    c. increase preload.
    d. maintain current coronary circulation.

14. The primary etiology of distributive shock is:
    a. arterial and venous dilatation.
    b. compromised cardiac contractility.
    c. decreased blood volume.
    d. obstructed blood flow.

15. Patients receiving fluid replacement should frequently be monitored for:
    a. adequate urinary output.
    b. changes in mental status.
    c. vital sign stability.
    d. all of the above.

16. The most commonly used colloidal solution to treat hypovolemic shock is:
    a. blood products.
    b. 5% albumin.
    c. 6% dextran.
    d. 6% hetastarch.

17. Vasoactive agents are effective in treating shock because of their ability to:
    a. decrease blood pressure.
    b. decrease stroke volume.
    c. increase cardiac output.
    d. increase cardiac preload.

18. A common vasoactive agent used to improve cardiac contractility is:
    a. dopamine.
    b. epinephrine.
    c. nitroprusside.
    d. phenylephrine.

19. The sequence of multiple organ failure (MOF) usually begins in the:
- a. heart.
- b. kidneys.
- c. liver.
- d. lungs.

20. A 40% mortality rate can be found with early stage MOF that is associated with:
- a. autocatabolism.
- b. a hypermetabolic phase.
- c. septic shock.
- d. all of the above.

Read the definitions of the terms related to shock and multisystem failure. Find each term in the scramblegram and circle it. Terms may be written in any direction. A sample is provided.

D	A	O	L	E	R	P	B	D	F	H	R
B	L	C	F	I	L	U	M	P	R	E	T
C	B	A	J	A	R	L	D	G	N	H	G
Y	U	D	K	S	E	M	J	I	L	F	K
L	M	G	W	F	B	O	N	E	D	N	O
M	I	S	P	T	G	N	S	G	N	U	L
A	N	D	T	C	R	A	R	M	I	H	I
I	V	I	A	D	H	Y	I	R	P	D	G
M	L	O	R	O	C	Y	P	J	R	K	U
E	A	L	T	P	X	E	L	S	I	O	R
X	C	L	B	A	I	D	M	N	D	M	I
O	S	O	K	M	W	E	S	O	E	P	A
P	V	C	O	I	L	M	A	H	K	I	F
Y	R	A	Q	N	F	A	N	T	O	C	P
H	T	R	C	E	S	E	P	T	I	C	J
C	K	G	P	N	W	T	U	C	M	B	K
F	H	J	M	E	S	B	M	E	D	I	A
H	A	D	G	K	O	R	H	L	O	B	F

Definition of Terms

1. A syndrome of inadequate blood flow to body tissues.

2. Nutrients, chemically broken down within the cell, are stored in this form.

3. This substance is responsible for the conversion of angiotensin I.

4. This hormone, secreted by the pituitary gland, causes the kidneys to retain fluid.

5. Insufficient oxygenation of the blood.

6. The degree of stretch of cardiac muscle before its contraction.

7. Urinary output less than 30 ml/hr.

8. A colloid that rapidly expands plasma volume.

9. A popular vasoactive agent that improves cardiac contractility.

10. The most common type of distributive shock.

11. A central line used to monitor venous pressure.

12. The most common side effect of fluid replacement in shock.

13. These solutions are used to expand intravascular volume in shock.

14. Multiple organ failure usually begins in this organ.

15. A vasodilator used to reduce the heart's demand for oxygen in conditions of shock.

Match the type of shock listed in Column II with its associated cause listed in Column I. An answer may be used more than once.

Column I

1. _____ valvular damage

2. _____ peritonitis

3. _____ burns

4. _____ bee sting allergy

5. _____ immunosuppression

6. _____ spinal cord injury

7. _____ dysrhythmias

8. _____ vomiting

9. _____ diuresis

10. _____ penicillin sensitivity

Column II

a. *hypovolemic*, owing to an internal fluid shift

b. *hypovolemic*, owing to an external fluid loss

c. *cardiogenic* of a noncoronary nature

d. *distributive* of a neurogenic nature

e. *distributive* of an anaphylactic nature

f. *distributive* of a septic nature

II. Critical Analysis Questions

Generating Solutions: Clinical Problem Solving

Read the following case study. Fill in the blanks or circle the correct answer.

CASE STUDY: Hypovolemic Shock

Mr. Mazda is a 57-year-old, 154-lb (70-kg) patient, who was received on the nursing unit from the recovery room after having a hemicolectomy for colon cancer. On initial assessment, Mr. Mazda was alert, yet anxious, his skin was cool, pale, and moist, and his abdominal dressings were saturated with bright red blood. Urinary output was 100 ml over 4 hours. The patient was receiving 1000 ml of LR. Vital signs were 80/60, 126, and 40 (baseline VS were 130/70, 84, 22). The nurse assessed that the patient was experiencing hypovolemic shock.

1. A nurse understands that hypovolemic shock will occur with an intravascular volume reduction of 15% to 25%. Therefore, the nurse determines that Mr. Mazda, who weighs 70 kg, has probably lost:
   a. 200 ml of blood.
   b. 500 ml of blood.
   c. 750 ml of blood.
   d. 1000 ml of blood.

2. The nurse knows to monitor vital signs every 5 to 15 minutes and to be concerned about the patient's pulse

   pressure of _____.

3. The nurse knows that the progressive pattern of changes in vital signs is more important than the exact readings. A _____ in pulse rate, followed by a _____ in blood pressure, is indicative of shock.

4. The nurse understands that a systolic reading of 80 mmHg is serious because a systolic reading below _____ mmHg, in a normotensive person, indicates well advanced shock.

5. Urinary output will be measured hourly. An output less than _____ ml/hr is indicative of decreased glomerular filtration.

6. Nursing interventions include notifying the physician, reinforcing the abdominal dressings, and treating the patient for shock by:

   a. administering fluids as ordered such as _____

   _____

   b. _____

   c. _____

   d. _____

   e. _____

16

Oncology: Nursing the Patient With Cancer

Chapter Overview

The diagnosis of cancer is a frightening experience that threatens patients and their families, associates, and communities. Even today, in an era of sophisticated research and an explosion of knowledge, the prognosis for many types of cancer is poor.

As health care providers coming into contact with cancer patients and their families, nurses are challenged to care for multisystem physical problems as well as for many emotional needs. Nurses have the additional obligation of educating patients about modifiable risk factors and the importance of early detection.

The role of the nurse is crucial in caring for the "person" behind the disease. The importance of keen assessment skills and sensitive care planning cannot be overemphasized.

FACT:

- *For information about cancer, call the National Cancer Institute at 1-800-4-CANCER.*

- *Scientists announce the discovery of the genes for cancer of the breast, prostate and colon* (Inquirer, *January 1, 1995, p. G1).*

I. Knowledge-Based Questions

Deduction and Interpretation

Read each question carefully. Circle your answer.

1. In the United States, cancer, as a cause of death, ranks:
   a. first.
   b. second.
   c. third.
   d. fourth.

2. The etiology of cancer can be associated with specific agents or factors such as:
   a. dietary and genetic factors.
   b. hormonal and chemical agents.
   c. viruses.
   d. all of the above.

3. David, age 67, is admitted for diagnostic studies to rule out cancer. He is white, has been employed as a landscaper for 40 years, and has a 36-year history of smoking one pack of cigarettes a day. David has three risk factors associated with the development of cancer. Choose the least significant risk factor among the following:
   a. age
   b. sex
   c. occupation
   d. race

4. Cancer cells can affect the immune system by:

    a. stimulating the release of T-cell lymphocytes into the circulation.

    b. suppressing the patient's natural defenses.

    c. mobilizing macrophages.

    d. all of the above.

5. To reduce nitrate intake because of possible carcinogenic action, the nurse suggests that a patient decrease his or her intake of:

    a. eggs and milk.

    b. fish and poultry.

    c. ham and bacon.

    d. green, leafy vegetables.

6. An endoscopic procedure can be used to remove an entire piece of suspicious tissue growth. The diagnostic biopsy method used for this procedure is known as:

    a. excisional.

    b. incisional.

    c. needle biopsy.

    d. staging.

7. A patient is admitted for an excisional biopsy of a breast lesion. The nurse should do all of the following *except:*

    a. clarify information provided by the physician.

    b. provide aseptic care to the incision postoperatively.

    c. provide time for the patient to discuss her concerns.

    d. counsel the patient about the possibility of losing her breast.

8. Surgery done to remove lesions that are likely to develop into cancer is known as:

    a. diagnostic.

    b. palliative.

    c. prophylactic.

    d. reconstructive.

9. An example of palliative surgery is a:

    a. colectomy.

    b. cordotomy.

    c. mastectomy.

    d. nephrectomy.

10. The *incorrect* rationale for the effectiveness of radiation therapy is its ability to:

    a. cause cell death.

    b. break the strands of the DNA helix.

    c. disrupt mitosis by slowing dividing cells.

    d. interrupt cellular growth when a nonsurgical approach is needed.

11. Radiation therapy for the treatment of cancer is administered over several weeks to:

    a. allow time for the patient to cope with the treatment.

    b. allow time for the repair of healthy tissue.

    c. decrease the incidence of leukopenia and thrombocytopenia.

    d. accomplish all of the above.

12. A patient with uterine cancer is being treated with internal radiation therapy. A primary nursing responsibility is to:

    a. explain to the patient that she will continue to emit radiation for approximately 1 week after the implant is removed.

    b. maintain as much distance as possible from the patient while in the room.

    c. alert family members that they should restrict their visiting to 5 minutes at any one time.

    d. wear a lead apron when providing direct patient care.

13. A major disadvantage of chemotherapy is that it:

    a. attacks cancer cells during their vulnerable phase.

    b. functions against disseminated disease.

    c. is systemic.

    d. targets normal body cells as well as cancer cells.

14. When a patient takes vincristine, a plant alkaloid, the nurse should assess for symptoms of toxicity affecting the:

    a. gastrointestinal system.

    b. nervous system.

    c. pulmonary system.

    d. urinary system.

15. Initial nursing action for extravasation of a chemotherapeutic agent includes all of the following *except:*

a. applying warm compresses to the phlebitic area.

b. immediately discontinuing the infusion.

c. injecting an antidote, if required.

d. placing ice over the site of infiltration.

16. Realizing that chemotherapy can result in renal damage, the nurse should:

a. encourage fluid intake to dilute the urine.

b. take measures to acidify the urine, and thus prevent uric acid crystallization.

c. withhold medication when the blood urea nitrogen level exceeds 20 mg/dl.

d. limit fluids to 1000 ml daily to prevent accumulation of the drugs' end products after cell lysis.

17. Allopurinol may be prescribed for a patient who is receiving chemotherapy to:

a. stimulate the immune system against the tumor cells.

b. treat drug-related anemia.

c. prevent alopecia.

d. lower serum and urine uric acid levels.

18. The use of hyperthermia as a treatment modality for cancer may cause:

a. fatigue, nausea, and vomiting.

b. hypotension, skin burn, and tissue damage.

c. thrombophlebitis, diarrhea, and peripheral neuropathies.

d. all of the above side effects.

19. Bacille Calmétte-Guerin (BCG) is a biologic response modifier that is a standard form of treatment for cancer of the:

a. bladder.

b. breast.

c. lungs.

d. skin.

20. The nurse should assess a cancer patient's nutritional status by:

a. weighing the patient daily.

b. monitoring daily calorie intake.

c. observing for proper wound healing.

d. doing all of the above.

21. A patient with lung cancer begins to exhibit signs of superior vena cava syndrome. These signs include:

a. elevated intracranial pressure, fluid retention, and dyspnea.

b. headache, tachycardia, and hypotension.

c. dehydration, coughing, and hypercalcemia.

d. all of the above.

22. An example of an oncologic emergency is the syndrome of inappropriate antidiuretic hormone (SIADH). Symptoms of this disorder include:

a. hypernatremia and decreased urinary sodium excretion.

b. weight gain, irritability, and nausea.

c. excessive fluid loss and cachexia.

d. decreased urine osmolality.

Match the type of neoplasm in Column II with its associated description listed in Column I.

Column 1

1. _B_ Cells bear little resemblance to the normal cells of the tissue from which they arose.

2. _A_ Rate of growth is usually slow.

3. _A_ Tumor tissue is encapsulated.

4. _B_ Tumor spreads by way of blood and lymph channels to other areas of the body.

5. _B_ Growth tends to recur when removed.

Column 2

a. Benign

b. Malignant

Read each statement carefully. Write your response in the space provided.

1. List in order of frequency the three leading causes of cancer deaths in the United States.

Men	Women
1 _____	1 _____
2 _____	2 _____
3 _____	3 _____

2. Distinguish between the terms *invasion* and *metastasis* as they relate to the spread of cancerous cells.

   Invasion: _____

   Metastasis: _____

3. List two significant tumor-specific antigens present in cancer cells that help with diagnosis and treatment:

   1. _____ 2. _____

4. At least _____ % of all cancers are thought to be related to the environment around us.

5. Three cruciferous vegetables that appear to reduce cancer risk are _____,

   _____, _____.

6. Describe what is meant by primary and secondary prevention of cancer, and provide an example of how nurses can participate in both types of prevention.

   Definition   **Example**

   Primary: _____   Primary: _____

   _____   _____

   Secondary: _____   Secondary: _____

   _____   _____

7. Distinguish between the three goals of cancer treatment.

   Cure: _____

   _____

   Control: _____

   _____

   Palliation: _____

   _____

8. Toxicity occurs with radiation therapy. For each heading in Column I list several examples of side effects in Column II.

   Column I   **Column II**

   1. Skin   1. a. _____

                                                  b. _____

                                                  c. _____

   2. Oral mucosal membrane   2. a. _____

                                                  b. _____

                                                  c. _____

                                                  d. _____

3. Stomach or colon

3. a. _____

   b. _____

   c. _____

   d. _____

4. Bone marrow–producing sites

4. a. _____

   b. _____

   c. _____

9. Describe the modes of action in the following classifications of chemotherapeutic agents.

Cell-cycle–specific: _____

Cell-cycle–nonspecific: _____

10. List five signs that indicate that an extravasation of an infusion of a cancer chemotherapeutic agent has occurred:

a. _____ c. _____ e. _____

b. _____ d. _____

11. Describe the role of hyperthermia in the treatment of cancer.

_____

_____

12. Describe the role of interferons in the treatment of cancer.

_____

_____

Match the drug category listed in Column II with an associated antineoplastic agent listed in Column I. An answer may be used more than once.

Column I

1. _____ vincristine

2. _____ 5-fluorouracil

3. _____ cisplatin

4. _____ estrogens

5. _____ thiotepa

6. _____ lomustine

7. _____ mitomycin

8. _____ amsacrine

9. _____ pentostatin

10. _____ paclitaxel (Taxol)

Column II

a. alkylating agent

b. nitrosourea

c. antimetabolite

d. antitumor antibiotic

e. plant alkaloid/natural product

f. hormonal agent

II. Critical Analysis Questions

Analyzing Comparisons

Read each analogy. Fill in the space provided with the best response.

1. Primary cancer prevention: preventing or reducing the risk of cancer :: Tertiary prevention: _____.

2. Staging of tumor cells: tumor size and existence of metastasis :: Grading: _____.

3. Allogenic bone marrow transplant: an unrelated donor :: Syngenic bone marrow transplant: _____.

4. Stomatitis: oral tissue inflammation :: Alopecia: _____.

5. Anorexia: loss of appetite :: Cachexia: _____.

Generating Solutions: Clinical Problem Solving

Read the following case study. Circle the correct answer.

CASE STUDY: Cancer of the Breast

Kim is a 45-year-old mother of four who, after a needle aspiration biopsy, is diagnosed as having a malignant breast tumor, stage III. She was scheduled for a modified radical mastectomy. On assessment, her breast tissue had a dimpling or "orange-peel" appearance. Nursing diagnoses included (a) fear and ineffective coping related to the diagnosis; and (b) disturbance in self-concept related to the nature of surgery.

1. Realizing that Kim's mother died of breast cancer, the nurse correlates the cause of Kim's diagnosis to:
   a. environmental factors.
   b. genetics.
   c. dietary factors.
   d. chemical agents.

2. To assist Kim in adapting to the loss of her breast, the nurse should assess her:
   a. attitude toward her body image.
   b. feelings of self-esteem.
   c. social and sexual values.
   d. attitudes and values regarding all of the above.

3. Kim's husband refuses to participate in any discussion about his wife's diagnosis. The nurse realizes that he is using the defense mechanism of:
   a. denial.
   b. depression.
   c. rationalization.
   d. repression.

4. Postoperatively Kim experiences severe incisional pain. The nurse realizes that Kim's perception of pain is possibly influenced by:
   a. tissue manipulation during surgery.
   b. apprehension regarding the prognosis of her condition.
   c. anger stemming from her change in body image.
   d. all of the above.

Kim is scheduled to begin radiation therapy, followed by chemotherapy with 5-fluorouracil.

5. Realizing the side-effects of radiation therapy, the nurse should prepare Kim for all of the following *except*:
   a. the possibility that her lungs may produce more mucus.
   b. that the skin at the treatment area may become red and inflamed.
   c. that she may tire more easily and require additional rest periods.
   d. that alopecia will occur as a result of the quickly growing hair follicles.

6. The nurse should teach Kim what she can do to protect her skin between radiation treatments. Measures include all of the following *except:*

    a. handling the area gently.

    b. avoiding irritation with soap and water.

    c. using a heat lamp once a day directed to the radiation site to promote tissue repair.

    d. wearing loose-fitting clothing.

After radiation therapy Kim begins a regimen of chemotherapy with 5-fluorouracil. Three weeks after treatment begins Kim develops a fever, sore throat, and cold symptoms.

7. The nurse knows that the symptoms could be due to all of the following *except:*

    a. hypercalcemia.

    b. bone marrow depression.

    c. altered nutrition.

    d. leukopenia.

8. Nursing assessment during Kim's chemotherapy includes observing for:

    a. evidence of stomatitis.

    b. renal and hepatic abnormalities.

    c. symptoms of infection owing to granulocytopenia.

    d. all of the above.

9. Kim is diagnosed as having thrombocytopenia. The nurse should assess for all of the following *except:*

    a. hematuria.

    b. fever.

    c. hematemesis.

    d. ecchymosis.

peau d'orange

17
Chronic Illness

Chapter Overview

Chronic illness affects all ages to varying degrees of severity and debility. It randomly strikes, predicated by genetic codes and predisposing factors. Its effects can be subtle or glaring. Regardless of cause, the results are similar; a compromised lifestyle with psychosocial and financial burdens. Only a few are able to balance the demands of chronic illness so activities of daily living and self-image are not compromised.

Nursing roles with the chronically ill are numerous. Central to all interventions and frameworks is the underlying commitment to maximize an individual's potential and support all efforts at health maintenance.

I. Knowledge-Based Questions

Deduction and Interpretation

Read each question carefully. Circle your answer.

1. The most prevalent chronic condition, according to the National Center for Health Statistics, is:
   a. arthritis.
   b. asthma.
   c. sinusitis.
   d. diabetes.

2. For individuals *younger than 18 years*, the chronic condition with the highest incidence is:
   a. acne.
   b. asthma.
   c. hay fever.
   d. chronic bronchitis.

3. For individuals *between 18 and 44 years*, the chronic condition with the highest incidence is:
   a. arthritis.
   b. chronic sinusitis.
   c. orthopedic deformity.
   d. migraine headache.

4. For individuals *between 45 and 64 years*, the chronic condition with the highest incidence is:
   a. arthritis.
   b. chronic sinusitis.
   c. hearing impairment.
   d. hypertension.

5. For individuals between *65 and 74 years*, the chronic condition with the highest incidence is:
   a. arthritis.
   b. cataracts.
   c. diabetes.
   d. ischemic heart disease.

6. For individuals *over 75 years*, the chronic condition with the highest incidence is:
   a. arthritis.
   b. cataracts.
   c. hypertension.
   d. visual impairment.

Mary Jo Boyer: Study Guide to Accompany Brunner & Suddarth's Textbook of Medical-Surgical Nursing, 8th ed. © 1996 Lippincott-Raven Publishers

7. With the "Trajectory Framework" as a model for chronic illness, the main target of care is the:
   a. individual.
   b. family.
   c. community.
   d. combination of all.

8. Within the Trajectory Framework, the phase that includes the diagnostic period is called the:
   a. pretrajectory phase.
   b. trajectory onset.
   c. crisis phase.
   d. acute onset.

Read each statement carefully. Write your response in the space provided.

1. List five habits of modern living that are related to the development of chronic conditions in genetically pre-disposed persons: (1) _____, (2) _____, (3) _____,

   (4) _____, and (5) _____.

2. List six common management problems related to chronic conditions:

   (1) _____, (3) _____, (5) _____,

   (2) _____, (4) _____, (6) _____.

3. Define the concept of *Trajectory Framework* as it relates to chronic illness:

   _____

   _____

4. Distinguish between the terms: Trajectory phasing _____

   _____

   Second trajectory scheme _____

   _____

5. Consider the Trajectory Nursing Model and the Nursing Process. Assessment: step one :: Intervention:

   _____.

II. Critical Analysis Questions

Recognizing Contradictions

Rewrite each statement correctly. Underline the key concepts.

1. Chronic illnesses decrease in frequency with age because individuals' immunologic systems adapt and over-come the impact.

2. Individuals with chronic illness will always function in a dependent role because they have a compromised system.

3. Orthopedic deformities are chronic disorders that are least prevalent in the United States, according to the National Center for Health Statistics.

4. A therapeutic way to manage chronic illness is to superimpose an "acute care framework" on a chronic con-dition so severe medical problems are not overlooked.

5. In the Trajectory Framework, medical aspects of illness are separated into their social and psychological com-ponents so that care can be targeted to specific areas.

18

Principles and Practices of Rehabilitation

Chapter Overview

Rehabilitation means the process of returning a person to a condition of optimum wellness. This need exists whenever an illness or disease alters a person's health status and someone has identified that rehabilitation is possible for improved health functioning. Once identified, rehabilitation goals can be met by the person alone, or by a health care provider. Rehabilitation begins as soon as the need exists, whether the person is in his or her home environment or in a clinical setting. Nurses need to be sensitive to early identification of rehabilitation needs based on detailed assessment. A course of therapy can then be prescribed, implemented, and evaluated.

I. Knowledge-Based Questions

Deduction and Interpretation

Read each question carefully. Circle your answer.

1. Rehabilitation, as an integral part of nursing, might begin:
   a. after the patient feels comfortable in the clinical setting.
   b. after the physician has prescribed rehabilitative goals.
   c. when an exercise program has been initiated.
   d. with initial patient contact.

2. A rehabilitation program for an elderly hip fracture patient must focus on the:
   a. impact of multiple system pathology on recovery.
   b. influence of mental status changes on health improvement.
   c. periodic physiologic evaluation of bone repair.
   d. value of all of the above factors.

3. The normal first emotional reactions to a disability are:
   a. anger and hostility.
   b. confusion and denial.
   c. depression and regression.
   d. grief and mourning.

4. Sexual problems faced by the disabled include:
   a. impaired self-image.
   b. lack of opportunities to form friendships.
   c. limited access to information about sexuality.
   d. all of the above.

5. A key member of the rehabilitation team is the:
   a. nurse.
   b. patient.
   c. physical therapist.
   d. physician.

Mary Jo Boyer: Study Guide to Accompany Brunner & Suddarth's Textbook of Medical-Surgical Nursing, 8th ed. © 1996 Lippincott-Raven Publishers

6. The PULSES profile uses six components to evaluate self-care independence. The assessment of bladder control would be documented under:

a. "E," excretory function.

b. "L," lower system functions.

c. "P," physical condition.

d. "S," sensory functions.

7. A nurse who wants to help a patient assume the side-lying position would:

a. align the lower extremities in a neutral position.

b. extend the legs with a firm support under the popliteal area.

c. place the uppermost hip slightly forward in a position of slight abduction.

d. position the trunk so that hip flexion is minimized.

8. Therapeutic exercises that are carried out by the patient with the nurse assisting are classified as:

a. active.

b. active assistive.

c. passive.

d. resistive.

9. Insufficient cerebral circulation can result from the use of the tilt table and can be identified by:

a. diaphoresis.

b. nausea.

c. tachycardia.

d. all of the above.

10. Weight-bearing on long bones is essential for preventing:

a. calcium loss.

b. potassium loss.

c. protein loss.

d. sodium loss.

11. Tissue ischemia associated with a decubitus ulcer results from:

a. dehydration and skin dryness.

b. excessive skin moisture.

c. inflammation and infection.

d. small nutrient vessel compression.

12. A patient at potential risk for skin breakdown is assessed by the nurse. A laboratory study the nurse should examine is one that measures:

a. hemoglobin.

b. serum glucose.

c. prothrombin time.

d. sedimentation rate.

13. A diet recommended for hypoproteinemia that "spares" protein is one high in:

a. carbohydrates.

b. fats.

c. minerals.

d. vitamins.

14. Wound healing depends on collagen formation, which depends on vitamin:

a. A.

b. C.

c. D.

d. K.

15. To initiate a schedule of bladder training, a nurse should:

a. encourage the patient to wait 30 minutes after drinking a measured amount of fluid before attempting to void.

b. give up to 2500 ml of fluid daily.

c. teach bladder massage to increase intra-abdominal pressure.

d. do all of the above.

16. Successful bowel training depends on:

a. a daily defecation time that is within 15 minutes of the same time every day.

b. an adequate intake of fiber-containing foods.

c. fluid intake between 2 and 4 L/day.

d. all of the above.

Match the explanations of range-of-motion techniques listed in Column II with their associated terms in Column I.

Column I

1. _____ adduction

2. _____ dorsiflexion

3. _____ extension

4. _____ inversion

5. _____ pronation

Column II

a. bending of the foot toward the leg

b. increasing the angle of a joint

c. moving away from the midline of the body

d. movement that turns the sole of the foot inward

e. movement toward the midline of the body

f. rotating the forearm so that the palm is down

Read each statement carefully. Write your response in the space provided.

1. Define the term *physiatrist*.

_____

2. List three complications commonly associated with a prolonged immobility.

(1) _____ (2) _____ (3) _____

3. Examples of orthotic devices include _____

_____

_____

4. A common hip complication for patients who are in bed for prolonged periods is _____ deformity of the hip.

5. Four factors that contribute to footdrop are: (1) _____ (2) _____

(3) _____ and (4) _____.

6. A joint should be moved through its range of motion _____ times, at least once a day.

7. For crutch-walking, the sequence for the four-point gait begins with the _____ crutch

and ends with the _____ foot.

8. Define the term *pressure sore*.

_____

9. Life-threatening complications of pressure sores include _____

_____.

10. Eschar covering an ulcer should be removed surgically because eschar _____

_____.

II. Critical Analysis Questions

Generating Solutions: Clinical Problem Solving

View Figure 18–5 and answer the clinically focused questions.

CLINICAL SITUATION: Impaired Skin Integrity

1. Define the term *pressure ulcer:* _____
   _____.

2. The initial sign of pressure is _____ caused by_____.

3. Look at Figure 18–5. Choose the two most susceptible surfaces for pressure ulcer formation:

   the _____ and the _____.

4. The least favorable position to use to shift body weight would be:
   a. prone.
   b. recumbent.
   c. semi-Fowler's.
   d. side-lying.

5. The patient should be repositioned:
   a. every 30 minutes.
   b. hourly.
   c. every 3 to 4 hours.
   d. once per shift.

6. Explain why a gel-type flotation pad and an air-fluidized bed reduce pressure.

   _____

   _____

   This logic is based on _____ law.

7. Look at Figure 18–5. Explain why the shearing force is increased when the head of the bed is raised, even if only by a few centimeters.

   _____

   _____

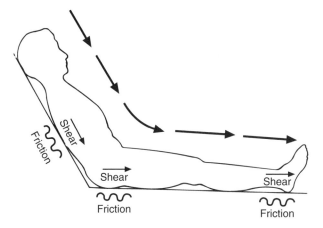

FIGURE 18–5 Mechanical forces contribute to pressure ulcer development. As the person slides down in bed, *friction* resists this movement. *Shearing* occurs when one layer of tissue slides over another, disrupting microcirculation of skin and subcutaneous tissue.

Read the following case studies. Circle the correct answer.

CASE STUDY: Traumatic Amputation Psychosocial Perspective

Oliver, a 42-year-old mechanical engineer, works at a major paper mill. While he was doing routine maintenance work, his foot slipped and he fell against an industrial paper cutter. He suffered a traumatic amputation of his left hand.

1. On admission to the emergency department the nurse expects Oliver's initial emotional reaction to be one of:
   a. adjustment and acceptance.
   b. anger and regression.
   c. denial and confusion.
   d. grief and depression.

2. If Oliver begins to mourn for his missing body part, the nurse should:
   a. emphasize all the abilities he has with his remaining hand.
   b. encourage him to cheer up.
   c. listen as he talks about his loss.
   d. remind him of his limited abilities, to reinforce reality.

3. The nurse notices that Oliver blames his loss on his family because he has rationalized that he had to work in a dangerous area to generate sufficient income to support his seven children and his dependent parents. A nursing care plan for Oliver should include:
   a. advising him about budgeting his income to minimize the stress associated with financial worries.
   b. allowing him to project his emotions.
   c. demonstrating self-assistive devices that will help him meet his activities of daily living.
   d. encouraging him to have a positive attitude toward his disability to facilitate his recovery.

4. After several weeks Oliver seems to be adjusting to his disability. Behaviors consistent with this period include:
   a. acceptance of his limitations.
   b. interest in obtaining information about his disability.
   c. redirecting his energies toward coping.
   d. all of the above.

CASE STUDY: Buck's Extension Traction

Patricia is 67 and has limited mobility as a result of a right hip fracture. She is in Buck's extension traction awaiting surgery.

1. During morning care the nurse suggests that Patricia attempt isometric exercises of her legs. This suggestion is based on the nurse's goal of:
   a. encouraging normal muscle function.
   b. maintaining muscle strength while immobilizing the joints.
   c. providing resistance to increase muscle strength.
   d. retaining as much joint range of motion as possible.

2. The nursing goals associated with therapeutic isometric exercises include all of the following *except:*
   a. enhanced joint mobility.
   b. improved patient well-being.
   c. increased strength of the musculature that controls the joints.
   d. prevention of venous stasis.

3. To assist Patricia with isometric exercises of her lower extremities, the nurse should teach her to:
   a. contract or tighten her thigh and calf muscles without moving her knees and hip joints, to hold for several seconds, and then to "let go."
   b. slowly move her legs through limited range of motion while the nurse stabilizes the proximal joint and supports the distal part.
   c. move her legs through their full range of motion while the nurse supports each distal part.
   d. put each leg through full range of motion while the nurse offers slight resistance to the movement.

Learner's Self-Evaluation Tool for End of Unit 4 Review

1. The most important concepts or facts I have learned from this unit are:

    1. _____

    2. _____

    3. _____

2. The most important reference page numbers for test review and clinical concepts are pages:

    _____   _____   _____

    _____   _____   _____

3. The concepts or facts that I do not fully understand are:

    _____

    _____

4. I will get the answer(s) to my questions by _____

    _____

    I will do this on _____ (date and time).

5. I believe my mastery of this unit to be:
    a. 100%   Great job! Good luck!
    b. 90%   2 hours of review recommended.
    c. 80%   4 hours of review recommended.
    d. <80%   Make an appointment with your instructor.

UNIT 5
Perioperative Concepts and Management

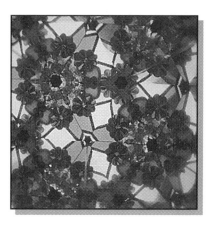

19

Preoperative Nursing Management

Chapter Overview

Preoperative nursing care begins with the nurse's initial contact with the surgical patient. The goal of the preoperative period is to identify individual needs so that accepted protocols of care can be modified. Assessment includes observing for alterations in normal physiologic functioning, determining specific nutritional needs, evaluating current pharmacotherapy, and identifying psychosocial patterns of behavior. This assessment process should result in a detailed nursing care plan. One area that must never be overlooked in the preoperative period is the initiation of a rehabilitation program.

I. Knowledge-Based Questions

Deduction and Interpretation

Read each question carefully. Circle your answer.

1. Hazards of surgery for the geriatric patient are directly related to the:
   a. number of coexisting health problems.
   b. type of surgical procedure.
   c. severity of the surgery.
   d. all of the above.

2. An example of a surgical procedure performed for *curative* effects is a(n):
   a. appendectomy.
   b. exploratory laparotomy.
   c. repair of multiple stab wounds.
   d. face lift.

3. Expected patient outcomes for relief of anxiety related to a surgical procedure include all of the following *except:*
   a. understands the nature of the surgery and voluntarily signs a consent.
   b. verbalizes an understanding of the preanesthetic medication.
   c. requests a visit with a member of the clergy.
   d. questions the anesthesiologist about anesthesia-related concerns.

4. Choose a statement that indicates that a patient is knowledgeable about his or her impending surgery. The patient:
   a. participates willingly in the preoperative preparation.
   b. discusses stress factors that are making him or her depressed.
   c. expresses concern about postoperative pain.
   d. verbalizes his or her fears to family.

 Mary Jo Boyer: Study Guide to Accompany Brunner & Suddarth's Textbook of Medical-Surgical Nursing, 8th ed. © 1996 Lippincott-Raven Publishers

5. Hidden fears may be indicated when a patient:
- a. avoids communication.
- b. repeatedly asks questions that have previously been answered.
- c. talks incessantly.
- d. does all of the above.

6. Choose the appropriate response to the statement "I'm so nervous about my surgery."
- a. "Relax, your recovery period will be shorter if you're less nervous."
- b. "Stop worrying. It only makes you more nervous."
- c. "You needn't worry. Your doctor has done this surgery many times before."
- d. "You seem nervous about your surgery."

7. Protein replacement for nutritional balance can be accomplished with a diet:
- a. high in carbohydrates.
- b. high in protein.
- c. low in fats.
- d. that includes all of the above.

8. Obesity is positively correlated to surgical complications of the:
- a. cardiovascular system.
- b. gastrointestinal system.
- c. pulmonary system.
- d. systems previously listed.

9. A significant mortality rate exists for those alcoholics who experience "delirium tremens" postoperatively. When caring for the alcoholic, the nurse should assess for symptoms of alcoholic withdrawal:
- a. within the first 12 hours.
- b. about 24 hours postoperatively.
- c. on the second or third day.
- d. 4 days after surgery.

10. The nurse should advise all surgical patients who smoke to stop smoking at least _____ week(s) before surgery.
- a. 1
- b. 2
- c. 3
- d. 4

11. Because liver disease is associated with a high surgical mortality, the nurse knows to alert the physician for a(an):
- a. blood ammonia of 180 µg/dl.
- b. LDH of 300 units.
- c. serum albumin of 5.0 g/dl.
- d. serum globulin of 2.8 g/dl.

12. Surgery would be contraindicated for a renal patient with a(an):
- a. BUN of 42 mg/dl.
- b. creatine kinase of 120 U/L.
- c. serum creatinine of 0.9 mg/dl.
- d. urine creatinine of 1.2 mg/dl.

13. The chief life-threatening hazard for surgical patients with uncontrolled diabetes is:
- a. dehydration.
- b. hypertension.
- c. hypoglycemia.
- d. glucosuria.

14. A nursing history of prior drug therapy is based on the particular concern(s) that:
- a. phenothiazines may increase the hypotensive action of anesthetics.
- b. thiazide diuretics may cause excessive respiratory depression during anesthesia.
- c. tranquilizers may cause anxiety and even seizures if withdrawn suddenly.
- d. all of the above potential complications could occur.

15. Assessment of a gerontologic patient reveals bilateral dimmed vision. This information alerts the nurse to plan for:
- a. a safe environment.
- b. restrictions of the patient's unassisted mobility activities.
- c. probable cataract extractions.
- d. referral to an ophthalmologist.

16. An informed consent is required for:
- a. closed reduction of a fracture.
- b. insertion of an intravenous catheter.
- c. irrigation of the external ear canal.
- d. urethral catheterization.

17. The nursing goal(s) of encouraging postoperative body movement is (are) to:
    a. contribute to optimal respiratory function.
    b. improve circulation.
    c. prevent venous stasis.
    d. promote all of the above activities.

18. Food and water are usually withheld beginning at midnight of the surgical day. However, if necessary, water may be given up to:
    a. 8 hours before surgery.
    b. 6 hours before surgery.
    c. 4 hours before surgery.
    d. 2 hours before surgery.

19. The primary goal in withholding food before surgery is to prevent:
    a. aspiration.
    b. distention.
    c. infection.
    d. obstruction.

20. The purpose of preoperative skin preparation is to:
    a. reduce the number of microorganisms.
    b. remove all resident bacteria.
    c. render the skin sterile.
    d. accomplish all of the above.

21. The *least* desirable method of hair removal is use of:
    a. electric clippers.
    b. a depilatory cream in nonsensitive patients.
    c. a razor with an extruded blade.
    d. scissors for long hair (more than 3 mm).

22. Purposes of preanesthetic medication include all of the following *except:*
    a. facilitation of anesthesia induction.
    b. lowering of the dose of the anesthetic agent used.
    c. potentiation of the effects of anesthesia.
    d. reduction of preoperative pain.

23. Anticholinergics, prescribed to reduce respiratory secretions, are used with caution in patients with:
    a. diabetes.
    b. glaucoma.
    c. hypertension.
    d. preoperative pain.

24. Preanesthetic medications need to be given approximately:
    a. 30 minutes before anesthesia.
    b. 1 hour before anesthesia.
    c. 2 hours before anesthesia.
    d. 3 hours before anesthesia.

25. Nursing measures after preanesthetic medications have been given include:
    a. keeping the patient in bed.
    b. maintaining a quiet environment.
    c. raising the side rails.
    d. all of the above.

For each drug classification below, list the potential effects of prior drug therapy on a patient's surgical course.

Drug Classification	Potential Effects of Drug Therapy
Adrenal steroids	_____
Diuretics	_____
Phenothiazines	_____
Antidepressants	_____
Insulin	_____
Antibiotics	_____

For each essential preoperative nursing intervention listed in Column I, write an appropriate nursing goal under Column II.

Column I: Nursing Activity	Column II: Nursing Goal
Restriction of nutrition and fluids	_____
Intestinal preparation	_____
Preoperative skin preparation (cleansing)	_____
Preoperative hair removal	_____
Urinary catheterization	_____
Administration of preoperative medications	_____
Transportation of patient to presurgical suite	_____

II. Critical Analysis Questions

Recognizing Contradictions

Rewrite each statement correctly. Underline the key concepts.

1. The majority of surgical procedures performed today require overnight hospitalization because "high-tech" interventions require intense postoperative monitoring.

2. The intraoperative phase of perioperative nursing ends when surgery is completed.

3. Cosmetic surgery is a type of elective surgery.

4. Vitamin K is an essential vitamin requirement for surgery because it is needed for collagen synthesis.

5. Corticosteroids should always be given up to the day before surgery so the immune system can fight off postoperative infection.

20

Intraoperative Nursing and Anesthesia

Chapter Overview

Intraoperative nursing management includes nursing care that begins before induction of anesthesia and continues throughout the operative period. Major areas of nursing focus are maintaining aseptic techniques and assessing the needs of an unconscious patient. The nurse functions as a patient advocate and modifies protocols of care as necessary. Open communication with the surgical team is essential to individualize care and give the patient the best possible start in his or her recovery period.

I. Knowledge-Based Questions

Deduction and Interpretation

Read each question carefully. Circle your answer.

1. The *circulating* nurse's responsibilities, in contrast to the *scrub* nurse's responsibilities, include:
   a. assisting the surgeon.
   b. monitoring aseptic practices.
   c. setting up the sterile tables.
   d. all of the above functions.

2. Preoperatively, an anesthesiologist is responsible for:
   a. assessing pulmonary status.
   b. inquiring about preexisting pulmonary infections.
   c. knowing the patient's history of smoking.
   d. all of the above.

3. The anesthesiologist classifies a person's physical status for anesthesia before surgery. A nurse should know that a preoperative classification of "good" refers to patients with:
   a. mild cardiac problems.
   b. minimal endocrine disturbances.
   c. moderate organic pathology.
   d. no systemic disturbances.

4. A nurse knows that perioperative risks increase with age because:
   a. ciliary action decreases, reducing the cough reflex.
   b. fatty tissue increases, prolonging the effects of anesthesia.
   c. liver size decreases, reducing the metabolism of anesthetics.
   d. all of the above biologic changes exist.

5. A general anesthetic can be administered:
   a. by inhalation.
   b. intravenously.
   c. rectally.
   d. by all of the above methods.

6. The nurse should know that, postoperatively, a general anesthetic is primarily eliminated by the:
   a. kidneys.
   b. lungs.
   c. skin.
   d. above routes.

7. An example of a stable and safe nondepolarizing muscle relaxant is:
   a. Anectine (succinylcholine chloride)
   b. Norcuron (vercuronium bromide)
   c. Pavulon (pancuronium bromide).
   d. Syncurine (decamethonium).

8. Postoperative nursing assessment for a patient who has received a depolarizing neuromuscular blocking agent includes careful monitoring of the:
   a. cardiovascular system.
   b. endocrine system.
   c. gastrointestinal system.
   d. genitourinary system.

9. A factor(s) involved in post-spinal–anesthesia headaches is(are) the:
   a. degree of patient hydration.
   b. leakage of spinal fluid from the subarchnoid space.
   c. size of the spinal needle used.
   d. combination of the above mechanisms.

10. Epinephrine is often used in combination with a local infiltration anesthetic because it:
    a. causes vasoconstriction.
    b. prevents rapid absorption of the anesthetic drug.
    c. prolongs the local action of the anesthetic agent.
    d. does all of the above.

11. A local infiltration anesthetic can last for up to:
    a. 1 hour.
    b. 3 hours.
    c. 5 hours.
    d. 7 hours.

12. If an operating room nurse is to assist a patient to the Trendelenburg position, she would place him:
    a. flat on his back with his arms next to his sides.
    b. on his back with his head lowered so the plane of his body meets the horizontal on an angle.
    c. on his back with his legs and thighs flexed at right angles.
    d. on his side with his uppermost leg adducted and flexed at the knee.

13. Recent research has indicated that inadvertent hypothermia in gerontologic patients can be effectively and inexpensively prevented by:
    a. placing the patient on a hyperthermia blanket.
    b. maintaining environmental temperature at 37° C.
    c. covering the top of the patient's head with an ordinary plastic shower cap during anesthesia.
    d. frequent massage of the extremities with warmed skin lotion.

14. A nurse caring for a patient at risk for malignant hyperthermia subsequent to general anesthesia would assess for the most frequent *earliest* sign of:
    a. hypertension.
    b. muscle rigidity ("tetany-like" movements).
    c. oliguria.
    d. tachycardia.

Read each statement carefully. Write your response in the space provided.

1. List four responsibilities of an RNFA: (1) _____, (2) _____, (3) _____, and (4) _____.

2. An older person undergoing surgery incurs increased cardiopulmonary risks. Identify a risk associated with each condition.

   Sudden hypotension _____

   Reduced vascular bed _____

   Reduced gas exchange _____

   Diminished ciliary action _____

3. The anesthetic most commonly used for general anesthesia by intravenous injection is: _____ _____, which can cause _____ as a serious, toxic side effect.

4. Spinal anesthesia is a conduction nerve block that occurs when a local anesthetic is injected into _____ _____.

5. What nursing assessment indicates that a patient has recovered from the effects of spinal anesthesia?

_____

II. Critical Analysis Questions

Recognizing Contradictions

Rewrite each statement correctly. Underline the key concepts.

1. A scrub nurse controls the environment, coordinates the activities of other personnel, and monitors the patient.

2. If there is any doubt about the sterility of an area, it is considered sterile.

3. A draped table is considered sterile from the top to the edge of the drapes.

4. Only the circulating nurse can extend an arm over the sterile area to deliver sterile supplies.

5. Older patients need more anesthetic agent to produce anesthesia because they eliminate anesthetic agents more quickly.

Generating Solutions: Clinical Problem Solving

Read the following case studies. Circle the correct answer.

CASE STUDY: General Anesthesia

Anne, age 34, is in excellent health and is scheduled for an open reduction of a fractured femur. The general anesthetic drugs to be used include enflurane and nitrous oxide.

1. The nurse knows that the advantages of enflurane (Ethrane) include all of the following *except:*
   a. fast recovery.
   b. low incidence of respiratory depression.
   c. potent analgesia.
   d. rapid induction.

2. The major disadvantage of nitrous oxide is its ability to cause:
   a. hypertension.
   b. hypoxia.
   c. liver damage.
   d. nausea and vomiting.

3. The major postoperative nursing assessment after administration of Ethrane is observation for:
   a. anuria.
   b. laryngospasm.
   c. respiratory depression.
   d. tachycardia.

CASE STUDY: Intravenous Anesthesia

Brian is scheduled to have a wisdom tooth extracted. The anesthetic agent of choice is thiopental sodium (Pentothal).

1. The nurse anticipates that the route of administration will be:
   a. by inhalation.
   b. by mask.
   c. intramuscular.
   d. intravenous.

2. The nurse is aware that after anesthetic administration, Brian will be unconscious in:
   a. 30 seconds.
   b. 60 seconds.
   c. 2 minutes.
   d. 3 minutes.

3. The chief danger with thiopental sodium is its:
   a. β-adrenergic blocking action.
   b. depressant action on the respiratory system.
   c. nephrotoxicity.
   d. rapid onset and prolonged duration.

21

Postoperative Nursing Management

Chapter Overview

During the postoperative period a nurse must be sufficiently skilled to "recover a patient." This means monitoring physiologic changes and laboratory data that indicate any deviation from the normal. It also involves being able to communicate with a semiconscious patient and reassure concerned family members. The recovery period is regarded as a critical care period, in which intense patient assessment is coupled with the performance of complex nursing skills. The dangers associated with the surgical period do not end until the patient is completely recovered. The postoperative nurse becomes the most important member of the recovery room team.

I. Knowledge-Based Questions

Deduction and Interpretation

Read each question carefully. Circle your answer.

1. Patients remain in the recovery room until they are fully recovered from anesthesia. This is evidenced by a(n):
   a. patient airway.
   b. reasonable degree of consciousness.
   c. stable blood pressure.
   d. indication that all of the above have occurred.

2. When a postanesthesia recovery (PAR) room scoring guide is used, a patient can be transferred out of the recovery room with a minimum score of:
   a. 5.
   b. 6.
   c. 7.
   d. 8.

3. With the PAR room scoring guide, a nurse would give a patient an admission cardiovascular score of 2 if systolic arterial pressure is _____% of the preanesthetic level.
   a. 80
   b. 75 to 60
   c. 60 to 50
   d. less than 50

4. The *primary* nursing goal in the immediate postoperative period is maintenance of pulmonary function and prevention of:
   a. laryngospasm.
   b. hyperventilation.
   c. hypoxemia and hypercapnia.
   d. pulmonary edema and embolism.

 Mary Jo Boyer: Study Guide to Accompany Brunner & Suddarth's Textbook of Medical-Surgical Nursing, 8th ed. © 1996 Lippincott-Raven Publishers

5. Unless contraindicated, any unconscious patient should be positioned:
a. flat on his back, without elevation of his head, to facilitate frequent turning and minimize pulmonary complications.
b. in semi-Fowler's position to promote respiratory function and reduce the incidence of orthostatic hypotension when the patient can eventually stand.
c. in Fowler's position, which most closely simulates a sitting position, thus facilitating respiratory as well as gastrointestinal functioning.
d. on his side with a pillow at his back and his chin extended, to minimize the dangers of aspiration.

6. A major postoperative nursing responsibility is assessing for cardiovascular function by monitoring:
a. arterial blood gases.
b. central venous pressure.
c. vital signs.
d. all of the above.

7. In the immediate postoperative period, a nurse should immediately report:
a. a systolic blood pressure lower than 90 mmHg.
b. a temperature reading between 97°F and 98°F.
c. respirations between 20 and 25 per minute.
d. all of the above assessments.

8. When vomiting occurs postoperatively, the most important nursing intervention is to:
a. measure the amount of vomitus to estimate fluid loss, to accurately monitor fluid balance.
b. offer tepid water and juices to replace lost fluids and electrolytes.
c. support the wound area so that unnecessary strain will not disrupt the integrity of the incision.
d. turn the patient's head to prevent aspiration of vomitus into the lungs.

9. Postoperative abdominal distention seems to be directly related to:
a. a temporary loss of peristalsis and gas accumulation in the intestines.
b. beginning food intake in the immediate postoperative period.
c. improper body positioning during the recovery period.
d. the type of anesthetic administered.

10. Postoperative thirst seems to result from dryness of the mouth directly related to the preoperative administration of:
a. anticholinergics.
b. anti-inflammatory agents.
c. barbiturates or sedatives.
d. narcotic analgesics.

11. Postoperatively, the nurse monitors urinary function. An abnormal outcome that should be reported to the physician is a 2-hour output:
a. less than 30 ml.
b. between 75 and 100 ml.
c. between 100 and 200 ml.
d. greater than 200 ml.

12. The characteristic sign of a paralytic ileus is:
a. abdominal tightness.
b. abdominal distention.
c. absence of peristalsis.
d. increased abdominal girth.

13. Nosocomial infections occur in:
a. 0% to 5% of surgical patients.
b. 10% to 15% of surgical patients.
c. 25% to 30% of surgical patients.
d. approximately 35% of surgical patients.

14. One of the most effective nursing procedures for reducing nosocomial infections is:
a. administration of prophylactic antibiotics.
b. aseptic wound care.
c. control of upper respiratory tract infections.
d. proper handwashing techniques.

15. The most common postoperative respiratory complication in elderly patients is:
a. pleurisy.
b. pneumonia.
c. hypoxemia.
d. pulmonary edema.

16. Most surgical patients are encouraged to be out of bed:
a. within 6 to 8 hours after surgery.
b. between 10 and 12 hours after surgery.
c. as soon as it is indicated.
d. on the second postoperative day.

17. The nurse recognizes that a clean-contaminated wound has a relative probability of infection of:
   a. 1% to 5%.
   b. 10% to 17%.
   c. 3% to 11%.
   d. more than 20%.

18. The proliferative stage of wound healing is characterized by:
   a. deposition of a fibrinoplatelet clot.
   b. histamine release and increased capillary permeability.
   c. fibroblast stimulation of collagen synthesis.
   d. scar formation.

19. A nurse wants to document the presence of granulation tissue in a healing wound. She describes the tissue as:
   a. necrotic and hard.
   b. pale yet able to blanch with digital pressure.
   c. pink to red and soft, and notes that it bleeds easily.
   d. white with long, thin areas of scar tissue.

20. A physician's admitting note lists a wound as healing by second intention. The nurse expects to see a:
   a. deep, open wound that was previously sutured.
   b. sutured incision with a little tissue reaction.
   c. wound with a deep wide scar that had been previously resutured.
   d. wound in which edges were not approximated.

21. A wound that has hemorrhaged has increased risk of infection because:
   a. reduced amounts of oxygen and nutrients are available.
   b. the tissue becomes less resilient.
   c. retrograde bacterial contamination may occur.
   d. dead space and dead cells provide a culture medium.

22. A nursing measure for evisceration is to:
   a. apply an abdominal binder snugly so that the intestines can be slowly pushed back into the abdomen.
   b. approximate the wound edges with adhesive tape so that the intestines can be gently pushed back into the abdomen.
   c. carefully push the exposed intestines back into the abdominal cavity.
   d. cover the protruding coils of intestines with sterile dressings moistened with sterile saline solution.

23. One of the major dangers associated with deep venous thrombosis is:
   a. pulmonary embolism.
   b. immobility because of calf pain.
   c. marked tenderness over the anteromedial surface of the thigh.
   d. swelling of the entire leg owing to edema.

24. Nursing measures to prevent thrombophlebitis include:
   a. assisting the patient with leg exercises.
   b. encouraging early ambulation.
   c. avoiding placement of pillows or blanket rolls under the knees.
   d. all of the above.

25. Nursing assessment to help confirm a diagnosis of pleurisy includes observation for signs and symptoms of:
   a. acute chest pain on the affected side, with pain more prominent on inspiration.
   b. a productive cough and a marked temperature elevation.
   c. chills, a high temperature, and respiratory embarrassment.
   d. crackles at the base of both lungs and a slight cough.

26. An indication that incontinence of retention is occurring is that:
   a. a person is unable to hold more than 10 ml of urine in his bladder.
   b. a person constantly dribbles urine when the bladder is overdistended.
   c. the bladder is unable to hold urine because of frequent bladder sphincter spasms.
   d. 100 to 200 ml of urine is eliminated from the bladder every 2 to 3 hours.

Read each statement carefully. Write your response in the space provided.

1. The primary nursing priorities during immediate postoperative assessment are evaluation of

   _____

   _____

2. List five areas of concern for a recovery room nurse who has just received a patient from the operating room.

   (a) _____   (d) _____

   (b) _____   (e) _____

   (c) _____

3. Several psychological factors that can influence a patient's pain experience are:

   _____

   _____

   _____

4. Explain patient-controlled analgesia (PCA).

   _____

   _____

5. The return of peristalsis in the postoperative period can be determined by the presence of
   _____ and _____, both of
   which are assessed by the nurse.

6. Explain why the postoperative complications of atelectasis and hypostatic pneumonia are reduced as a result
   of early ambulation. _____

   _____

7. Name three criteria that must be met before a postoperative patient can be given fluids:

   (a) _____ ,   (c) _____ ,

   (b) _____ .

8. Name four organisms found to cause nosocomial infections:

   (a) _____   (c) _____

   (b) _____   (d) _____

9. Describe the correct way to apply and remove adhesive tape during a surgical dressing change.

   _____

   _____

10. Explain the differences among the three classifications of hemorrhage.

    Primary: _____

    Intermediary: _____

    _____

    Secondary: _____

    _____

II. Critical Analysis Questions

Supporting Arguments

Read each situation. Offer logical supporting arguments for your response.

1. Mr. Flynn's pain medication was frequently delayed because his staff nurses were busy with other patients. As a nursing supervisor, you stressed the necessity of preventing or managing postoperative pain knowing that there is a positive correlation between pain experience and the frequency of complications. Support your argument by filling in these blank spaces.

Pain stimulates _____ which increases _____

_____

Noxious impulses stimulate

_____ which increases _____

and

_____

Hypothalmic stress responses increase _____

which can lead to _____ and

and _____

_____

Benedetti (1992) found that _____ can be _____

more frequent and _____ _____ greater with inadequate

postoperative control.

Recognizing Contradictions

Rewrite each statement correctly. Underline the key concepts.

1. Nurses need to think "pain control," rather than "pain prevention," when administering postoperative narcotics because of the potential for drug addiction.

2. Pain intensity is considered most severe for lower abdominal surgery.

3. Signs of hypervolemia include: hypotension, tachycardia, oliguria and CVP < 4 cmH$_2$O.

4. A contaminated wound is characterized by the presence of devitalized tissue.

5. Sutures should always remain in place for 2 weeks to allow time for skin approximation.

Generating Solutions: Clinical Problem Solving

Read the following case studies. Circle the correct answer.

CASE STUDY: Hypopharyngeal Obstruction

Daena is unconscious when she is transferred to the recovery room. She has experienced prolonged anesthesia, and all her muscles are relaxed.

1. During the initial assessment the nurse diagnosed hypopharyngeal obstruction. This difficulty is signaled by:
   a. choking.
   b. cyanosis.
   c. irregular respirations.
   d. all of the above.

2. To treat hypopharyngeal obstruction, the nurse would:
   a. flex the neck and pull the lower jaw down toward the chest.
   b. hyperextend the neck and push forward on the angle of the lower jaw.
   c. raise the head and open the mouth as far as possible.
   d. rotate the head to either side and unclench the teeth.

3. The nurse knows that the *most accurate* way to determine whether Daena is breathing is to:
   a. auscultate for breath sounds.
   b. inspect for diaphragmatic movement.
   c. palpate for thoracic changes.
   d. place her palm over Daena's nose and mouth.

4. The anesthesiologist chose to leave a plastic airway in Daena's mouth. The nurse knows that an airway should not be removed:
   a. without a physician's order.
   b. until the patient's secretions have been aspirated.
   c. until signs indicate that reflexes are returning.
   d. until arterial blood gas measurements indicate adequate PO_2 levels.

CASE STUDY: Wound Healing

Elizabeth is returned from the recovery room to a patient care area after a routine cholecystectomy.

1. The nurse expects that the inflammatory phase of wound healing should last for about:
   a. 1 day.
   b. 3 days.
   c. 5 days.
   d. 7 days.

2. The nurse is aware that both sides of the wound should approximate within:
   a. 2 to 12 hours.
   b. 12 to 23 hours.
   c. 24 to 48 hours.
   d. 60 to 72 hours.

3. Those clinical manifestations associated with the inflammatory phase of wound healing that the nurse would expect to see postoperatively are:
   a. pain.
   b. redness.
   c. warmth.
   d. all of the above.

4. Nursing measures to promote adequate tissue oxygenation during the *inflammatory phase* of wound healing include:
   a. applying warm compresses to the incision every 4 hours for 2 to 3 days to stimulate vasodilation.
   b. encouraging coughing and deep breathing to enhance pulmonary and cardiovascular functions.
   c. helping Elizabeth stay in bed for 4 to 6 days to prevent unnecessary strain on the suture line.
   d. leaving soiled dressings in place to prevent airborne microorganisms from entering the wound and setting up a localized infection.

View Figure 21–4 and answer the clinically focused questions.

CLINICAL SITUATION: Phlebothrombosis

1. Look at (A) and explain what the nurse is doing: _____

_____

2. Describe how the nurse would assess for a positive Homans' sign: _____

_____

3. Describe what phlebothrombosis is: _____

_____

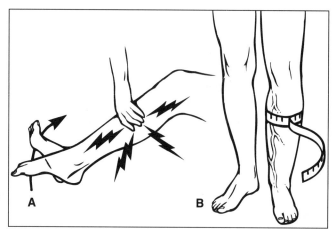

FIGURE 21-4

4. Look at (B) and explain why a tape measure is around the calf muscle. _____

_____

Learner's Self-Evaluation Tool for End of Unit 5 Review

1. The most important concepts or facts I have learned from this unit are:

    1. _____

    2. _____

    3. _____

2. The most important reference page numbers for test review and clinical concepts are pages:

    _____   _____   _____

    _____   _____   _____

3. The concepts or facts that I do not fully understand are:

_____

_____

4. I will get the answer(s) to my questions by _____

_____

    I will do this on _____ (date and time).

5. I believe my mastery of this unit to be:

    a.   100%   Great job! Good luck!

    b.   90%   2 hours of review recommended.

    c.   80%   4 hours of review recommended.

    d.   <80%   Make an appointment with your instructor.

UNIT 6
Oxygen–Carbon Dioxide Exchange and Respiratory Function

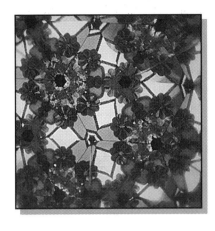

22

Assessment of Respiratory Function

Chapter Overview

Illness may be accompanied by ventilatory–perfusion abnormalities. Therefore, nurses need a thorough knowledge of lung anatomy and physiology to assess pulmonary dysfunction. Nurses also need to be knowledgeable about various diagnostic studies and tests. In addition to assessment, nursing responsibilities include assisting patients with various procedures, implementing a plan of care to meet individual pulmonary needs, incorporating principles of respiratory rehabilitation into health-teaching programs, and evaluating each patient's response to therapy.

I. Knowledge-Based Questions

Deduction and Interpretation

Read each question carefully. Circle your answer.

1. The exchange of oxygen and carbon dioxide from the alveoli into the blood occurs by:
   a. active transport.
   b. diffusion.
   c. osmosis.
   d. pinocytosis.

2. Gas exchange between the lungs and blood, and between the blood and tissues, is called:
   a. active transport.
   b. respiration.
   c. ventilation.
   d. cellular respiration.

3. The divisions of the lung lobe proceed in the following order, beginning at the main stem bronchi:
   a. lobar bronchi, bronchioles, segmented bronchi, subsequent bronchi
   b. segmented bronchi, subsegmented bronchi, lobar bronchi, bronchioles
   c. lobar bronchi, segmented bronchi, subsegmented bronchi, bronchioles
   d. subsegmented bronchi, lobar bronchi, bronchioles, segmented bronchi

4. The left lung, in contrast to the right lung, has:
   a. one less lobe.
   b. one more lobe.
   c. the same number of lobes.
   d. two more lobes.

5. The lungs are enclosed in a serous membrane called the:
   a. diaphragm.
   b. mediastinum.
   c. pleura.
   d. xiphoid process.

 Mary Jo Boyer: Study Guide to Accompany Brunner & Suddarth's Textbook of Medical-Surgical Nursing, 8th ed. © 1996 Lippincott-Raven Publishers

6. The purpose of the cilia is to:
   a. produce mucus.
   b. phagocytize bacteria.
   c. contract smooth muscle.
   d. move the mucous blanket to the larynx.

7. Choose the part of the respiratory tract that is not considered part of the gas-exchange airways.
   a. Bronchioles
   b. Respiratory bronchioles
   c. Alveolar duct
   d. Alveolar sacs

8. Choose the alveolar cell(s) that secrete surfactant.
   a. Type I cell
   b. Type II cell
   c. Type III cell
   d. Type I and type II cells

9. Airflow into the lungs during inspiration depends on all of the following *except:*
   a. contraction of the muscles of respiration.
   b. enlargement of the thoracic cavity.
   c. lowered intrathoracic pressure.
   d. relaxation of the diaphragm.

10. The pulmonary circulation is considered a:
    a. high-pressure, high-resistance system.
    b. low-pressure, low-resistance system.
    c. high-pressure, low-resistance system.
    d. low-pressure, high-resistance system.

11. Uneven perfusion of the lung is primarily due to:
    a. pulmonary artery pressure.
    b. gravity.
    c. alveolar pressure.
    d. all of the above.

12. A nurse caring for a patient with a pulmonary embolism understands that a high ventilation–perfusion ratio may exist. This means that:
    a. perfusion exceeds ventilation.
    b. there is an absence of perfusion and ventilation.
    c. ventilation exceeds perfusion.
    d. ventilation matches perfusion.

13. A nurse understands that a safe, but abnormal, level of oxygen saturation provides for adequate tissue saturation, but allows no reserve for situations that threaten ventilation. A safe yet abnormal oxygen saturation level is:
    a. 40 mmHg.
    b. 75 mmHg.
    c. 80 mmHg.
    d. 95 mmHg.

14. The central chemoreceptors respond to:
    a. changes in PaO_2.
    b. changes in the pH of the blood.
    c. changes in the PO_2 of the cerebrospinal fluid.
    d. changes in the pH of the cerebrospinal fluid.

15. When taking a respiratory history, the nurse should assess:
    a. previous history of lung disease in the patient or family.
    b. occupational and environmental influences.
    c. smoking and exposure to allergies.
    d. all of the above.

16. The nurse inspects the thorax of a patient with advanced emphysema. The nurse expects chest configuration change consistent with a deformity known as:
    a. barrel chest.
    b. funnel chest.
    c. kyphoscoliosis.
    d. pigeon chest.

17. Breath sounds that originate in the smaller bronchi and bronchioles that are high-pitched, sibilant, and musical are called:
    a. wheezes.
    b. rhonchi.
    c. rales.
    d. crackles.

18. Bacterial pneumonia can be indicated by the presence of:
    a. green purulent sputum.
    b. thick yellow sputum.
    c. thin mucoid sputum.
    d. rusty sputum.

19. Nursing assessment for a patient with chest pain includes:
    a. determining if there is a relationship between pain and the patient's posture.
    b. evaluating the effect of the phases of respiration on pain.
    c. looking for factors that precipitate the pain.
    d. all of the above.

20. Chest pain described as knifelike on inspiration would most likely be diagnostic of:
    a. bacterial pneumonia.
    b. bronchogenic carcinoma.
    c. lung infarction.
    d. pleurisy.

21. Hemoptysis, a symptom of cardiopulmonary disorders, is characterized by all of the following *except:*
    a. a coffeeground appearance.
    b. an alkaline pH.
    c. a sudden onset.
    d. bright red bleeding mixed with sputum.

22. A patient exhibits cyanosis when _____ g/dl of hemoglobin is unoxygenated.
    a. 0.77
    b. 2.3
    c. 15.0
    d. 5.0

23. The arterial blood gas measurement that best reflects the adequacy of alveolar ventilation is the:
    a. PaO_2.
    b. $PaCO_2$.
    c. pH.
    d. SaO_2.

24. A physician wants a study of diaphragmatic motion because of suspected pathology. He would most likely order a:
    a. barium swallow.
    b. bronchogram.
    c. fluoroscopy.
    d. tomogram.

25. The nurse should advise the prebronchoscope patient that he will:
    a. have his nose sprayed with a topical anesthetic.
    b. have to fast before the procedure.
    c. receive preoperative medication.
    d. experience all of the above.

26. Nursing directions to a patient from whom a sputum specimen is to be obtained should include all of the following *except* directing him to:
    a. initially clear his nose and throat.
    b. spit surface mucus and saliva into a sterile specimen container.
    c. take a few deep breaths before coughing.
    d. use diaphragmatic contractions to aid in the expulsion of sputum.

27. Nursing instructions for a patient who is scheduled for a perfusion lung scan should include informing him that:
    a. a mask will be placed over his nose and mouth during the test.
    b. he will be expected to lie under the camera.
    c. the imaging time will amount to 20 to 40 minutes.
    d. all of the above will occur.

II. Critical Analysis Questions

Generating Solutions: Clinical Problem Solving

Read the following case studies. Circle the correct answer.

CASE STUDY: Bronchoscopy

Mr. Kecklin is scheduled for a bronchoscopy for the diagnostic purpose of locating a pathologic process.

1. Because a bronchoscopy was ordered, the nurse knows that the suspected lesion was not in the:
   a. bronchus.
   b. larynx.
   c. pharynx.
   d. trachea.

2. Nursing measures before the bronchoscopy include:
   a. obtaining an informed consent.
   b. supplying information about the procedure.
   c. withholding food and fluids for 6 hours before the test.
   d. all of the above.

3. The nurse is aware that possible complications of bronchoscopy include all of the following *except:*
   a. aspiration.
   b. gastric perforation.
   c. infection.
   d. pneumothorax.

4. After the bronchoscopy Mr. Kecklin must be observed for:
   a. dyspnea.
   b. hemoptysis.
   c. tachycardia.
   d. all of the above.

5. After the bronchoscopy Mr. Kecklin:
   a. can be given ice chips and fluids after he demonstrates that he can perform the gag reflex.
   b. should immediately be given a house diet to alleviate his hunger resulting from the required fast.
   c. should initially be given iced ginger ale to prevent vomiting and possible aspiration of stomach contents.
   d. will need to remain NPO for 6 hours to prevent pharyngeal irritation.

CASE STUDY: Thoracentesis

Mrs. Lomar is admitted to the clinical area for a thoracentesis. The physician wants to remove excess air from the pleural cavity.

1. Nursing responsibilities before the thoracentesis should include:
   a. informing Mrs. Lomar about pressure sensations that will be experienced during the procedure.
   b. making sure that chest roentgenograms ordered in advance have been completed.
   c. seeing that the consent form has been explained and signed.
   d. all of the above.

2. For the thoracentesis, the patient is assisted to any of the following positions *except:*
   a. lying on the unaffected side with the bed elevated 30 to 40 degrees.
   b. lying prone with the head of the bed lowered 15 to 30 degrees.
   c. sitting on the edge of the bed with her feet supported and her arms and head on a padded overbed table.
   d. straddling a chair with her arms and head resting on the back of the chair.

3. Nursing intervention includes exposing the entire chest even though the thoracentesis site is normally in the midclavicular line between the:
   a. first and second intercostal spaces.
   b. second and third intercostal spaces.
   c. third and fourth intercostal spaces.
   d. fourth and fifth intercostal spaces.

4. Nursing observations after the thoracentesis include assessment for:
   a. blood-tinged mucus.
   b. signs of hypoxemia.
   c. tachycardia.
   d. all of the above.

5. A chest x-ray film is usually ordered after the thoracentesis to rule out:
   a. pleurisy.
   b. pneumonia.
   c. pneumothorax.
   d. pulmonary edema.

23

Management of Patients With Conditions of the Upper Respiratory Tract

Chapter Overview

Each of us has, at some time, experienced upper airway discomforts, either from the common cold or from severe respiratory tract infections. When we cannot breathe or swallow without congestion or pain, our whole body reacts. The nurse needs to be sensitive to systemic as well as localized responses when developing a plan of care so that the patient's total needs can be met. The need for physical rest must be considered equally as important as the need for pain relief, hydration, and ventilation. The focus of nursing implementation, therefore, must be the total patient, even though the alteration is localized in the upper respiratory airway.

I. Knowledge-Based Questions

Deduction and Interpretation

Read each question carefully. Circle your answer.

1. Nursing measures associated with the uncomplicated common cold include all of the following *except:*
   a. administering prescribed antibiotics to decrease the severity of the viral infection.
   b. informing the patient about the symptoms of secondary infection, the major complication of a cold.
   c. suggesting adequate fluid intake and rest.
   d. teaching people that the virus is contagious for 2 days before symptoms appear and during the first part of the symptomatic phase.

2. Acyclovir, an antiviral agent, is recommended for:
   a. herpes simplex infection.
   b. rhinitis.
   c. sinusitus.
   d. bronchitis.

3. The herpes virus, which remains latent in cells of the lips or nose, usually subsides spontaneously in:
   a. 5 days.
   b. 1 week.
   c. 10 to 14 days.
   d. 3 to 4 weeks.

4. Nursing suggestions for a patient with acute or chronic sinusitis include:
   a. adequate fluid intake.
   b. increased humidity.
   c. local heat applications to promote drainage.
   d. all of the above.

Mary Jo Boyer: Study Guide to Accompany Brunner & Suddarth's Textbook of Medical-Surgical Nursing, 8th ed. © 1996 Lippincott-Raven Publishers

5. About 60% of cases of acute sinusitis are caused by bacterial organisms. The antibiotic of choice is:

   a. amoxicillin–clavulanate (Augmentin)
   b. acyclovir.

   c. erythromycin.
   d. cefotetan.

6. Health teaching for viral rhinitis includes advising the patient to:

   a. blow his nose gently to prevent spread of the infection.
   b. blow through both nostrils to equalize the pressure.

   c. rest, to promote overall comfort.
   d. do all of the above.

7. Acute pharyngitis of a bacterial nature is most commonly caused by:

   a. group A *Streptococcus*.
   b. gram-negative *Klebsiella*.

   c. *Pseudomonas*.
   d. *Staphylococcus aureus*.

8. A complication(s) of acute pharyngitis is(are):

   a. mastoiditis.
   b. nephritis.

   c. rheumatic fever.
   d. all of the above.

9. Nursing management for a patient with acute pharyngitis includes:

   a. applying an ice collar for symptomatic relief of a severe sore throat.
   b. encouraging bed rest during the febrile stage of the illness.

   c. suggesting a liquid or soft diet during the acute stage of the disease.
   d. all of the above measures.

10. The most common organism associated with tonsillitis and adenoiditis is:

   a. group A *Streptococcus*.
   b. gram-negative *Klebsiella*.

   c. Psuedomonas.
   d. *Staphylococcus aureus*.

11. Potential complications of enlarged adenoids include all of the following *except*:

   a. bronchitis.
   b. nasal obstruction.

   c. allergies.
   d. acute otitis media.

12. To assess for an upper respiratory tract infection, the nurse should *palpate:*

   a. the frontal and maxillary sinuses.
   b. the trachea.

   c. the neck lymph nodes.
   d. all of the above areas.

13. To assess for an upper respiratory tract infection, the nurse should *inspect:*

   a. the nasal mucosa.
   b. the frontal sinuses.

   c. the tracheal mucosa.
   d. all of the above.

14. Airway clearance in a patient with an upper airway infection is facilitated by all of the following *except:*

   a. decreasing systemic hydration.
   b. humidifying inspired room air.

   c. positional drainage of the affected area.
   d. administering prescribed vasoconstrictive medications.

15. Nursing intervention for a patient with a fractured nose includes all of the following *except:*

   a. applying cold compresses to decrease swelling and control bleeding.
   b. assessing respirations to detect any interference with breathing.

   c. observing for any clear fluid drainage from either nostril.
   d. packing each nostril with a cotton pledget to minimize bleeding and help maintain the shape of the nose during fracture setting.

16. Surgical reduction of nasal fractures is usually performed _____ after the fracture.

   a. within 24 hours
   b. 7 to 10 days

   c. 2 to 3 weeks
   d. 2 months

17. The glottis is also known as the:

   a. larynx.
   b. cricoid cartilage.

   c. "Adam's apple."
   d. opening between the vocal chords.

18. To correctly perform the Heimlich maneuver, a person should forcefully apply pressure against the victim's:
   a. abdomen.
   b. diaphragm.
   c. lungs.
   d. trachea.

19. An *early sign* of intrinsic cancer of the larynx is:
   a. affected voice sounds.
   b. burning of the throat when hot liquids are ingested.
   c. enlarged cervical nodes.
   d. dysphagia.

20. Assessment of a patient admitted for laryngeal carcinoma includes:
   a. palpation of the frontal and maxillary sinuses to detect infection or inflammation.
   b. palpation of the neck for swelling.
   c. inspection of the nasal mucosa for polyps.
   d. all of the above techniques.

21. A patient with a total laryngectomy would no longer have:
   a. natural vocalization.
   b. protection of the lower airway from foreign particles.
   c. a normal effective cough.
   d. all of the above mechanisms.

22. Patient education for a laryngectomy includes:
   a. advising that large amounts of mucus can be coughed up through the stoma.
   b. cautioning about preventing water from entering the stoma.
   c. telling the patient to expect a diminished sense of taste and smell.
   d. doing all of the above.

II. Critical Analysis Questions

Generating Solutions: Clinical Problem Solving

Read the following case studies. Fill in the blanks or circle the correct answer.

CASE STUDY: Epistaxis

Gilberta, a 14-year-old high school student, is sent with her mother to the emergency department of a local hospital for uncontrolled epistaxis.

1. Describe what the school nurse should tell Gilberta to manage the bleeding site while being transported to the hospital.

   _____

   _____

2. Initial nursing measures in the emergency room that can be used to stop the nasal bleeding include:
   a. compressing the soft outer portion of the nose against the midline septum continuously for 5 to 10 minutes.
   b. keeping Gilberta in the upright position with her head tilted forward to prevent swallowing and aspiration of blood.
   c. telling her to breathe through her mouth and to refrain from talking.
   d. all of the above.

3. The nurse expects that emergency medical treatment may include insertion of a cotton pledget moistened with:
   a. an adrenergic blocking agent.
   b. aqueous epinephrine.
   c. protamine sulfate.
   d. vitamin K.

4. The nurse is aware that nasal packing used to control bleeding can be left in place:
   a. no longer than 2 hours.
   b. an average of 12 hours.
   c. an average of 24 hours.
   d. anywhere from 2 to 6 days.

CASE STUDY: Tonsillectomy and Adenoidectomy

Isabel, a 14-year-old, just had a tonsillectomy and adenoidectomy. The staff nurse assists her with her transport from the recovery area to her room.

1. Based on her knowledge about tonsillar disease, the nurse knows that Isabel must have experienced symptoms that required surgical intervention. Clinical manifestations may have included:
   a. hypertrophy of the tonsils.
   b. repeated attacks of otitis media.
   c. suspected hearing loss secondary to otitis media.
   d. all of the above.

2. The nurse assesses Isabel's postoperative vital signs and checks for the most significant postoperative complication of:
   a. epiglottis.
   b. eustachian tube perforation.
   c. hemorrhage.
   d. oropharyngeal edema.

3. The nurse maintains Isabel in the recommended postoperative position of:
   a. prone with her head on a pillow and turned to the side.
   b. reverse Trendelenburg with the neck extended.
   c. semi-Fowler's with the neck flexed.
   d. supine with her neck hyperextended and supported with a pillow.

4. Isabel is to be discharged the same day of her tonsillectomy. The nurse makes sure that her family knows to:
   a. encourage her to eat a house diet to build up her resistance to infection.
   b. offer her only clear liquids for 3 days, to prevent pharyngeal irritation.
   c. offer her soft foods for several days to minimize local discomfort and supply her with necessary nutrients.
   d. supplement her diet with orange and lemon juices because of the need for vitamin C to heal tissues.

CASE STUDY: Laryngectomy

Jerome, a 52-year-old widower, is admitted for a laryngectomy owing to a malignant tumor.

1. Before developing a care plan, the nurse needs to know if Jerome's voice will be preserved. The surgical procedure that would not damage the voice box is a:
   a. partial laryngectomy.
   b. supraglottic laryngectomy.
   c. thyrotomy.
   d. total laryngectomy.

2. Jerome is scheduled for a total laryngectomy. Preoperative education includes:
   a. informing him that there are ways he will be able to carry on a conversation without his voice.
   b. making sure that he knows he will require a permanent tracheal stoma.
   c. reminding him that he will not be able to sing, whistle, or laugh.
   d. all of the above.

3. Postoperative nutrition is usually maintained by way of a nasogastric catheter. The nurse needs to tell Jerome that oral feedings usually begin after.
   a. 24 hours.
   b. 2 to 3 days.
   c. 5 to 6 days.
   d. 1 week.

4. Postoperative nursing measures to promote respiratory effectiveness include:
   a. assisting with turning and early ambulation.
   b. positioning Jerome in semi- to high Fowler's position.
   c. reminding him to cough and take frequent deep breaths.
   d. all of the above.

5. Jerome needs to know that the laryngectomy tube will be removed when:
   a. esophageal speech has been perfected.
   b. he requests that it be removed.
   c. oral feedings are initiated.
   d. the stoma is well healed.

24

Management of Patients With Conditions of the Chest and Lower Respiratory Tract

Chapter Overview

Pulmonary infections, whether minor or life-threatening, result in systemic as well as localized responses to the causative agent. Nursing interventions address individual needs based on each patient's prior state of health, current defense mechanisms, and recommended goals of treatment. Infectious agents are especially virulent to patients with chronic pulmonary disorders. Chronic lung disease requires a multidisciplinary approach to patient care.

The nurse of today needs to be cognizant of respiratory pathophysiology and chest conditions in order to develop and implement a plan of care for acutely ill and chronically debilitated patients (*e.g.*, those with infections or chest trauma).

I. Knowledge-Based Questions

Deduction and Interpretation

Read each question carefully. Circle your answer.

1. The most common clinical syndrome resulting from mycoplasmal pneumonia infection is:
   a. bronchiolitis.
   b. tracheobronchitis.
   c. bronchitis.
   d. lung abscess.

2. Nursing management for a person diagnosed as having tracheobronchitis includes:
   a. applying moist heat to the chest to relieve soreness and pain.
   b. encouraging the patient to remain in bed.
   c. using cool-vapor therapy to relieve laryngeal and tracheal irritation.
   d. all of the above.

3. The most common cause of death from infectious diseases in the United States is:
   a. atelectasis.
   b. pulmonary embolus.
   c. pneumonia.
   d. tracheobronchitis.

4. Characteristics of the tuberculosis mycobacterium include all of the following *except* that it:
   a. can be transmitted only by droplet nuclei.
   b. is able to lie dormant within the body for years.
   c. is acid-fast.
   d. survives in anaerobic conditions.

 Mary Jo Boyer: Study Guide to Accompany Brunner & Suddarth's Textbook of Medical-Surgical Nursing, 8th ed. © 1996 Lippincott-Raven Publishers

5. For the tubercle bacillus to multiply and initiate a tissue reaction in the lungs, it must be deposited in:
   a. the alveoli.
   b. the bronchi.
   c. the trachea.
   d. all of the above tissues.

6. Diagnostic confirmation of a lung abscess is made by:
   a. chest x-ray.
   b. bronchoscopy.
   c. sputum culture.
   d. evaluating all of the above studies.

7. The most diagnostic clinical symptom(s) of pleurisy is(are):
   a. dullness or flatness on percussion over areas of collected fluid.
   b. dyspnea and coughing.
   c. fever and chills.
   d. stabbing pain during inspiration.

8. A pleural effusion results in fluid accumulation in the pleural space that is greater than:
   a. 5 ml.
   b. 10 ml.
   c. 15 ml.
   d. 20 ml.

9. Chronic obstructive pulmonary disease (COPD) includes the following disorders:
   a. chronic bronchitis and bronchiectasis.
   b. emphysema and asthma.
   c. chronic bronchitis and asthma.
   d. all four respiratory disorders.

10. COPD is believed to affect over _____ % of the adult population.
    a. 10
    b. 15
    c. 20
    d. 25

11. Nursing assessment of a patient with bronchospasm associated with chronic obstructive pulmonary disease would include assessment for:
    a. compromised gas exchange.
    b. decreased airflow.
    c. wheezes.
    d. all of the above.

12. For a patient with chronic bronchitis, the nurse expects to see the major clinical symptoms(s) of:
    a. chest pain during respiration.
    b. dyspnea and a productive cough.
    c. fever, chills, and diaphoresis.
    d. tachypnea and tachycardia.

13. The nurse should be alert for a complication of bronchiectasis that results from a combination of retained secretions and obstruction. This complication is known as:
    a. atelectasis.
    b. emphysema.
    c. pleurisy.
    d. pneumonia.

14. The *most common* respiratory cause of disability under Medicare is:
    a. aspiration of food particles.
    b. bronchiectasis.
    c. emphysema.
    d. pulmonary embolism.

15. The major cause of emphysema is:
    a. air pollution.
    b. allergens.
    c. infectious agents.
    d. smoking.

16. The primary presenting symptom of emphysema is:
    a. chronic cough.
    b. dyspnea.
    c. tachypnea.
    d. wheezing.

17. Bronchodilators are prescribed in emphysema primarily because they:
    a. improve gas exchange.
    b. interfere with mucosal edema.
    c. reduce airway obstruction.
    d. participate in all the above functions.

18. Obstruction of the airway in the patient with asthma is caused by all of the following *except:*
    a. thick mucus.
    b. swelling of bronchial membranes.
    c. destruction of the alveolar wall.
    d. contraction of muscles surrounding the bronchi.

19. The major symptom(s) of asthma is(are):
    a. cough.
    b. dyspnea.
    c. wheezing.
    d. all three are major.

20. The nurse understands that a patient with *status asthmaticus* is most likely to evidence symptoms of:
    a. metabolic acidosis.
    b. metabolic alkalosis.
    c. respiratory acidosis.
    d. respiratory alkalosis.

21. Acute respiratory failure occurs when oxygen tension falls below _____ mm Hg (hypoxemia).
    a. 50
    b. 60
    c. 75
    d. 80

22. The following calculation, $PAO_2 = FIO_2 (P_B - 47) - \frac{(PaCO_2)}{(0.8)}$, is used to determine:
    a. dead space ventilation.
    b. arterial oxygen tension.
    c. shuting.
    d. alveolar oxygen tension.

23. Neuromuscular blockers are given to patients who are on ventilators in acute respiratory failure to accomplish all of the following *except:*
    a. maintain positive end-expiratory pressure (PEEP).
    b. maintain better ventilation.
    c. increase the respiratory rate.
    d. keep the patient from fighting the ventilator.

24. Clinical manifestations directly related to cor pulmonale include all of the following *except:*
    a. ascites.
    b. diminished peripheral pulses.
    c. distended neck veins.
    d. leg edema.

25. To assess for a positive Homans' sign, the nurse should:
    a. dorsiflex the foot while the leg is elevated to check for calf pain.
    b. elevate the patient's legs for 20 minutes and then lower them slowly while checking for areas of inadequate blood return.
    c. extend the leg, plantar flex the foot, and check for the patency of the dorsalis pedis pulse.
    d. lower the patient's legs and massage the calf muscles to note any areas of tenderness.

26. Nursing measures to assist in the prevention of pulmonary embolism include all of the following *except:*
    a. a liberal fluid intake.
    b. assisting the patient to do leg elevations above the level of the heart.
    c. encouraging the patient to dangle his legs over the side of the bed for 30 minutes, four times a day.
    d. the use of elastic stockings, especially when decreased mobility would promote venous stasis.

27. Anticoagulation with heparin attempts to maintain the partial thromboplastin time (PTT) at _____ times normal.
    a. 1.0 to 1.3
    b. 1.5 to 2.0
    c. 2.0 to 2.5
    d. 2.0 to 3.0

28. There seems to be a positive correlation between sleep apnea and:
    a. a history of frequent upper respiratory tract infections.
    b. body position during sleep.
    c. chronic obstructive lung disease.
    d. obesity and age.

29. As a cause of death among men in the United States, lung cancer ranks:
    a. first.
    b. second.
    c. third.
    d. fourth.

30. The cellular type of lung cancer that has the poorest prognosis is:
    a. adenocarcinoma.
    b. epidermoid.
    c. large cell (undifferentiated).
    d. small cell (oat cell).

31. Paradoxical chest movement is associated with the following chest disorder:
  a. pneumothorax.
  b. flail chest.
  c. adult respiratory distress syndrome (ARDS).
  d. tension pneumothorax.

II. Critical Analysis Questions

Generating Solutions: Clinical Problem Solving

Read the following case studies. Circle the correct answer.

CASE STUDY: Bacterial Pneumonia

Theresa, a 36-year-old single parent, lives in a small twin house with her two daughters. She is a waitress and is diagnosed as having bacterial pneumonia.

1. The nurse is informed that Theresa has the most common strain of bacterial pneumonia. The nurse suspects that the infecting agent is:
  a. *Haemophilis influenzae.*
  b. *Klebsiella.*
  c. *Proteus.*
  d. *Streptococcus pneumoniae.*

2. All of the following are manifestations of bacterial pneumonia *except:*
  a. a rapidly rising fever.
  b. bradycardia.
  c. stabbing chest pain.
  d. tachypnea.

3. The nurse expects that Theresa will be medicated with the usual antibiotic of choice, which is:
  a. cephalosporin.
  b. clindamycin.
  c. erythromycin.
  d. penicillin G.

4. The nurse is aware that Theresa may develop arterial hypoxemia because:
  a. bronchospasm causes alveolar collapse, which decreases the surface area necessary for perfusion.
  b. mucosal edema occludes the alveoli, thereby producing a drop in alveolar oxygen.
  c. venous blood is shunted from the right to the left side of the heart.
  d. all of the above are true.

5. Theresa is expected to respond to antibiotic therapy:
  a. within 6 hours.
  b. between 1 and 2 days.
  c. by the fourth day.
  d. after 7 days.

6. Nursing management includes assessment for a complication(s) such as:
  a. atelectasis.
  b. hypotension and shock.
  c. pleural effusion.
  d. all of the above.

CASE STUDY: Bronchitis

Lois, who has had emphysema for 25 years, is admitted to the hospital with a diagnosis of bronchitis.

1. During assessment the nurse notes the presence of a "barrel chest," which she knows is due to a:
  a. compensatory expansion of the bronchial airway.
  b. decrease in intrapleural pressure.
  c. loss of lung elasticity.
  d. progressive increase in vital capacity.

2. The nurse recognizes the need to be alert for the major presenting symptom of emphysema, which is:
  a. bradypnea.
  b. dyspnea.
  c. expiratory wheezing.
  d. fatigue.

3. Arterial blood gas measurements that are consistent with a diagnosis of emphysema are:
  a. pH, 7.32; PaO_2, 70 mmHg; $PaCO_2$, 50 mmHg.
  b. pH, 7.37; PaO_2, 90 mmHg; $PaCO_2$, 42 mmHg.
  c. pH, 7.39; PaO_2, 80 mmHg; $PaCO_2$, 35 mmHg.
  d. pH, 7.40; PaO_2, 85 mmHg; $PaCO_2$, 42 mmHg.

hypoxia
hypercapnia

111

4. Lois is being medicated with a bronchodilator to reduce airway obstruction. Nursing actions include observing for the side effect(s) of:
a. dysrhythmias.
b. central nervous system excitement.
c. tachycardia.
d. all of the above.

5. Diaphragmatic breathing is recommended for Lois because it does all of the following *except:*
a. decrease respiratory rate.
b. decrease tidal volume.
c. increase alveolar ventilation.
d. reduce functional residual capacity.

6. Oxygen is prescribed for Lois. The nurse knows that the most effective delivery system is:
a. a rebreathing bag that delivers an oxygen concentration above 60%.
b. an oxygen mask set at 8 L/min.
c. a nasal cannula set at 6 L/min.
d. a Venturi mask that delivers a predictable oxygen flow at about 24%.

CASE STUDY: Adult Respiratory Distress Syndrome

Anne, age 71 and single, is admitted to the unit with a diagnosis of adult respiratory distress syndrome (ARDS). She has been receiving treatment at home for viral pneumonia and appeared to be improving until yesterday.

1. During assessment the nurse notes symptoms positively correlated with ARDS that include:
a. dysrhythmias and hypotension.
b. contraction of the accessory muscles of respiration.
c. tachypnea and tachycardia.
d. all of the above.

2. The nurse also observes symptoms of cerebral hypoxia that include:
a. drowsiness.
b. confusion.
c. irritability.
d. all of the above.

3. The nurse observes that Anne is receiving oxygen by way of a nasal cannula at 6 L/min. The nurse knows that Anne's FIO_2 is:
a. 24%.
b. 34%.
c. 44%.
d. 54%.

4. Indications for ventilator support for ARDS include all of the following *except:*
a. PaO_2 less than 70 mmHg.
b. PCO_2 greater than 60 mmHg.
c. respiratory rate greater than 35 beats per minute.
d. vital capacity equal to 60 ml/kg of body weight.

5. It is decided that Anne needs a ventilator to help her breathe. Her physician prescribes positive end-expiratory pressure (PEEP). When PEEP is used,
a. compliance is improved.
b. shunting is decreased.
c. small airway closure is prevented.
d. all of the above occur.

CASE STUDY: Pulmonary Embolism

Sandy, a 37-year-old who was recovering from multiple fractures sustained in a car accident, was admitted to the intensive care unit for treatment of a pulmonary embolism. Before admission she was short of breath after walking up a flight of stairs.

1. On the basis of Sandy's medical history, the nurse suspects that a predisposing condition may have been:
a. hypercoagulability.
b. postoperative immobility.
c. venous stasis.
d. all of the above factors.

2. As part of her assessment information, the nurse knows that the majority of pulmonary emboli originate in the:
a. deep leg veins.
b. lung tissue.
c. pelvic area.
d. right atrium of the heart.

3. The most common symptom of pulmonary embolism is:
a. chest pain.
b. dyspnea.
c. fever.
d. hemoptysis.

4. Based on Sandy's diagnosis, the nurse knows to look for a decrease in
   a. alveolar dead space.
   b. cardiac output.
   c. pulmonary arterial pressure.
   d. right ventricular work load of the heart.

5. A primary nursing problem for Sandy would be:
   a. atelectasis.
   b. bradycardia.
   c. dyspnea.
   d. hypertension.

6. The nurse knows that Sandy's diagnosis was probably confirmed by a(n):
   a. bronchogram.
   b. chest roentgenogram.
   c. electrocardiogram.
   d. lung scan.

25

Respiratory Care Modalities

Chapter Overview

Respiratory therapy measures are vital adjuncts to the medical management of patients with pulmonary disorders. Nurses have to be alert to patient symptoms that indicate a need for pulmonary support measures. They also need to be knowledgeable about the physics of selected delivery systems, as well as the scientific rationale supporting various practices. Evaluating the effectiveness of therapy is also a vital nursing role.

Patients undergoing thoracic surgery present a unique challenge to nursing. Preoperatively, alveolar ventilation should be improved and respiratory secretions decreased as much as possible. Patients need to practice the technique of deep breathing, coughing, and splinting of the future incision site. Postoperatively, the patient needs vigilant cardiopulmonary assessment and monitoring. Adequate ventilation, pain control, positioning, ambulation, hydration, and management of chest drainage will all be part of the total nursing care.

Rehabilitation, begun with admission, should be continued during the postoperative period. The rehabilitative goal is to return the patient to his or her highest functioning capacity. Before discharge these patients need specific health education concerning activity levels and the avoidance of respiratory irritants.

I. Knowledge-Based Questions

Deduction and Interpretation

Read each question carefully. Circle your answer.

1. Hypoxemia can be detected by noting a decrease in:
   a. Pao_2.
   b. PAo_2.
   c. pH.
   d. Pco_2.

2. A patient with bradycardia and hypotension would most likely exhibit:
   a. anemic hypoxia.
   b. circulatory hypoxia.
   c. histotoxic hypoxia.
   d. hypoxic hypoxia.

3. Carbon monoxide poisoning results in:
   a. anemic hypoxia.
   b. histoxic hypoxia.
   c. hypoxic hypoxia.
   d. stagnant hypoxia.

4. In assessing a patient with a need for oxygen therapy, a nurse needs to look for a clinical sign(s) such as:
   a. abnormal color (pallor).
   b. blood pressure changes.
   c. disturbed consciousness.
   d. all of the above.

5. Oxygen therapy administered to a pulmonary patient who retains carbon dioxide:
a. can cause a dangerous rise in $PaCO_2$ levels.
b. can suppress ventilation.
c. should bring the patient's PO_2 level to 60 to 70 mmHg.
d. is able to accomplish all of the above mechanisms.

6. When oxygen therapy is being used, "no smoking" signs are posted because oxygen:
a. is combustible.
b. is explosive.
c. prevents the dispersion of smoke particles.
d. supports combustion.

7. A patient has been receiving 100% oxygen therapy by way of a nonrebreather mask for several days. He complains of tingling in his fingers and shortness of breath. He is extremely restless and states that he has pain beneath his breastbone. The nurse should suspect:
a. oxygen-induced hypoventilation.
b. oxygen toxicity.
c. oxygen-induced atelectasis.
d. all of the above.

8. Oxygen concentrations of 70% can usually be delivered with the use of a(n):
a. nasal cannula.
b. oropharyngeal catheter.
c. partial rebreathing mask.
d. Venturi mask.

9. The method of oxygen administration primarily used for patients with chronic obstructive pulmonary disease is a(n):
a. nasal cannula.
b. oropharyngeal catheter.
c. nonrebreathing mask.
d. Venturi mask.

10. Intermittent positive-pressure breathing differs from incentive spirometry in all the following ways *except* that it:
a. is a mechanical aid to lung expansion.
b. is used to encourage hyperinflation.
c. produces a forced flow of air into the lungs during inhalation.
d. provides for the breathing of air or oxygen.

11. To help a patient use a mininebulizer, the nurse should do all of the following *except* encourage him to:
a. hold his breath at end inspiration for a few seconds.
b. cough frequently.
c. take rapid, deep breaths.
d. frequently evaluate his progress.

12. To assist a patient with the use of an incentive spirometer, the nurse should:
a. make sure the patient is in a flat, supine position.
b. tell the patient to try not to cough during and after each session because it will cause pain.
c. set an unrealistic goal so that the patient will try to maximize effort.
d. encourage the patient to take approximately 10 breaths per hour between treatments, while awake.

13. A nursing action(s) associated with postural drainage include(s):
a. encouraging the patient to cough after the procedure.
b. auscultating the lungs before and after the procedure.
c. encouraging the patient to exhale through pursed lips.
d. all of the above.

14. When using percussion to aid in secretion removal, the nurse should avoid the:
a. sternum and spine.
b. liver and kidneys.
c. spleen and female breast area.
d. above areas.

15. Percussion is accomplished by continuing the process for:
a. 3 to 5 minutes while the patient uses diaphragmatic breathing.
b. 10 to 15 minutes while the patient uses diaphragmatic breathing.
c. 3 to 5 minutes while the patient breathes normally.
d. 10 to 15 minutes while the patient breathes normally.

16. When you vibrate the patient's chest, you vibrate:
   a. during inhalation.
   b. during inhalation and exhalation.
   c. while he is exhaling.
   d. while he is holding his breath.

17. The purpose of pursed lips during exhalation is to:
   a. prolong exhalation.
   b. slow down the respiratory rate to allow for maximum lung expansion during inspiration.
   c. widen the airways.
   d. do all of the above.

18. Signs of an upper airway obstruction include:
   a. drawing in of the upper chest, sternum, and intercostal spaces.
   b. prolonged contraction of the abdominal muscles.
   c. tracheal tug.
   d. all of the above.

19. The suggested sequence of nursing actions for management of an *upper airway obstruction* are:
   a. clear airway, extend head, lift chin, use cross-finger technique, and perform a Heimlich maneuver.
   b. extend head, lift chin, clear airway, and perform Heimlich.
   c. extend head, clear airway, lift chin, and insert airway.
   d. lift chin, clear airway, and perform Heimlich.

20. Nursing management of a patient with an endotracheal tube includes:
   a. ensuring oxygen administration with high humidity.
   b. repositioning the patient every 2 hours.
   c. suctioning the oropharynx, as needed.
   d. all of the above.

21. When suctioning secretions from a tracheostomy tube, it is helpful to first instill:
   a. less than 1 ml of sterile normal saline solution.
   b. 1 to 2 ml of sterile normal saline solution.
   c. 3 to 5 ml of sterile normal saline solution.
   d. 6 to 8 ml of sterile normal saline solution.

22. When suctioning a tracheostomy tube, the nurse needs to remember that each aspiration *should not* exceed:
   a. 15 seconds.
   b. 30 seconds.
   c. 45 seconds.
   d. 60 seconds.

23. Choose the blood gas sequence that indicates a need for mechanical ventilation.
   a. Decreasing PO_2, decreasing PCO_2, normal pH
   b. Increasing PO_2, decreasing PCO_2, increasing pH
   c. Decreasing PO_2, increasing PCO_2, decreasing pH
   d. Increasing PO_2, decreasing PCO_2, decreasing pH

24. The most commonly used ventilator in use today is the:
   a. chest cuirass.
   b. time-cycled ventilator.
   c. pressure-cycled ventilator.
   d. volume-cycled ventilator.

25. With positive-pressure ventilation, positive intrathoracic pressure:
   a. increases venous return and decreases cardiac output.
   b. decreases venous return and increases cardiac output.
   c. decreases venous return and decreases cardiac output.
   d. increases venous return and increases cardiac output.

26. The term used to describe thoracic surgery in which an entire lung is removed is:
   a. lobectomy.
   b. pneumonectomy.
   c. segmentectomy.
   d. wedge resection.

27. Preoperatively, the patient who is scheduled for thoracic surgery needs to know that postoperatively:
   a. chest tubes and drainage bottles may be necessary.
   b. he will be turned frequently and asked to cough and breathe deeply.
   c. oxygen will be administered to facilitate breathing if the need arises.
   d. all of the above treatments will be incorporated into a plan of care.

28. The water seal used in a Pleur-Evac chest drainage system is effective if the water seal chamber is filled to the level of:
   a. 0.5 cmH$_2$O.
   b. 1.0 cmH$_2$O.
   c. 1.5 cmH$_2$O.
   d. 2.0 cmH$_2$O.

Complete the chart.

Look at the following figure of a three-bottle chest drainage system and Pleur-Evac drainage system and label the figure using the terms provided.

Water seal
Manometer bottle
Tube that leads to wall suction
Tube that provides for air escape
Drainage collection chambers
Tube that provides a water seal
Tube that regulates vacuum in the system
Fluid collection bottle

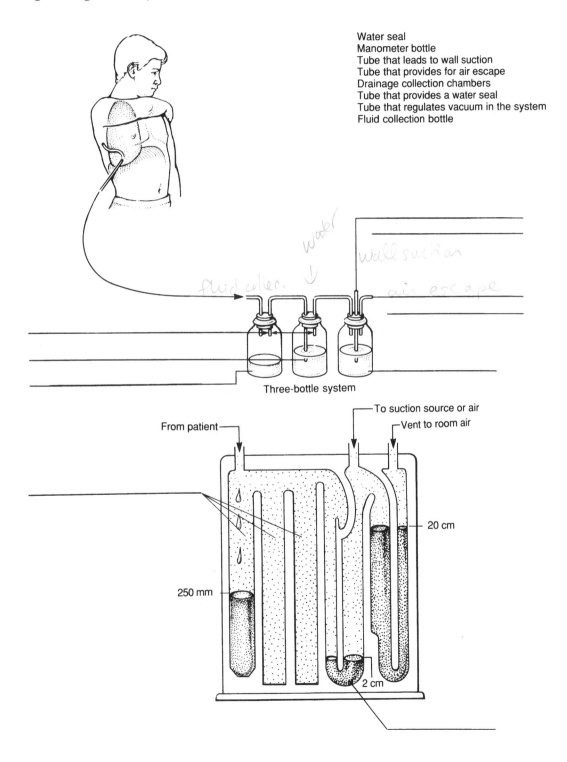

Three-bottle system

From patient
To suction source or air
Vent to room air
20 cm
250 mm
2 cm

II. Critical Analysis Questions

Generating Solutions: Clinical Problem Solving

Read the following case studies. Circle the correct answer.

CASE STUDY: Pneumonectomy: Preoperative Concerns

Mrs. Miley, a 66-year-old widow, is admitted to the clinical area as a preoperative patient scheduled for a pneumonectomy for lung cancer.

1. Nursing assessment during the admission history and physical examination includes obtaining data about the patient's:
   a. breathing patterns during exertion.
   b. cardiac status during exercise.
   c. smoking history.
   d. history relevant to all of the above.

2. The nurse knows that medical clearance for surgery is based primarily on evaluation of the:
   a. cardiopulmonary system.
   b. endocrine system.
   c. neurologic system.
   d. renal–urinary system.

3. A battery of preoperative tests are ordered. The nurse evaluates the serum creatinine level because it reflects:
   a. cardiac status.
   b. endocrine status.
   c. pulmonary function.
   d. renal function.

4. The nurse knows that Mrs. Miley's functional lung capacity can be assessed by evaluating:
   a. arterial blood gases.
   b. blood urea nitrogen levels.
   c. chest x-rays.
   d. serum protein levels.

CASE STUDY: Pneumonectomy: Postoperative Concerns

Mrs. Miley was returned to the clinical area after being in the intensive care unit. She is recovering from a right pneumonectomy.

1. The major postoperative nursing objective is to:
   a. maintain a patent airway.
   b. provide for maximum remaining lung expansion.
   c. provide rehabilitative measures.
   d. recognize early indicators of complications.

2. Mrs. Miley had a central venous pressure line in place. Readings were to be taken to detect:
   a. hypothermia.
   b. hypovolemia.
   c. hypoxemia.
   d. hypoxia.

3. Pulmonary edema is a potential danger owing to the possible rapid infusion of intravenous fluids and a reduced vascular bed. An early symptom(s) of pulmonary edema is(are):
   a. dyspnea.
   b. frothy sputum.
   c. crackles (rales).
   d. all of the above.

4. The nurse should always be alert for signs of impending respiratory insufficiency, which would include all of the following *except:*
   a. bradycardia.
   b. dyspnea.
   c. hypertension.
   d. tachypnea.

CASE STUDY: Ventilator Patient

Mr. Brown, a 25-year-old man with a drug overdose, has been maintained on a volume-cycled ventilator for 3 weeks.

1. A major nursing assessment for Mr. Brown would be:
   a. breath sounds.
   b. nutritional needs.
   c. psychological status.
   d. spontaneous ventilatory efforts.

2. Positive-pressure ventilation can alter cardiac function. The nurse assesses for indicators of hypoxia and hypoxemia, which would include all of the following *except:*
   a. bradycardia and bradypnea.
   b. diaphoresis and oliguria.
   c. restlessness and confusion.
   d. transient hypertension.

3. A primary nursing intervention for Mr. Brown is maintaining optimal gas exchange. This can be accomplished by:
   a. conservative use of analgesics so that pain is relieved, yet the respiratory drive is not decreased.
   b. daily monitoring of fluid balance to prevent fluid overload.
   c. frequent repositioning to diminish the pulmonary effects of immobility.
   d. all of the above measures.

4. The nurse wants to determine early if Mr. Brown is "bucking" his ventilator (breathing out during the ventilator's mechanical inspiratory phase) so that she can initiate preventive measures if necessary. The nurse should assess for signs and symptoms related to:
   a. hypercarbia.
   b. hypoxia.
   c. inadequate minute volume.
   d. all of the above.

CASE STUDY: Weaning from Ventilator

Mr. O'Day, a 71-year-old trauma victim, is to be weaned from his ventilator.

1. Before weaning, Mr. O'Day's ventilatory capacity should be such that he:
   a. can maintain an inspiratory force of at least – 20 cmH$_2$O pressure.
   b. had a tidal volume of 3 to 4 ml/lb of body weight.
   c. is able to generate a minimum vital capacity of 10 to 15 ml/kg of body weight.
   d. is capable of all of the above.

2. Criteria to determine if Mr. O'Day's endotracheal tube could be removed include:
   a. active pharyngeal and laryngeal gag reflexes.
   b. adequate spontaneous ventilation.
   c. voluntary cough mechanisms.
   d. all of the above.

3. Mr. O'Day will be weaned from oxygen when he can breathe room air and maintain at PaO$_2$ in the range of:
   a. 40 to 60 mmHg.
   b. 50 to 70 mmHg.
   c. 60 to 80 mmHg.
   d. 70 to 100 mmHg.

Complete the following nursing care plan.

David is a 25-year-old who had chest tubes inserted after a pneumothorax sustained during an automobile accident. You are assigned to care for him on his first postoperative day.

Nursing Diagnosis:

Immediate Goal(s):

Intermediate Goal(s):

Long-term Goal(s):

Nursing Interventions   *Expected Outcomes*

Learner's Self-Evaluation Tool for End of Unit 6 Review

1. The most important concepts or facts I have learned from this unit are:

1. _____

2. _____

3. _____

2. The most important reference page numbers for test review and clinical concepts are pages:

_____   _____   _____

_____   _____   _____

3. The concepts or facts that I do not fully understand are:

_____

_____

4. I will get the answer(s) to my questions by _____

_____

I will do this on _____ (date and time).

5. I believe my mastery of this unit to be:

a. 100%   Great job! Good luck!

b. 90%   2 hours of review recommended.

c. 80%   4 hours of review recommended.

d. <80%   Make an appointment with your instructor.

UNIT 7
Cardiovascular, Circulatory, and Hematologic Function

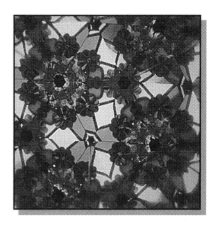

26
Assessment of Cardiovascular Function

Chapter Overview

Heart disease is currently the primary cause of death in the United States. Even with increased emphasis on consumer education about modifiable risk factors, compliance with an altered lifestyle has not been seen as positively correlated with a person's level of knowledge. As future nurses, your major impact will be in the areas of assessment, diagnosis, and health teaching.

A major asset in the battle against heart disease is the ever-increasing sophistication of diagnostic tests and procedures. Nurses will need to maintain competence in understanding various studies, interpreting data, and supporting the patient and his or her family during the period of cardiovascular assessment.

I. Knowledge-Based Questions

Deduction and Interpretation

Read each question carefully. Circle your answer.

1. The coronary arteries arise from the:
   a. aorta near the origin of the left ventricle.
   b. pulmonary artery at the apex of the right ventricle.
   c. pulmonary vein near the left atrium.
   d. superior vena cava at the origin of the right atrium.

2. The pacemaker for the entire myocardium is the:
   a. atrioventricular junction.
   b. bundle of His.
   c. Purkinje fibers.
   d. sinoatrial node.

3. The intrinsic pacemaker rate of ventricular myocardial cells is:
   a. more than 80 beats per minute.
   b. 60 to 80 beats per minute.
   c. 40 to 60 beats per minute.
   d. fewer than 40 beats per minute.

4. So that blood may flow from the right ventricle to the pulmonary artery, all of the following conditions must be met *except* that:
   a. the atrioventricular valves must be closed.
   b. the pulmonic valve must be open.
   c. right ventricular pressure must be less than pulmonary arterial pressure.
   d. right ventricular pressure must rise with systole.

5. Heart rate is stimulated by all of the following *except:*
   a. excess thyroid hormone.
   b. increased levels of circulating catecholamines.
   c. the sympathetic nervous system.
   d. the vagus nerve.

 Mary Jo Boyer: Study Guide to Accompany Brunner & Suddarth's Textbook of Medical-Surgical Nursing, 8th ed. © 1996 Lippincott-Raven Publishers

6. Stroke volume of the heart is determined by the:
   a. degree of cardiac muscle strength (precontraction).
   b. intrinsic contractility of the cardiac muscle.
   c. pressure gradient against which the muscle ejects blood during contraction.
   d. all of the above factors.

7. A nonmodifiable risk factor for atherosclerosis is:
   a. stress.
   b. obesity.
   c. positive family history.
   d. hyperlipidemia.

8. The difference between the systolic and the diastolic pressure is called the:
   a. pulse pressure.
   b. auscultatory gap.
   c. pulse deficit.
   d. Korotkoff sound.

9. If the sphygmomanometer cuff is too small for the patient, the blood pressure reading will probably be:
   a. falsely elevated.
   b. falsely decreased.
   c. an accurate reading.
   d. significantly different with each reading.

10. The first heart sound is generated by:
    a. closure of the aortic valve.
    b. closure of the atrioventricular valves.
    c. opening of the atrioventricular valves.
    d. opening of the pulmonic valve.

11. Exercise stress testing is a noninvasive procedure that can be used to assess certain aspects of cardiac function. After the test the patient is instructed to:
    a. rest for a time.
    b. avoid stimulants.
    c. avoid extreme temperature changes.
    d. do all of the above.

12. Postcatheterization nursing measures for a patient who has had a cardiac catheterization include:
    a. assessing the peripheral pulses in the affected extremity.
    b. checking the insertion site for hematoma formation.
    c. evaluating temperature and color in the affected extremity.
    d. all of the above.

Read each statement carefully. Write your response in the space provided.

1. Distinguish between the function of the atrioventricular and the semilunar valves.

   _____

   _____

2. Briefly explain depolarization as it relates to cardiac physiology.

   _____

   _____

3. Estimate cardiac output for an adult heart rate of 76 beats per minute and an average stroke volume of 70 ml per beat.

   _____

   _____

4. Describe Starling's law of the heart.

   _____

   _____

5. List several physiologic effects on the cardiovascular system that are associated with the aging process.

   _____

   _____

6. List several purposes of cardiac catheterization.

_____

_____

7. Describe selective angiography.

_____

_____

8. Describe echocardiography.

_____

_____

_____

9. Discuss the implications of a low central venous pressure reading.

_____

_____

10. Identify possible complications of pulmonary artery monitoring.

_____

_____

Complete the following crossword puzzle using terminology associated with coronary atherosclerosis.

Down

1. A principal blood lipid

2. A risk factor that causes pulmonary damage

4. The functional lesion of atherosclerosis

5. Biochemical substances, soluble in fat, that accumulate within a blood vessel

6. A risk factor that is endocrine in origin

9. A risk factor associated with a type A personality

10. A risk factor related to weight gain

14. A recommended dietary restriction

Across

3. For persons of this sex, the incidence of coronary heart disease increases steadily with age

6. Influences amount of fat ingested

7. A symptom of myocardial ischemia

8. An unmodifiable risk factor

11. Myocardial manifestation of coronary artery disease

12. A risk factor related to patterns of daily activity

13. A part of blood vessels

15. A lifestyle habit that is considered a modifiable risk factor for heart disease

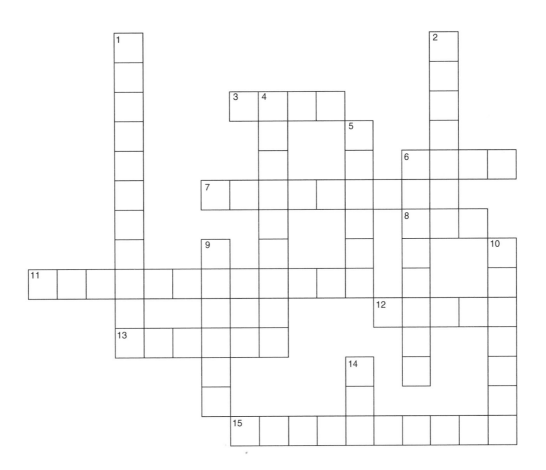

II. Critical Analysis Questions

Analyzing Comparisons

Read each analogy. Fill in the space provided with the best response.

1. The pulmonary artery : lungs :: aorta:_____.

2. Epicardium : outer layer of cells lining the heart ::_____:
   the heart muscle itself.

3. Apical area of the heart : fifth intercostal space :: Erb's point:

   _____.

4. The first heart sound : closure of the mitral and tricuspid valves :: the second heart sound : closure
   of_____.

5. Murmurs : malfunctioning valves :: friction rubs: _____.

125

Generating Solutions: Clinical Problem Solving

Look at the following illustration from Table 26–1 on page 595 depicting the pain pathway of myocardial infarction and angina pectoris. Answer the associated questions.

Myocardial Infarction   **Angina Pectoris**

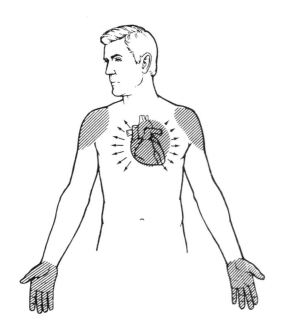 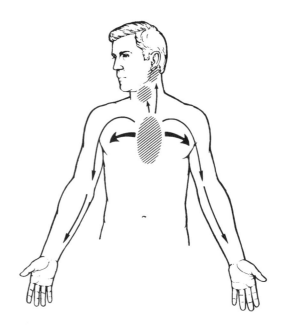

Name nursing assessment data
that are relevant to record/report
about the pain location, character, radiation, and duration.

Describe relevant precipitating
events that would help with
collaborative diagnosis.

Describe relevant nursing
interventions based on pain
assessment.

27

Management of Patients With Dysrhythmias and Conduction Problems

Chapter Overview

Complications related to cardiac disorders indicate that heart function is inadequate. Dysrhythmias, pulmonary edema, cardiac failure, cardiogenic shock, and thromboembolic episodes are responsible for many of the deaths from heart disease.

Increasingly, management of cardiac patients requires expertise in cardiovascular theory, knowledge about new drug regimens, competency in complex nursing skills, an ability to deal with seriously ill patients, and the empathy needed to support concerned loved ones.

I. Knowledge-Based Questions

Deduction and Interpretation

Read each question carefully. Circle your answer.

1. The heart is under the control of the autonomic nervous system. Stimulation of the parasympathetic system results in:
   a. slowed heart rate.
   b. lowered blood pressure.
   c. reduction in the force of contraction.
   d. all of the above.

2. Characteristics of sinus bradycardia include all of the following, *except* that:
   a. a P wave precedes every QRS complex.
   b. every QRS complex is normal.
   c. the rate is 40 to 60 beats per minute.
   d. the rhythm is altered.

3. Paroxysmal atrial tachycardia is characterized by a heart rate:
   a. of 100 beats per minute.
   b. between 100 and 150 beats per minute.
   c. between 150 and 250 beats per minute.
   d. more than 250 beats per minute.

4. *Atrial fibrillation* is associated with a heart rate up to:
   a. 300 beats per minute.
   b. 400 beats per minute.
   c. 500 beats per minute.
   d. 600 beats per minute.

5. *Ventricular bigeminy* refers to a conduction defect in which:
   a. conduction is primarily from the atrioventricular (AV) node.
   b. every other beat is premature.
   c. rhythm is regular but fast.
   d. the rate is between 150 and 250 beats per minute.

6. With ventricular tachycardia,
 a. conduction originates in the ventricle.
 b. electrical defibrillation is used immediately.
 c. the P wave usually is normal.
 d. the ventricular rate is twice the normal atrial rate.

7. Ventricular fibrillation is associated with an absence of:
 a. heartbeat.
 b. palpable pulse.
 c. respirations.
 d. all of the above.

8. First-degree AV block is characterized by:
 a. a variable heart rate, usually fewer than 60 beats per minute.
 b. an irregular rhythm.
 c. delayed conduction, producing a prolonged PR interval.
 d. P waves hidden with the QRS complex.

9. Cardioversion is used to terminate dysrhythmias. With cardioversion the:
 a. amount of voltage used should exceed 400 watt-seconds.
 b. electrical impulse can be discharged during the T wave.
 c. machine should be set to deliver a shock during the QRS complex.
 d. above statements are all true.

10. When electrical defibrillation is used,
 a. between 20 and 25 lbs of pressure should be exerted on each paddle in order to ensure good skin contact.
 b. the defibrillator should discharge at 100 W-sec/k of body weight.
 c. the discharge shock needs to be timed to the T wave.
 d. all of the above are necessary.

11. Candidates for automatic implantable cardioverter defibrillation (AICD) are patients at high risk who have:
 a. experienced syncope secondary to ventricular tachycardia.
 b. survived sudden cardiac death.
 c. sustained ventricular tachycardia.
 d. experienced one or more of the above.

12. The nurse needs to teach the patient with an automatic implantable cardioverter defibrillator that he must:
 a. avoid magnetic fields such as metal detection booths.
 b. call for emergency assistance if he feels dizzy.
 c. record events that trigger a shock sensation.
 d. be compliant with all of the above.

13. When assessing vital signs in a patient with a permanent pacemaker, the nurse needs to know the:
 a. date and time of insertion.
 b. location of the generator.
 c. model number.
 d. pacer rate.

Read each statement carefully. Write your response in the space provided.

1. Distinguish between the physiologic properties of the cardiac muscle (excitability, automaticity, conductivity, and contractility).

_____

_____

_____

2. Describe normal electrical conduction through the heart.

_____

_____

_____

3. Name several causes of sinus tachycardia.

_____

_____

4. Describe the placement on a person's chest of the electrode paddles used for defibrillation.

_____

_____

_____

5. Describe the difference between demand and fixed pacemakers.

_____

_____

II. Critical Analysis Questions

Generating Solutions: Clinical Problem Solving

Graph Analysis

Analyze the following QRS complexes and answer the questions.

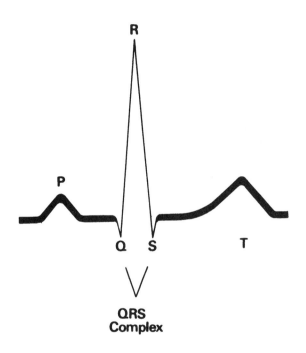

1. Look at the above graphic recording of cardiac electrical activity. For each action below, choose a wave deflection that corresponds to it and write the appropriate letter(s) on the line provided.

a. _____ ventricular muscle repolarization

b. _____ time required for impulse to travel through the atria and the conduction system to the Purkinje fibers

c. _____ atrial muscle depolarization

d. _____ ventricular muscle depolarization

e. _____ early ventricular repolarization of the ventricles

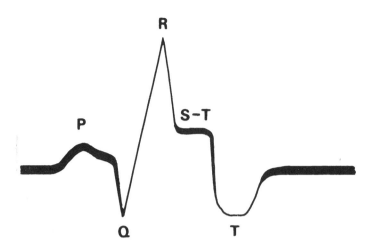

2. Consider the above graphic recording and identify three alterations that are consistent with the myocardial ischemia and infarction, hours to days after the attack.

a. _____   c. _____

b. _____

Analyze the graphic recording for each of the following dysrhythmias and describe the altered deflection.

1. Figure 27–7.

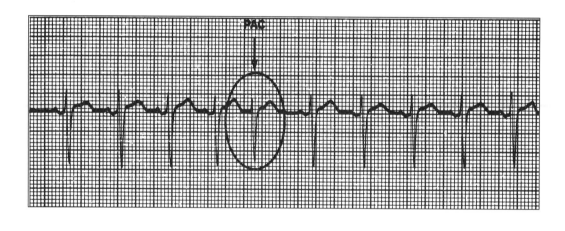

_____

_____

_____

2. Figure 27–11.

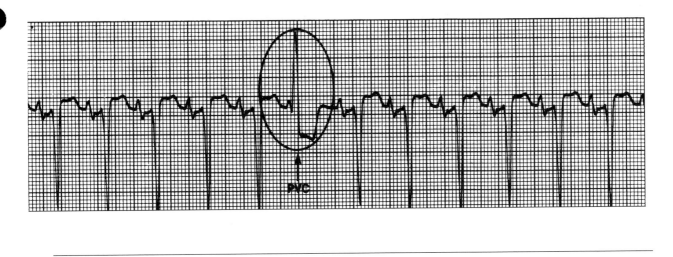

_____

_____

_____

28

Management of Patients With Cardiac Disorders and Related Complications

Chapter Overview

Heart disease is a major cause of morbidity and mortality in the United States today, with coronary artery disease continuing to be a major threat to health, even in younger and middle-aged adults whose lifestyles and dietary habits lead to major cardiac problems. Cardiac disease requires a multisystem approach to management (medical, nursing, nutritional, and pharmacologic). The patient becomes the recipient and co-manager of his or her care, who can, by compliance, minimize the symptoms and tremendously improve the quality of life. To do this, it is necessary to accept limitations and modify a lifestyle. Nurses need to be familiar with the symptoms and treatment modalities to help prevent, treat, and manage patient care problems.

I. Knowledge-Based Questions

Deduction and Interpretation

Read each question carefully. Circle your answer.

1. The *most common* heart disease in the United States is:
   a. angina pectoris.
   b. coronary atherosclerosis.
   c. myocardial infarction.
   d. valvular heart disease.

2. Lumen narrowing with atherosclerosis is caused by:
   a. atheroma formation on the intima.
   b. scarred endothelium.
   c. thrombus formation.
   d. all of the above.

3. Primary hyperlipidemia is characterized as:
   a. a hereditary disorder.
   b. the most common of the phenotypes.
   c. a manifestation of alcoholism.
   d. a disorder related to diabetes mellitus.

4. The pain of angina pectoris is primarily produced by:
   a. coronary vasoconstriction.
   b. movement of thromboemboli.
   c. myocardial ischemia.
   d. the presence of atheromas.

5. A common side effect of nitroglycerin is:
   a. musculoskeletal weakness.
   b. hypertension.
   c. bradycardia.
   d. headache.

 Mary Jo Boyer: Study Guide to Accompany Brunner & Suddarth's Textbook of Medical-Surgical Nursing, 8th ed. © 1996 Lippincott-Raven Publishers

6. Patient education includes telling someone who takes nitroglycerin sublingually that he should go quickly to the nearest emergency room if he has taken _____ tablet(s) at 5-minute intervals, without relief.
   a. more than 1.
   b. 2 or more.
   c. 3 or more.
   d. greater than 4.

7. The scientific rationale supporting the administration of β-adrenergic blockers is the drug's ability to:
   a. block sympathetic impulses to the heart.
   b. elevate blood pressure.
   c. increase myocardial contractility.
   d. induce bradycardia.

8. An antidote for propranolol hydrochloride (a β-adrenergic blocker) for bradycardia is:
   a. digoxin.
   b. atropine.
   c. protamine sulfate.
   d. sodium nitroprusside.

9. The need for surgical intervention of coronary artery disease is determined by the:
   a. amount of stenosis in the coronary arteries.
   b. myocardial area served by the stenotic artery.
   c. occurrence of previous infarction related to the affected artery.
   d. all of the above.

10. A candidate for percutaneous transluminal coronary angioplasty (PTCA) is a patient with coronary artery disease who has:
    a. compromised left ventricular function.
    b. had angina longer than 3 years.
    c. at least 70% occlusion of a major coronary artery.
    d. questionable left ventricular function.

11. A goal of dilation in PTCA is an increase in the artery's lumen size by at least:
    a. 20%.
    b. 35%.
    c. 60%.
    d. 85%.

12. The nurse expects a postoperative PTCA patient to be discharged:
    a. the same day as surgery.
    b. within 24 hours of the procedure.
    c. 3 days later.
    d. after 1 week.

13. Possible postoperative PTCA complications that a nurse needs to be alert to assess for clinical symptoms are:
    a. abrupt closure of the artery.
    b. arterial dissection.
    c. coronary artery spasm.
    d. all of the above.

14. One of the most important and immediate postoperative PTCA complications that the nurse needs to assess for is:
    a. bleeding.
    b. depression.
    c. hypertension.
    d. hypoventilation.

15. A candidate for coronary artery bypass grafting must meet the following criteria:
    a. blockage that cannot be treated by PTCA.
    b. >60% blockage in the left coronary artery.
    c. unstable angina.
    d. all of the above.

16. According to the critical care pathway outlined for CABP, the nurse knows that postoperative teaching must occur before discharge on the _____ day.
    a. third
    b. fifth
    c. seventh
    d. tenth

17. The most common site of myocardial infarction is the:
    a. left atrium.
    b. left ventricle.
    c. right atrium.
    d. right ventricle.

18. Choose an *incorrect statement* about myocardial infarction pain. It is:
    a. relieved by rest and inactivity.
    b. substernal in location.
    c. sudden in onset and prolonged in duration.
    d. viselike and radiates to the shoulders and arms.

19. Myocardial cell damage can be reflected by high levels of cardiac enzymes. The most sensitive indicator of all cardiac enzymes is:
   a. alkaline phosphatase.
   b. creatine kinase.
   c. lactic dehydrogenase.
   d. serum aspartate transaminase (glutamic oxaloacetic transaminase).

20. The cardiac enzyme that occurs, peaks, and takes the longest to return to normal, thus *not being a reliable indicator* of acute myocardial damage is:
   a. creatine kinase.
   b. alkaline phosphatase.
   c. creatine kinase isoenzyme.
   d. lactic dehydrogenase.

21. The most common vasodilator used to treat myocardial pain is:
   a. amyl nitrite.
   b. Inderal.
   c. nitroglycerine.
   d. Pavabid HCL.

22. Tissue plasminogen activator is a thrombolytic agent that:
   a. must be administered by the intracoronary route.
   b. entails the serious risk of allergic reactions.
   c. has a serious potential to cause systemic bleeding.
   d. is a naturally occurring enzyme.

23. An intravenous analgesic frequently administered to relieve chest pain associated with myocardial infarction is:
   a. meperidine hydrochloride.
   b. hydromorphone hydrochloride.
   c. morphine sulfate.
   d. codeine sulfate.

24. According to the critical care pathway for an acute myocardial infarction, the nurse needs to prepare the patient for discharge by the _____ day.
   a. fourth
   b. sixth
   c. eighth
   d. tenth

25. Pulmnoary edema is characterized by:
   a. elevated left ventricular end-diastolic pressure.
   b. a rise in pulmonary venous pressure.
   c. increased hydrostatic pressure.
   d. all of the above alterations.

26. A recommended position for a patient in acute pulmonary edema is:
   a. prone, to encourage maximum rest, thus decreasing respiratory and cardiac rates.
   b. semi-Fowler's, to facilitate breathing and promote pooling of blood in the sacral area.
   c. Trendelenburg, to drain the upper airways of congestion.
   d. upright with the legs down, to decrease venous return.

27. Morphine is given in acute pulmonary edema to redistribute the pulmonary circulation to the periphery by decreasing:
   a. peripheral resistance.
   b. pulmonary capillary pressure.
   c. transudation of fluid.
   d. all of the above.

28. Hemodynamic monitoring by means of a multilumen pulmonary artery catheter can provide detailed information about:
   a. preload.
   b. afterload.
   c. cardiac output.
   d. all of the above.

29. Nursing measures in hemodynamic monitoring include assessing for localized ischemia owing to inadequate arterial flow. The nurse should:
   a. assess the involved extremity for color and temperature.
   b. check for capillary filling.
   c. evaluate pulse rate.
   d. do all of the above.

30. The treatment of cardiac failure is directed at:
   a. decreasing oxygen needs of the heart.
   b. increasing the cardiac output by strengthening muscle contraction or decreasing peripheral resistance.
   c. reducing the amount of circulating blood volume.
   d. all of the above.

31. An example of a potassium-sparing diuretic that might be prescribed for a person with congestive heart failure is:
  a. Aldactone.
  b. Diuril.
  c. Esidrix.
  d. Lasix.

32. Cardiogenic shock is pump failure that primarily occurs as the result of:
  a. coronary artery stenosis.
  b. left ventricular damage.
  c. myocardial ischemia.
  d. right atrial flutter.

33. Classic signs of cardiogenic shock include all of the following *except:*
  a. bradycardia.
  b. cerebral hypoxia.
  c. hypotension.
  d. oliguria.

34. A clinical manifestation of pericardial infusion is:
  a. widening pulse pressure.
  b. a decrease in venous pressure.
  c. shortness of breath.
  d. an increase in blood pressure.

35. The most reliable sign of cardiac arrest is:
  a. absence of carotid pulsation.
  b. cessation of respirations.
  c. dilation of the pupils.
  d. inaudible heart sounds.

36. Brain damage occurs with cessation of circulation after an approximate interval of:
  a. 2 minutes.
  b. 4 minutes.
  c. 6 minutes.
  d. 8 minutes.

37. The drug of choice during cardiopulmonary resuscitation to suppress ventricular dysrhythmias is:
  a. atropine.
  b. epinephrine.
  c. lidocaine.
  d. morphine.

Match the type of congestive failure listed in Column II with its associated pathophysiology in Column I.

Column I

1. _____ fatigability

2. _____ dependent edema

3. _____ pulmonary congestion predominates

4. _____ distended neck veins

5. _____ ascites

6. _____ dyspnea from fluid in alveoli

7. _____ orthopnea

8. _____ hepatomegaly

9. _____ cough which may be blood-tinged

10. _____ nocturia

Column II

a. left-sided cardiac failure

b. right-sided cardiac failure

II. Critical Analysis Questions

Supporting Arguments

Offer a supporting rationale for your response.

1. Explain, supported with a scientific base to your rationale, why cigarette smoking contributes to the severity of coronary heart disease for each of these three factors:

   Factor   ***Scientific Rationale***

   a. increased CO levels   a. _____

                                        _____

   b. increased catecholamines   b. _____

                                        _____

   c. increased platelet adhesion   c. _____

                                        _____

2. Argue in support of using calcium channel blockers for treatment of angina._____

   _____

   _____

Generating Solutions: Clinical Problem Solving

Read the following case studies. Circle the correct answer.

CASE STUDY: Angina Pectoris

Ermelina, a 64-year-old retired secretary, is admitted to the medical–surgical area for management of chest pain caused by angina pectoris.

1. The nurse knows that the basic cause of angina pectoris is believed to be:
   a. dysrhythmias triggered by stress.
   b. insufficient coronary blood flow.
   c. minute emboli discharged through the narrowed lumen of the coronary vessels.
   d. spasms of the vessel walls owing to excessive secretion of epinephrine (adrenaline).

2. The medical record lists a probable diagnosis of chronic, stable angina. The nurse knows that Ermelina's pain:
   a. has increased progressively in frequency and duration.
   b. is incapacitating.
   c. never occurs at rest and is predictable.
   d. usually occurs at night and may be relieved by sitting upright.

3. Ermelina has nitroglycerin at her bedside to take prn. The nurse knows that nitroglycerin acts in all of the following ways *except* by:
   a. causing venous pooling throughout the body.
   b. constricting arterioles to lessen peripheral blood flow.
   c. dilating the coronary arteries to increase oxygen supply.
   d. lowering systemic blood pressure.

4. Ermelina took a nitroglycerin tablet at 10:00 AM, after her morning care. It did not relieve her pain, so she repeated the dose. Ten minutes later and still in pain, she calls the nurse, who:

   a. administers a prn dose of diazepam (Valium), tries to calm her, and recommends that she rest in a chair with her legs dependent to encourage venous pooling.

   b. assists her to the supine position, gives her oxygen at 6 L/min, and advises her to rest in bed.

   c. helps her to a comfortable position, gives her oxygen at 2 L/min, and calls her physician.

   d. suggests that she double her previous dose in 5 minutes and try to sleep, to decrease her body's need for oxygen.

CASE STUDY: Decreased Myocardial Tissue Perfusion

Mr. Lillis, a 46-year-old bricklayer, is brought to the emergency department by ambulance with a suspected diagnosis of myocardial infarction. He appears ashen, is diaphoretic, and tachycardiac, and has severe chest pain. The nursing diagnosis is decreased cardiac output, related to decreased myocardial tissue perfusion.

1. The nurse knows that the most critical time period for his diagnosis is:

   a. the first hour after symptoms begin.

   b. within 24 hours of the onset of symptoms.

   c. within the first 48 hours after the attack.

   d. between the third and fifth day after the attack.

2. The nurse needs to look for symptoms associated with one of the major causes of sudden death during the first 48 hours, which is:

   a. cardiogenic shock.

   b. pulmonary edema.

   c. pulmonary embolism.

   d. ventricular rupture.

3. Mr. Lillis is transferred to a telemetry unit after 6 days in the cardiac care unit, where he was treated for an anterior wall myocardial infarction. The nurse expects Mr. Lillis to be able to do all of the following *except:*

   a. isometric exercises.

   b. participate in self-care activities.

   c. sit in a chair several times a day.

   d. walk within his room.

4. The nurse is aware that ischemic tissue remains sensitive to oxygen demands because scar formation is not seen until the:

   a. second week.

   b. third week.

   c. sixth week.

   d. eighth week.

5. Mr. Lillis needs to be advised that myocardial healing will not be complete for about:

   a. 2 months.

   b. 4 months.

   c. 6 months.

   d. 8 months.

6. For discharge planning, Mr. Lillis is advised to:

   a. avoid large meals.

   b. exercise daily.

   c. restrict caffeine-containing beverages.

   d. do all of the above.

29

Management of Patients With Structural, Infectious, or Inflammatory Cardiac Disorders

Chapter Overview

Preoperatively and postoperatively, the cardiovascular surgical patient needs intense cardiopulmonary management, since the organs vital to survival have been compromised. Cardiopulmonary assessment needs to be all-inclusive, and any indicator of a potential complication needs to be evaluated. Frequently the management of such patients requires the combined efforts of an interdisciplinary team, consisting of a physician, a nurse, a respiratory therapist, an occupational therapist, a psychologist, a social worker, and a nutritionist.

I. Knowledge-Based Questions

Deduction and Interpretation

Read each question carefully. Circle your answer.

1. Incomplete closure of the tricuspid valve results in a backward flow of blood from the:
   a. aorta to the left ventricle.
   b. left atrium to the left ventricle.
   c. right atrium to the right ventricle.
   d. right ventricle to the right atrium.

2. The pathophysiology of mitral stenosis is consistent with:
   a. aortic stenosis.
   b. left ventricular failure.
   c. right atrial hypertrophy.
   d. all of the above.

3. Severe aortic stenotic disease is consistent with all of the following *except:*
   a. increased cardiac output.
   b. left ventricular hypertrophy.
   c. pulmonary edema.
   d. right-sided heart failure.

4. The presence of a water-hammer pulse (quick, sharp strokes that suddenly collapse) is diagnostic for:
   a. aortic insufficiency.
   b. mitral insufficiency.
   c. tricuspid insufficiency.
   d. tricuspid stenosis.

5. The most common valvuloplasty procedure is the:
   a. balloon valvuloplasty.
   b. annuloplasty.
   c. chordoplasty.
   d. commissurotomy.

 Mary Jo Boyer: Study Guide to Accompany Brunner & Suddarth's Textbook of Medical-Surgical Nursing, 8th ed. © 1996 Lippincott-Raven Publishers

6. Xenographs, used for valve replacement, have a viability of about:
   a. 2 years.   c. 8 years.
   b. 4 years.   d. 12 years.

7. The most commonly occurring cardiomyopathy is:
   a. congestive.   c. idiopathic.
   b. hypertrophic.   d. restrictive.

8. Probably the most helpful diagnostic test to identify cardiomyopathy is:
   a. serial enzyme studies.   c. echocardiogram.
   b. cardiac catheterization.   d. phonocardiogram.

9. Rheumatic endocarditis is an inflammatory reaction to:
   a. group A *Streptococcus.*   c. *Serratia marcescens.*
   b. *Pseudomonas aeruginosa.*   d. *Staphylococcus aureus.*

10. The causative microorganism responsible for sequelae such as rheumatic endocarditis is identified by:
   a. a throat culture.   c. roentgenography.
   b. an echocardiogram.   d. serum analysis.

11. Clinical manifestations of infective endocarditis may include:
   a. embolization.   c. heart murmurs.
   b. focal neurologic lesions.   d. all of the above.

12. The characteristic sign of pericarditis is:
   a. a friction rub.   c. fever.
   b. dyspnea.   d. hypoxia.

13. A serious consequence of pericarditis is:
   a. cardiac tamponade.   c. hypertension.
   b. decreased venous pressure.   d. left ventricular hypertrophy.

Read each statement carefully. Write your response in the space provided.

1. Describe the valve prolapse syndrome.

_____

_____

2. Explain how left ventricular hypertrophy develops from mitral insufficiency.

_____

_____

3. Briefly describe the pathophysiology of endocarditis, beginning with the formation of a vegetation.

_____

_____

4. Briefly describe the pathophysiology of myocarditis.

_____

_____

_____

5. Describe the anatomic landmark for auscultation of a pericardial friction rub.

_____

_____

Match the pathophysiology listed in Column II with the valvular disorder listed in Column I.

Column I

1. _____ mitral valve prolapse

2. _____ mitral stenosis

3. _____ mitral regurgitation

4. _____ aortic valve stenosis

5. _____ aortic regurgitation

Column II

a. leaflet malformation prevents complete closure

b. can be caused by rheumatic endocarditis

c. characterized by "water-hammer" pulse

d. blood seeps backward into left atrium

e. thickening and contracture of mitral valve cusps

II. Critical Analysis Questions

Generating Solutions: Clinical Problem Solving

Read the following case study. Fill in the blanks below or circle the correct answer.

CASE STUDY: Infective Endocarditis

Mr. Fontana, a 60-year-old executive, is admitted to the hospital with a diagnosis of *infective endocarditis.* Pertinent history includes a previous diagnosis of mitral valve prolapse. A physical examination at his physician's office before admission reveals complaints of anorexia, joint pain, intermittent fever, and a 10-lb weight loss in the past 2 months.

1. The nurse knows, prior to assessment, that Mr. Fontana's vague clinical symptoms are characteristic of an infectious disease that arises from one of three conditions:

   (a) _____, (b) _____, or

   (c) _____.

2. While examining Mr. Fontana during the admission assessment, the nurse notes conjunctival hemorrhages with pale centers. These are known as:
   a. Roth's spots.
   b. Osler's nodes.
   c. Janeway's lesions.
   d. Heberden's nodes.

3. The nurse also assesses for central nervous system manifestations of the infectious disease. She looks for

   symptoms such as: (a) _____,

   (b) _____, (c) _____,

   and (d) _____.

4. The primary objective of medical management is:

   _____

5. Serial blood cultures identified *Streptococcus viridans* as the causative organism, and parenteral antibiotic treatment was initiated. The nurse expects that Mr. Fontana will probably remain on the antibiotic intravenous infusion for:
   a. 7 days.
   b. 2 weeks.
   c. 4 to 6 weeks.
   d. 8 to 12 weeks.

6. Even with successful treatment, organ damage can occur. Cardiac complications may include:

(a)_____,(b) _____, or

(c)_____, and (d) _____.

7. Mr. Fontana needs to be advised that prophylactic antibiotic therapy is also recommended for:

    a. tooth extraction.

    b. bronchoscopy.   d. all of the above.

   c. cystoscopy.

30

Management of the Cardiac Surgery Patient

Chapter Overview

Preoperatively and postoperatively, the cardiovascular surgical patient needs intense cardiopulmonary management, since the organs vital to survival have been compromised. Cardiopulmonary assessment needs to be all-inclusive, and any indication of a potential complication needs to be evaluated. Frequently the management of such patients requires the combined effect of an interdisciplinary team consisting of a physician, a nurse, a respiratory therapist, an occupational therapist, a psychologist or a social worker, and a nutritionist.

I. Knowledge-Based Questions

Deduction and Interpretation

Read each question carefully. Circle your answer.

1. Heart transplantation has become a therapeutic option for patients with end-stage heart disease, primarily owing to the development of the immunosuppressant:
   a. azathioprine.
   b. cimetidine.
   c. cyclosporine.
   d. muromonab.

2. A transplanted heart must be implanted within _____ hours of being harvested from the donor.
   a. 4
   b. 8
   c. 12
   d. 24

3. Heart transplant patients have a 5-year survival rate of:
   a. 25%.
   b. 40%.
   c. 65%.
   d. 90%.

4. Based on assessment data, potential collaborative problems may include:
   a. anxiety.
   b. angina.
   c. cardiac arrest.
   d. all of the above.

5. One of the most important preoperative nursing diagnoses is:
   a. body-image disturbance.
   b. fear.
   c. impaired physical mobility.
   d. pain.

6. During the preoperative period, cardiac patients need to be taught how to:
   a. breathe deeply and cough.
   b. perform foot exercises.
   c. use the incentive spirometer or the intermittent positive-pressure breathing machine.
   d. do all of the above.

 Mary Jo Boyer: Study Guide to Accompany Brunner & Suddarth's Textbook of Medical-Surgical Nursing, 8th ed. © 1996 Lippincott-Raven Publishers

7. Preoperatively, cardiac patients need to know that postoperatively they will remain intubated and will be assisted to breathe by mechanical ventilation for the average time of:
a. 12 hours.
b. 36 hours.
c. 48 hours.
d. 72 hours.

8. A characteristic sign(s)of postcardiotomy psychosis is (are):
a. disorientation and paranoid delusions.
b. transient perceptual illusions.
c. visual and auditory hallucinations.
d. all of the above are considered significant signs.

9. Postoperative assessment for hypokalemia is necessary if the serum potassium level drops to:
a. 3.0 mEq/L.
b. 3.5 mEq/L.
c. 4.0 mEq/L.
d. 4.5 mEq/L.

10. Nursing assessment for postoperative hypovolemia as a result of blood loss includes all of the following *except:*
a. a central venous pressure reading of 3 cm H_2O.
b. a heart rate of 50 beats per minute.
c. arterial hypotension.
d. low left atrial pressure.

11. The nurse determines that renal function is compromised owing to decreased cardiac output. An indicator would be:
a. urine output of 80 ml/hr.
b. urine specific gravity of 1.005.
c. urine osmolality of 750 mOsm/kg.
d. capillary refill < 1.0 second.

12. Postoperative chest drainage should be recorded hourly. Cause for alarm in the first 4 to 6 hours would be drainage of:
a. 50 ml/hr.
b. 150 ml/hr.
c. 200 ml/hr.
d. 250 ml/hr.

13. Nursing assessment for a diagnosis of cardiac tamponade includes all of the following *except:*
a. decreased heart rate.
b. decreased urinary output.
c. muffled heart sounds.
d. neck vein distention.

14. Nursing measures to prevent postoperative embolization include:
a. applying antiembolism stockings.
b. discouraging leg-crossing.
c. instituting passive exercises followed by active exercises to promote circulation.
d. all of the above.

Read each statement carefully. Write your response in the space provided.

1. List the five most common indications for heart transplantation:

1. _____   4. _____
2. _____   5. _____
3. _____

2. The most common surgical procedure for cardiac transplantation is the:

_____.

3. List four intraoperative complications of cardiac surgery:

1. _____   3. _____
2. _____   4. _____

4. Postcardiac surgery patients need to be observed for symptoms of hypoxia, such as:

1. _____   4. _____
2. _____   5. _____
3. _____   6. _____

5. Identify the three most common dysrhythmias that occur during the postoperative period:

1. _____,   3. _____,

2. _____

II. Critical Analysis

Generating Solutions: Clinical Problem Solving

Read the following case study. Fill in the blanks or circle the correct answer.

CASE STUDY: Cardiac Surgery Patient

Mrs. Effgen is a 56-year-old grandmother who lives alone and is scheduled for cardiac surgery in the morning. She had most of her preoperative evaluation completed before admission.

1. A history and physical will include a physiological and psychosocial health assessment. List three areas under psychosocial information that are of particular importance.

1. _____

2. _____

3. _____

2. As a nurse, you know that preoperative patient information must include letting the patient and her family know that surgery can affect alterations in the cardiac output of six major systems which are:

1. _____   4. _____

2. _____   5. _____

3. _____   6. _____

3. List four major types of fear most frequently expressed by preoperative surgical patients:

1. _____

2. _____

3. _____

4. _____

4. The primary nursing diagnosis for this patient is:

_____

5. In the immediate postoperative period, hypokalemia is evidenced by an alteration on the ECG strip. Therefore, the nurse should assess for a (an):
  a. inverted T wave.
  b. peaked T wave.
  c. prolonged QT interval.
  d. widened QRS complex.

6. Characteristic signs of postoperative psychosis are:
  a. disorientation and paranoid delusions.
  b. transient perceptual illusions.
  c. visual and auditory hallucinations.
  d. all of the above.

7. Cardiac tamponade is a postoperative complication of decreased cardiac output. It is primarily related to an alteration in:
  a. preload.
  b. afterload.
  c. heart rate.
  d. contractility.

8. Identify five nursing activities that should be used to prevent postoperative venous stasis:

1. _____   4. _____

2. _____   5. _____

3. _____

9. Postoperative assessment includes the knowledge that *postpericordiotomy syndrome* occurs in _____ of patients.

10. The most common cause of decreased cardiac output after cardiac surgery is:

_____.

31

Assessment and Management of Patients With Vascular Disorders and Problems of Peripheral Circulation

Chapter Overview

Circulatory disorders are frequently a person's first indication that cardiovascular disease is present. Pain and disability are usually associated with alterations in circulation. A patient's lifestyle will probably change, and he or she will have to adapt to the reality of a life-threatening condition or a chronic, progressively deteriorating disorder. Nursing interventions will have to meet the challenge of treating active symptoms, along with helping the patient cope with self-image changes. Many patients will have to adapt to nutritional modifications or prolonged pharmacologic therapy.

I. Knowledge-Based Questions

Deduction and Interpretation

Read each question carefully. Circle your answer.

1. The most important factor in regulating the caliber of blood vessels, which determines resistance to flow, is:
   a. hormonal secretion.
   b. independent arterial wall activity.
   c. the influence of circulating chemicals.
   d. the sympathetic nervous system.

2. Clinical manifestations of *acute venous insufficiency* include all of the following *except:*
   a. cool and cyanotic skin.
   b. initial absence of edema.
   c. sharp pain that may be relieved by the elevation of the extremity.
   d. full superficial veins.

3. With *peripheral arterial insufficiency,* leg pain during rest can be reduced by:
   a. elevating the limb above heart level.
   b. lowering the limb so that it is dependent.
   c. massaging the limb after application of cold compresses.
   d. placing the limb in a plane horizontal to the body.

 Mary Jo Boyer: Study Guide to Accompany Brunner & Suddarth's Textbook of Medical-Surgical Nursing, 8th ed. © 1996 Lippincott-Raven Publishers

4. Saturated fats are strongly implicated in the causation of atherosclerosis. Saturated fats include all of the following *except:*
 a. corn oil.
 b. eggs and milk.
 c. meat and butter.
 d. solid vegetable oil.

5. The American diet is known to be high in fat. The amount of calories typically supplied by fat in most diets is:
 a. 20% of the total caloric intake.
 b. 40% of the total caloric intake.
 c. 60% of the total caloric intake.
 d. 80% of the total caloric intake.

6. Buerger's disease is characterized by all of the following *except:*
 a. arterial thrombus formation and occlusion.
 b. lipid deposits in the arteries.
 c. redness or cyanosis in the limb when it is dependent.
 d. venous inflammation and occlusion.

7. The most outstanding symptom of Buerger's disease is:
 a. a burning sensation.
 b. cramping in the feet.
 c. pain.
 d. paresthesia.

8. The most common cause of all thoracic aortic aneurysms is:
 a. a congenital defect in the vessel wall.
 b. atherosclerosis.
 c. infection.
 d. trauma.

9. Diagnosis of a thoracic aortic aneurysm is done primarily by:
 a. computed tomography.
 b. sonography.
 c. x-ray.
 d. all of the above.

10. A nurse who suspects the presence of an abdominal aortic aneurysm should look for the presence of:
 a. a pulsatile abdominal mass.
 b. low back pain.
 c. lower abdominal pain.
 d. all of the above.

11. To save a limb affected by occlusion of a major artery, surgery must be initiated before necrosis develops, which is usually:
 a. within the first 4 hours.
 b. between 6 and 10 hours.
 c. between 12 and 24 hours.
 d. within 1 to 2 days.

12. Raynaud's disease is a form of:
 a. arterial vessel occlusion caused by multiple emboli that develop in the heart and are transported through the systemic circulation.
 b. arteriolar vasoconstriction, usually on the fingertips, that results in coldness, pain, and pallor.
 c. peripheral venospasm in the lower extremities owing to valve damage resulting from prolonged venous stasis.
 d. phlebothrombosis related to prolonged vasoconstriction resulting from overexposure to the cold.

13. Hypertension is defined as persistent blood pressure levels in which the systolic pressure is above _____ and the diastolic above _____.
 a. 110/60
 b. 120/70
 c. 130/80
 d. 140/90

14. The percentage of patients with hypertension who discontinue their drug therapy within 1 year of its initiation is estimated to be:
 a. 15%.
 b. 30%.
 c. 50%.
 d. 75%.

15. When administering anticoagulant therapy, the nurse needs to monitor the clotting time to make certain that it is within the therapeutic range of:
 a. one to two times the normal control.
 b. two to three times the normal control.
 c. 3.5 times the normal control.
 d. 4.5 times the normal control.

16. When caring for a patient who has started anticoagulant therapy with warfarin (Coumadin), the nurse knows not to expect therapeutic benefits for:

a. at least 12 hours.
b. the first 24 hours.
c. 2 to 3 days.
d. 1 week.

17. A nurse should teach a patient with chronic venous insufficiency to do all of the following *except:*

a. avoid constricting garments.
b. elevate the legs above the heart level for 30 minutes every 2 hours.
c. sit as much as possible, to rest the valves in the legs.
d. sleep with the foot of the bed elevated about 6 inches.

18. Nursing measures to promote a clean leg ulcer include:

a. applying wet-to-dry saline solution dressings, which when changed would remove necrotic debris.
b. flushing out necrotic material with hydrogen peroxide.
c. using an ointment that would treat the ulcer by enzymatic debridement.
d. all of the above.

19. A varicose vein is caused by:

a. phlebothrombosis.
b. an incompetent venous valve.
c. venospasm.
d. venous occlusion.

20. Clinical manifestations of deep vein obstruction include:

a. edema and pain.
b. pigmentation changes.
c. ulcerations.
d. all of the above.

21. Postoperative nursing management for vein ligation and stripping include all of the following *except:*

a. dangling the legs over the side of the bed for 10 minutes every 4 hours for the first 24 hours.
b. elevating the foot of the bed to promote venous blood return.
c. maintaining elastic compression of the leg continuously for about 1 week.
d. starting the patient ambulating 24 to 48 hours after surgery.

22. Coumadin (warfarin) is used for the treatment of lymphedema because it:

a. decreases the tissue colloidal oncotic pressure, thereby allowing interstitial fluid to move back into the capillaries.
b. promotes platelet aggregation, which increases the plasma osmotic pressure, which in turn pulls fluid out of the interstitial spaces.
c. reduces blood viscosity, thereby promoting the transudation of interstitial fluid into the capillary.
d. does all of the above.

Match the type of vessel insufficiency listed in Column II with its associated symptoms listed in Column I.

Column I

1. _____ intermittent claudication
2. _____ paresthesia
3. _____ dependent rubor
4. _____ cold, pale extremity
5. _____ ulcers of lower legs and ankles
6. _____ muscle fatigue and cramping
7. _____ diminished or absent pulses
8. _____ reddish blue discoloration with dependency

Column II

a. arterial insufficiency
b. venous insufficiency

II. Critical Analysis Questions
Analyzing Comparisons

Analyze the two formulas below and explain the hemodynamics represented by each.

1. Flow = $\Delta P/R$ (blood flow):

_____

_____

2. $R = 8\,nL/\pi r^4$ (resistance):

_____

_____

Read each analogy. Fill in the space provided with the best response.

3. Norepinephrine: vasoconstriction :: _____ vasodilation.

4. Left-sided heart failure :: blood accumulation in the lungs :: right-sided heart failure:

_____.

5. Arteriosclerosis: "hardening of the arteries" :: atherosclerosis :_____.

Generating Solutions: Clinical Problem Solving

Read the following case studies. Circle the correct answer.

CASE STUDY: Peripheral Arterial Occlusive Disease

Fred, a 43-year-old construction worker, has a history of hypertension. He smokes two packs of cigarettes a day, is nervous about the possibility of being unemployed, and has difficulty coping with stress. His current concern is calf pain during minimal exercise that decreases with rest.

1. The nurse assesses Fred's symptoms as being associated with peripheral arterial occlusive disease. The nursing diagnosis is probably:
   a. alteration in tissue perfusion related to compromised circulation.
   b. dysfunctional use of extremities related to muscle spasms.
   c. impaired mobility related to stress associated with pain.
   d. impairment in muscle use associated with pain on exertion.

2. The nurse knows that the specific symptom of peripheral arterial occlusion disease is:
   a. intermittent claudication.
   b. phlebothrombosis.
   c. postphlebitis syndrome.
   d. thrombophlebitis.

3. Additional symptoms to support the nurse's diagnosis include all of the following *except:*
   a. blanched skin appearance when the limb is elevated.
   b. diminished distal pulsations.
   c. reddish blue discoloration of the limb when it is dependent.
   d. warm and rosy coloration of the extremity after exercise.

4. The nurse knows that in health teaching she should suggest methods to increase arterial blood supply, which include:
   a. a planned program involving systematic lowering of the extremity below heart level.
   b. Buerger-Allen exercises.
   c. graded extremity exercises.
   d. all of the above.

CASE STUDY: Essential Hypertension

Georgia is diagnosed as having essential hypertension at 30 years of age when serial blood pressure recordings showed her average reading to be 170/100 mm Hg. Georgia is a grade school teacher in a depressed socioeconomic area and has been obese for 10 years.

1. The nurse knows that essential hypertension:
   a. can be managed only with drug therapy.
   b. has no identifiable cause.
   c. is positively correlated with diabetes mellitus.
   d. is secondary to parenchymal renal disease.

2. The kidneys help maintain the hypertensive state in essential hypertension by:
   a. increasing their elimination of sodium in response to aldosterone secretion.
   b. releasing renin in response to decreased renal perfusion.
   c. secreting acetylcholine, which stimulates the sympathetic nervous system to constrict major vessels.
   d. doing all of the above.

3. Renal pathology associated with essential hypertension can be identified by:
   a. a urine output greater than 2000 ml/24 hr.
   b. a urine specific gravity of 1.005.
   c. hyponatremia and decreased urine osmolality.
   d. increased blood urea nitrogen and creatinine levels.

4. Georgia is prescribed spironolactone (Aldactone), 50 mg once every day. The nurse knows that spironolactone:
   a. blocks the reabsorption of sodium, thereby increasing urinary output.
   b. inhibits renal vasoconstriction, which prevents the release of renin.
   c. interferes with fluid retention by inhibiting aldosterone.
   d. prevents the secretion of epinephrine from the adrenal medulla.

5. Health education for Georgia includes advising her to:
   a. adhere to her dietary regimen.
   b. become involved in a regular program of exercise.
   c. take her medication as prescribed.
   d. do all of the above.

Complete the outline below, which depicts the pathophysiology of atherosclerosis, beginning with the direct results of atherosclerosis in the arteries and ending with fibrotic tissue formation.

Pathophysiology of Atherosclerosis

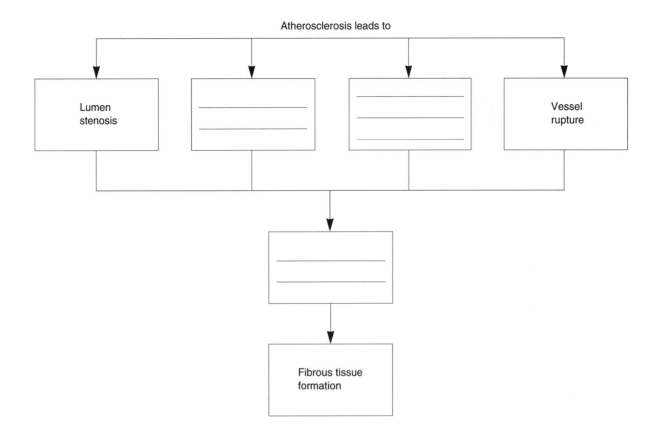

Atherosclerosis leads to

| Lumen stenosis | _____ _____ | _____ _____ _____ | Vessel rupture |

_____
_____

Fibrous tissue formation

32

Assessment and Management of Patients With Hematologic Disorders

Chapter Overview

Hematologic disorders can be temporary or chronic, and acute, benign, or malignant. Because blood is vital to every cell, any abnormality results in a localized or systemic response. Symptoms may range from nondescriptive fatigue in hemolytic anemia to semiconsciousness in Hodgkin's disease. Accurate assessment and diagnosis are necessary to develop individual nursing care plans because many manifestations of hematologic disorders are insidious.

I. Knowledge-Based Questions

Deduction and Interpretation

Read each question carefully. Circle your answer.

1. A nurse who cares for a patient who has experienced bone marrow aspiration or biopsy should be aware of the most serious hazard of:
   a. hemorrhage.
   b. infection.
   c. shock.
   d. splintering of bone fragments.

2. A person can usually tolerate a gradual reduction in hemoglobin until the level reaches:
   a. 5.0 to 5.5 g/dl.
   b. 4.0 to 4.5 g/dl.
   c. 3.0 to 3.5 g/dl.
   d. 2.0 to 2.5 g/dl.

3. A nurse should know that a diagnosis of hemolytic anemia is associated with all of the following *except* a(n):
   a. abnormality in the circulation of plasma.
   b. decrease in the reticulocyte count.
   c. defect in the erythrocyte.
   d. elevated indirect bilirubin.

4. The cause of aplastic anemia may:
   a. be related to drugs, chemicals, or radiation damage.
   b. be idiopathic.
   c. result from certain infections.
   d. be related to all of the above.

5. A clinical manifestation of aplastic anemia is:
   a. adenopathy.
   b. hepatosplenomegaly.
   c. normocytic red blood cells.
   d. thrombocytopenia owing to bleeding.

6. For a patient diagnosed as having an iron-deficiency anemia, the nurse should recommend an increased intake of:
a. fresh citrus fruits.
b. milk and cheese.
c. organ meats.
d. whole-grain breads.

7. The recommended parenteral route for administering iron preparations for anemia is by:
a. deep gluteal intramuscular injection, using a Z-track method.
b. intermittent infusion.
c. intramuscular injection in the deltoid so that muscle contraction can help dissipate the medication.
d. subcutaneous injection with weekly site rotation.

8. Absence of intrinsic factor is associated with a vitamin B_{12} deficiency because the vitamin cannot bind to be transported for absorption in the:
a. duodenum.
b. ileum.
c. jejunum.
d. stomach.

9. A diagnostic sign of pernicious anemia is:
a. a smooth, sore red tongue.
b. exertional dyspnea.
c. pale mucous membranes.
d. weakness.

10. The *Schilling* test is used to diagnose:
a. aplastic anemia.
b. iron-deficiency anemia.
c. megaloblastic anemia.
d. pernicious anemia.

11. A nurse expects an adult patient with sickle cell anemia to have a hemoglobin value of:
a. near 3 g/dl.
b. near 5 g/dl.
c. between 5 and 7 g/dl.
d. between 7 and 10 g/dl.

12. Sickle-shaped erythrocytes cause:
a. cellular blockage in small vessels.
b. decreased organ perfusion.
c. tissue ischemia and infarction.
d. all of the above.

13. A person with sickle cell trait would:
a. be advised to avoid fluid loss and dehydration.
b. be protected from crisis under ordinary circumstances.
c. experience hemolytic jaundice.
d. have chronic anemia.

14. Polycythemia vera is characterized by bone marrow overactivity, resulting in the clinical manifestation(s) of:
a. angina.
b. claudication.
c. thrombophlebitis.
d. all of the above.

15. The common feature of the leukemias is:
a. a compensatory polycythemia stimulated by thrombocytopenia.
b. an unregulated accumulation of white cells in the bone marrow, which replace normal marrow elements.
c. increased blood viscosity, resulting from an overproduction of white cells.
d. reduced plasma volume in response to a reduced production of cellular elements.

16. Nursing assessment for a patient with leukemia should include observation for:
a. fever and infection.
b. dehydration.
c. petechiae and ecchymoses.
d. all of the above.

17. The major cause of death in patients with leukemia is believed to be:
a. anemia.
b. dehydration.
c. embolis.
d. infection.

18. Multiple myeloma:
a. can be diagnosed by roentgenograms that show bone lesion destruction.
b. is a malignant disease of plasma cells that affects bone and soft tissue.
c. is suspected in any person who evidences albuminuria.
d. is associated with all of the above.

19. In the normal blood-clotting cycle, the final formation of a clot will occur:
a. during the platelet phase.
b. during the vascular phase.
c. when fibrin reinforces the platelet plug.
d. when the plasmin system produces fibrinolysis.

20. Bleeding and petechiae do not usually occur with thrombocytopenia until the platelet count falls below 50,000/mm^3. The normal value for blood platelets is:
a. between 50,000 and 100,000/mm^3.
b. between 100,000 and 150,000/mm^3.
c. between 150,000 and 350,000/mm^3.
d. greater than 350,000/mm^3.

21. Hemophilia is a hereditary bleeding disorder that:
a. has a higher incidence among males.
b. is associated with joint bleeding, swelling, and damage.
c. is related to a genetic deficiency of a specific blood-clotting factor.
d. is associated with all of the above.

22. Hypoprothrombinemia, in the absence of gastrointestinal or biliary dysfunction, may be caused by a deficiency in vitamin:
a. A.
b. B$_{12}$.
c. C.
d. K.

23. A potential blood donor would be rejected if he had:
a. a history of infectious disease exposure within the past 2 to 4 months.
b. close contact with a hemodialysis patient within the past 6 months.
c. donated blood within the past 3 to 6 months.
d. received a blood transfusion 9 to 12 months before the blood donation time.

24. The recommended minimum hemoglobin level for a woman to donate blood is:
a. 8.0 g/dl.
b. 10.5 g/dl.
c. 12.5 g/dl.
d. 14 g/dl.

25. A unit of blood obtained from a donor can be stored at 1° to 6°C (33.8° to 42.8°F) for:
a. 7 days.
b. 14 days.
c. 21 to 35 days.
d. 42 days.

Read each statement carefully. Write your response in the space provided.

1. The volume of blood in humans is about _____ L.

2. Blood is produced in the: _____, and _____.

3. Red bone marrow, the site of active blood cell production, is confined in adults to the _____, _____, and _____.

4. The principal function of the erythrocyte is to: _____

_____.

5. Each 100 ml of blood should normally contain _____ g of hemoglobin.

6. The average life span of a circulating red blood cell is _____ days.

7. The major function of leukocytes is to _____.

8. Plasma proteins consist primarily of _____, and

_____.

9. The two most common areas used for bone marrow aspirations for an adult are
_____ and _____.

10. Distinguish between primary and secondary polycythemia.

_____

_____

II. Critical Analysis Questions

Generating Solutions: Clinical Problem Solving

Read the following case studies. Circle the correct answer.

CASE STUDY: Hodgkin's Disease

Ian, a 24-year-old graduate student, was recently diagnosed as having Hodgkin's disease. He sought medical attention because of an annoying pruritus and a small enlargement on the right side of his neck.

1. Ian's disease is classified as Hodgkin's paragranuloma. The nurse knows that this classification is associated with:
   a. a minimal degree of cellular differentiation in the affected node(s).
   b. an excessive production of the Reed-Sternberg cell, the diagnostic atypical cell of Hodgkins's disease.
   c. nodular sclerosis, which reflects advanced malignancy.
   d. replacement of the involved lymph nodes by tumor cells.

2. A positive diagnosis of Hodgkin's disease depends on:
   a. enlarged, firm, and painful lymph nodes.
   b. histologic analysis of an enlarged lymph node.
   c. progressive anemia.
   d. the presence of generalized pruritus.

3. Ian's diagnosis of stage I Hodgkin's disease implies that the disease:
   a. has disseminated diffusely to one or more extrahepatic sites.
   b. involves multiple nodes and is confined to one side of the diaphragm.
   c. is limited to a single node or a single intralymphatic organ or site.
   d. is present above and below the diaphragm and may include spleen involvement.

4. The nurse expects that Ian's course of treatment will involve:
   a. a combination of chemotherapy and radiation.
   b. a drug regimen of nitrogen mustard, vincristine, and a steroid.
   c. chemotherapy with vincristine alone.
   d. radiotherapy to the specific node over a space of 4 weeks.

CASE STUDY: Transfusion

Jerry is to receive 1 unit of packed red cells because he has a hemoglobin level of 8 g/dl and a diagnosis of gastrointestinal bleeding.

1. Before initiating the transfusion the nurse needs to check:
   a. for the abnormal presence of gas bubbles and cloudiness in the blood bag.
   b. that the blood has been typed and cross-matched.
   c. that the recipient's blood numbers match the donor's blood numbers.
   d. all of the above.

2. Administration technique should include all of the following *except:*

   a. adding 50 to 100 ml of 0.9% NaCl to the packed cells to dilute the solution and speed up delivery of the transfusion.

   b. administering the unit in combination with dextrose in water if the patient needs additional carbohydrates.

   c. administering the unit of blood over 1 to 2 hours.

   d. squeezing the bag of blood every 20 to 30 minutes during administration to mix the cells.

3. The nurse is aware that a transfusion reaction, if it occurs, will probably occur:

   a. 1 to 2 minutes after the infusion begins.

   b. during the first 15 to 30 minutes of the transfusion.

   c. after half the solution has been infused.

   d. several hours after the infusion, when the body has assimilated the new blood components into the general circulation.

4. If a transfusion reaction occurs, the nurse should:

   a. call the physician and wait for directions based on the specific type of reaction.

   b. stop the transfusion immediately and keep the vein patent with a saline or dextrose solution.

   c. slow the infusion rate and observe for an increase in the severity of the reaction.

   d. slow the infusion and request a venipuncture for retyping to start a second transfusion.

Learner's Self-Evaluation Tool for End of Unit 7 Review

1. The most important concepts or facts I have learned from this unit are:

   1. _____

   2. _____

   3. _____

2. The most important reference page numbers for test review and clinical concepts are pages:

   _____ _____ _____

   _____ _____ _____

3. The concepts or facts that I do not fully understand are:

   _____

   _____

4. I will get the answer(s) to my questions by _____

   _____

   I will do this on _____ (date and time).

5. I believe my mastery of this unit will be:

   a.   100%   Great job! Good luck!

   b.   90%   2 hours of review recommended.

   c.   80%   4 hours of review recommended.

   d.   <80%   Make an appointment with your instructor.

UNIT 8
Digestive and Gastrointestinal Function

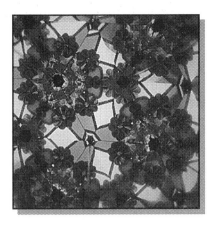

33

Assessment of Digestive and Gastrointestinal Function

Chapter Overview

A sense of health or wellness implies that our bodies are maintaining internal stability in relation to intrinsic and extrinsic stimuli. All systems combine in this effort to establish a sense of balance. Of all the major body systems, the digestive and gastrointestinal systems seem to be most subject to autonomous control. People can directly influence their functioning because they can choose what they eat and drink. They can also control the elimination process by self-medication with over-the-counter drugs. They can treat their indigestion, constipation, and diarrhea.

When caring for patients with digestive or gastrointestinal dysfunction, it is vital to give them the information they need to make knowledgeable decisions about symptoms and to instruct them in how to manage self-care and when to seek professional help.

I. Knowledge-Based Questions

Deduction and Interpretation

Read each question carefully. Circle your answer.

1. Reflux of food into the esophagus from the stomach is prevented by contraction of the:
   a. ampulla of Vater.
   b. cardiac sphincter.
   c. ileocecal valve.
   d. pyloric sphincter.

2. The digestion of starches begins in the mouth with the secretion of:
   a. lipase.
   b. pepsin.
   c. ptyalin.
   d. trypsin.

3. The stomach is acidic at a pH of approximately:
   a. 1.0.
   b. 3.5.
   c. 5.0.
   d. 7.5.

4. Intrinsic factor is a gastric secretion necessary for the intestinal absorption of vitamin:
   a. B_1.
   b. B_{12}.
   c. C.
   d. K.

5. Pancreatic secretions into the duodenum:
a. are stimulated by hormones released in the presence of chyme as it passes through the duodenum.
b. have an alkaline effect on intestinal contents.
c. increase the pH of the food contents.
d. do all of the above.

6. Bile, which emulsifies fat, enters the duodenum through the:
a. cystic duct.
b. common bile duct.
c. common hepatic duct.
d. pancreatic duct.

7. Secretin is a gastrointestinal hormone that:
a. causes the gallbladder to contract.
b. influences contraction of the esophageal and pyloric sphincters.
c. regulates the secretion of gastric acid.
d. stimulates the secretion of bicarbonate in pancreatic juice.

8. Tissue cells use carbohydrate in the form of:
a. fructose.
b. galactose.
c. glucose.
d. sucrose.

9. The time it usually takes for food to enter the colon is:
a. 2 or 3 hours after a meal is eaten.
b. 4 or 5 hours after a meal is eaten.
c. 6 or 7 hours after a meal is eaten.
d. 8 or 9 hours after a meal is eaten.

10. Obstruction of the gastrointestinal tract leads to:
a. increased force of intestinal contraction.
b. distention above the point of obstruction.
c. pain and a sense of bloating.
d. all of the above.

11. A nurse who is investigating a patient's statement about duodenal pain should assess the:
a. epigastric area and consider possible radiation of pain to the right subscapular region.
b. hypogastrium in the right or left lower quadrant.
c. left lower quadrant.
d. periumbilical area, followed by the right lower quadrant.

?

12. Abdominal pain associated with indigestion is usually:
a. described as crampy or burning.
b. in the left lower quadrant.
c. less severe after an intake of fatty foods.
d. relieved by the intake of coarse vegetables, which stimulate peristalsis.

13. Consequences of diarrhea include all of the following *except:*
a. acidosis.
b. decreased bicarbonate.
c. electrolyte imbalance.
d. hyperkalemia.

14. A gastric analysis with stimulation that results in an excess of gastric acid being secreted could be diagnostic of:
a. chronic atrophic gastritis.
b. a duodenal ulcer.
c. gastric carcinoma.
d. pernicious anemia.

15. Before a gastroscopy the nurse should inform the patient that:
a. he must fast for 6 to 8 hours before the examination.
b. his throat will be sprayed with a local anesthetic.
c. after gastroscopy, he will not be given anything to eat or drink until his gag reflex returns.
d. all of the above will be necessary.

16. A flexible sigmoidoscope permits examination of the lower bowel for:
a. 5 to 10 inches.
b. 10 to 15 inches.
c. 16 to 20 inches.
d. 25 to 35 inches.

17. Magnetic resonance imaging (MRI) is contraindicated for patients who have:
a. pacemakers.
b. artificial heart valves.
c. implanted insulin pumps.
d. all of the above.

18. Patient preparation for esophageal manometry requires the withholding of specific medication such as:
    a. anticholinergics.
    b. calcium channel blockers.
    c. sedatives.
    d. all of the above.

19. The nurse knows when examining the consistency of a stool specimen, that a greasy, gray-colored specimen may be indicative of:
    a. biliary obstruction.
    b. chronic ulcerative colitis.
    c. obstipation.
    d. steatorrhea.

20. Choose the diagnostic test for gastrointestinal cancer that is recommended before age 50.
    a. Colonoscopy
    b. Digital rectal examination
    c. Proctosigmoidoscopy
    d. Stool for occult blood

Match the major digestive enzyme in Column II with its associated digestive action listed in Column I.

Column I

1. _____ helps convert protein into amino acids

2. _____ facilitates the production of dextrins and maltose

3. _____ digests protein and helps form polypeptides

4. _____ digests carbohydrates and helps form fructose

5. _____ glucose is a product of this enzyme's action

6. _____ helps form galactose

Column II

a. amylase

b. maltase

c. sucrase

d. lactase

e. pepsin

f. trypsin

34

Management of Patients With Ingestive Problems and Upper Gastrointestinal Disorders

Chapter Overview

Because food has many psychosocial as well as physiologic connotations, any condition that interferes with ingestion or digestion can negatively influence a person's self-perception and overall sense of well-being. Nursing care plans must be holistic in their development and implementation. Outcome criteria should reflect the numerous variables that influence individual food preferences, the frequency of meals, and the quality of food consumed daily.

I. Knowledge-Based Questions

Deduction and Interpretation

Read each question carefully. Circle your answer.

1. The floor of the mouth, a common area for oral cancer, is assessed for the characteristic sign(s) of a(n):
   a. indurated ulcer.
   b. warty growth.
   c. white or red plaque.
   d. all of the above.

2. The oral cavity of a person with acquired immunodeficiency syndrome (AIDS) should be assessed for:
   a. oral candidiasis.
   b. hairy leukoplakia.
   c. oral herpes simplex.
   d. all of the above possible manifestations.

3. Actinic cheilitis is a lip lesion that results from sun exposure and can lead to squamous cell carcinoma. It is evidenced by:
   a. erythema.
   b. fissuring. ✓
   c. white hyperkeratosis.
   d. all of the above.

4. The most common disease of oral tissue is:
   a. candidiasis.
   b. gingivitis.
   c. herpes simplex.
   d. periodontitis.

5. The most common lesion of the mouth is:
  a. aphthous stomatitis.
  b. candidiasis.
  c. leukoplakia buccalis.
  d. lichen planus.

6. The ingestion of fluoridated water effectively prevents and reduces the incidence of dental caries. Fluoride intake is recommended until:
  a. all primary teeth have emerged.
  b. 5 or 6 years of age.
  c. all secondary teeth are present.
  d. 10 years of age.

7. A patient taking anticoagulants should take vitamin K before a dental procedure for:
  a. 1 day.
  b. 2 days.
  c. 3 days.
  d. 4 days.

8. A patient who receives dentures should be taught that it takes _____ for gum tissue to adapt.
  a. less than 1 month
  b. 6 to 8 weeks
  c. about 3 months
  d. 3 to 4 months

9. Postoperative nursing care for drainage of a dentoalveolar or periopical abscess includes all of the following *except:*
  a. soft diet after 24 hours
  b. fluid restriction for the first 48 hours because the gums are swollen and painful.
  c. external heat by pad or compress to hasten the resolution of the inflammatory swelling.
  d. warm saline mouthwashes every 2 hours while awake.

10. Preventive orthodontics for malocclusion is started at age:
  a. 3.
  b. 5.
  c. 7.
  d. 9.

11. Neoplasms of the salivary glands:
  a. are normally malignant and are treated by surgical excision.
  b. commonly recur, and recurrences are more malignant than the original tumor.
  c. may be quiescent for years before rapidly increasing in size.
  d. are characterized by all of the above.

12. The most common site for cancer of the oral cavity is the:
  a. lip.
  b. mouth.
  c. pharynx.
  d. tongue.

13. After a radical neck dissection a patient is placed in Fowler's position to:
  a. decrease venous pressure on the skin flaps.
  b. facilitate swallowing.
  c. increase lymphatic drainage.
  d. accomplish all of the above.

14. Postoperatively, a finding that should be immediately reported is:
  a. temperature of 99°F.
  b. pain.
  c. stridor.
  d. localized wound tenderness.

15. A nurse who is caring for a patient who has had radical neck surgery notices an abnormal amount of serosanguineous secretions in the wound suction unit during the first postoperative day. An expected normal amount of drainage is:
  a. between 40 and 80 ml.
  b. approximately 80 to 120 ml.
  c. between 120 and 160 ml.
  d. greater than 160 ml.

16. Postoperatively, the nurse observes excessive drooling. She assesses for damage to the:
  a. facial nerve.
  b. hypoglossal nerve.
  c. spinal accessory nerve.
  d. auditory nerve.

17. A major potential complication is hemorrhage from the:
  a. brachial artery.
  b. carotid artery.
  c. innominate artery.
  d. vertebral artery.

18. Usually the first symptom associated with esophageal disease is:
    a. dysphagia.
    b. malnutrition.
    c. pain.
    d. regurgitation of food.

19. The nurse suspects that a patient who presents with the symptom of food "sticking" in the lower portion of the esophagus may have the motility disorder known as:
    a. achalasia.
    b. diffuse spasm.
    c. gastroesophageal reflex.
    d. hiatal hernia.

20. A hiatal hernia involves a(n):
    a. extension of the esophagus through the diaphragm.
    b. involution of the esophagus, which causes a severe stricture.
    c. protrusion of the upper stomach into the lower portion of the thorax.
    d. twisting of the duodenum through an opening in the diaphragm.

21. Intervention for a person who has swallowed strong acid includes all of the following *except*:
    a. administering an irritant that will stimulate vomiting.
    b. aspirating secretions from the pharynx if respirations are affected.
    c. neutralizing the chemical.
    d. washing the esophagus with large volumes of water.

22. Cancer of the esophagus occurs primarily in:
    a. black men over 50 years of age.
    b. black women after menopause.
    c. white men 30 to 40 years old.
    d. white women over 60 years of age.

23. A common postoperative complication of esophageal surgery for cancer is:
    a. aspiration pneumonia.
    b. hemorrhage.
    c. incompetence of the suture line, resulting in fluid seepage.
    d. the dumping syndrome.

Match the abnormality listed in Column II with its associated symptomatology of the lip, mouth or gums listed in Column I.

Column I

1. _____ ulcerated and painful white papules.

2. ___G___ reddened area or rash associated with itching.

3. ___E___ painful, inflamed, swollen gums.

4. _____ white overgrowth of horny layer of epidermis

5. _____ shallow ulcer with a red border and white or gray center

6. ___B___ hyperkeratotic white patches usually in buccal mucosa

7. ___C___ reddened circumscribed lesion that ulcerates and becomes encrusted.

8. ___H___ white patches with rough hairlike projections

Column II

a. actinic chelitis

b. leukoplakia

c. chancre

d. canker sore

e. gingivitis

f. lichen planus

g. contact dermatitis

h. hairy leukoplakia

II. Critical Analysis Questions

Generating Solutions: Clinical Problem Solving

Read the following case study. Fill in the blanks or circle the correct answer.

CASE STUDY: Mandibular Fracture

William, a 17-year-old student, suffered a mandibular fracture while playing football. He is scheduled for jaw repositioning surgery.

1. Preoperatively, the nurse assures William that the surgical procedure for treatment of a mandibular fracture has improved greatly over the last few years. Describe the difference in the procedure that you would explain preoperatively to William.

   _____

   _____

2. Postoperatively, the nurse should immediately position William:
   a. flat on his back to facilitate lung expansion during inspiration.
   b. on his side with his head slightly elevated to prevent aspiration.
   c. supine with his head to the side to promote the drainage of secretions.
   d. with his head lower than his trunk to prevent aspiration of fluids.

3. Postoperatively, the nurse's primary goal is to maintain:
   a. adequate nutrition.
   b. an open airway.
   c. jaw immobilization.
   d. oral hygiene.

4. What would you tell the patient to explain why nasogastric suctioning is needed?

   _____

   _____

5. For emergency use, which of the following should be available at the head of the bed?
   a. A nasogastric suction tube
   b. A nasopharyngeal suction catheter
   c. A wire cutter or scissors
   d. An oxygen cannula

6. A recommended *initial* postoperative diet for William would be:
   a. bland pureed.
   b. clear liquid.
   c. full liquid.
   d. semisoft.

7. William must be instructed *not to chew food* until the _____ postoperative week.
   a. third
   b. fourth
   c. fifth
   d. eighth

8. What essential item must be sent home with William when he is discharged?

   _____

35

Gastrointestinal Intubation and Special Nutritional Management

Chapter Overview

Occasionally gastrointestinal intubation is necessary to help meet a patient's nutritional needs. A nurse who is caring for a patient who is intubated needs to be familiar with the mechanics of tube maintenance as well as with the caloric distribution of various supplemental feedings. A patient's psychosocial needs must be part of any care plan, since the socialization surrounding eating influences everyone.

I. Knowledge-Based Questions

Deduction and Interpretation

Read each question carefully. Circle your answer.

1. The Levin tube, a commonly used nasogastric tube, has circular markings at specific points. The tube should be inserted to:
   a. a length of 50 cm (20 in.).
   b. a point that equals the distance from the nose to the xiphoid process.
   c. the midpoint between a 50-cm marking and the distance measured from the tip of the nose to the xiphoid process.
   d. the distance determined by measuring from the tragus of the ear to the xiphoid process.

2. When continuous or intermittent suction is used with a nasogastric tube, the goal is to have the amount of suction in the gastric mucosa reduced to:
   a. 25 mm Hg.
   b. 50 mm Hg.
   c. 80 mm Hg.
   d. 120 mm Hg.

3. It is essential for the nurse who is managing a gastric sump tube to:
   a. maintain intermittent or continuous suction at a rate >120 mm Hg.
   b. keep the vent lumen above the patient's midline to prevent gastric content reflux.
   c. irrigate only through the vent lumen.
   d. do all of the above activities.

4. A nasoenteric tube used for decompression is the:
 a. Cantor tube.
 b. Moss tube.
 c. Nutriflex tube.
 d. Sengstaken–Blakemore.

5. Nasoenteric tubes usually remain in place until:
 a. bowel sounds are present.
 b. flatus is passed.
 c. peristalsis is resumed.
 d. all of the above mechanisms occur.

6. A commonly used, double-lumen, decompression tube is the:
 a. Cantor tube.
 b. Harris tube.
 c. Levin tube.
 d. Mieler–Abbott tube.

7. A nurse prepares a patient for insertion of the Dubbhoff nasoenteric tube. The nurse positions the patient:
 a. in high Fowler's position.
 b. flat in bed.
 c. on his right side.
 d. in semi-Fowler's with his head turned to the left.

8. A nasoenteric tube can be safely advanced 2 to 3 in. every:
 a. hour.
 b. 2 hours.
 c. 4 hours.
 d. 8 hours.

9. Osmosis is the process whereby:
 a. particles disperse throughout a liquid medium to achieve an equal concentration throughout.
 b. particles move from an area of greater concentration to an area of lesser concentration to establish equilibrium.
 c. water moves through a membrane from a dilute solution to a more concentrated solution to achieve equal osmolality.
 d. water moves through a membrane from an area of higher osmolality to an area of lesser osmolality to establish equilibrium.

10. The dumping syndrome occurs when high-carbohydrate foods are administered over a period of less than 20 minutes. A nursing measure to prevent or minimize the dumping syndrome is to administer the feeding:
 a. at a warm temperature to decrease peristalsis.
 b. by bolus to prevent continuous intestinal distention.
 c. with about 100 ml of fluid to dilute the high carbohydrate concentration.
 d. with the patient in semi-Fowler's position to decrease transit time influenced by gravity.

11. Residual content is checked before each tube feeding. A feeding would be delayed and the patient reassessed if the residual were:
 a. about 50 ml.
 b. between 50 and 80 ml.
 c. about 100 ml.
 d. greater than 150 ml.

12. To induce positive nitrogen balance, a tube feeding is delivered at a rate of about:
 a. 50 ml/hr.
 b. 100 to 150 ml/hr.
 c. 200 ml/hr.
 d. greater than 150 ml/hr.

13. Gastrostomy feedings are preferred to nasogastric feedings in the comatose patient because the:
 a. gastroesophageal sphincter is intact, lessening the possibility of regurgitation.
 b. digestive process occurs more rapidly as a result of the feeding's not having to pass through the esophagus.
 c. feedings can be administered in the recumbent position.
 d. patient cannot experience the deprivational stress of not swallowing.

14. Initial fluid nourishment after a gastrostomy usually consists of:
 a. distilled water.
 b. 10% glucose and tap water.
 c. milk.
 d. high-calorie liquids.

15. When administering a bolus gastrostomy feeding, the receptacle should be held no higher than _____ in. above the abdominal wall.
 a. 9
 b. 18
 c. 27
 d. 36

16. The basic hyperalimentation solution consists of:
a. 10% glucose.
b. 25% glucose.
c. 35% glucose.
d. 50% glucose.

17. The preferred route for infusion of total parenteral nutrition solution is the:
a. brachial vein.
b. jugular vein.
c. subclavian vein.
d. superior vena cava.

18. Patients who are receiving total parenteral nutrition should be observed for signs of hyperglycemia, which would include:
a. headache.
b. lassitude.
c. nausea.
d. all of the above.

II. Critical Analysis Questions

Generating Solutions: Clinical Problem Solving

Read the following case studies. Fill in the blanks or circle the correct answer.

CASE STUDY: Cantor Tube

Martin, a 69-year-old widower who lives alone, has been diagnosed as having an obstruction of the small intestine. The physician has requested nursing assistance for insertion of a Cantor tube.

1. Before insertion of the Cantor tube, the nurse should:
a. assist Martin to high Fowler's position and help him hyperextend his neck.
b. explain the purpose of the tube.
c. screen Martin to ensure privacy.
d. do all of the above.

2. Martin needs to be informed that the procedure may involve:
a. having him hold ice chips in his mouth for a few minutes.
b. mouth breathing or panting during passage of the tube.
c. the spraying of his oropharynx with tetracaine (Pontocaine) to dull the nasal passages and gag reflex.
d. all of the above.

3. After the tube has passed the pyloric sphincter, nursing responsibilities include advancing the tube:
a. 1 in. every hour.
b. 1 in. every 4 hours.
c. 2 to 3 in. every hour.
d. 2 to 3 in. every 4 hours.

4. The nurse knows that tube placement can be verified by checking the pH of aspirated secretions. If the tube were in the intestines, the pH reading would be approximately:
a. 5.4.
b. 6.8.
c. 7.0.
d. 8.2.

5. Fluid volume deficit is a potential problem with nasoenteric intubation. Indicators of fluid volume deficit include all of the following *except:*
a. the body temperature of 102°F.
b. dry mucous membranes.
c. lethargy and exhaustion.
d. oliguria.

CASE STUDY: The Dumping Syndrome

Nancy is a 37-years-old, 5 ft 7 in. tall, and weighs 140 lb. She receives 250 ml of Osmolite (liquid nutrition) over a 15-minute period every 4 hours through a nasogastric tube. Nancy has had esophageal surgery for carcinoma.

1. Nancy tells you, the nurse, that she has diarrhea. You suspect she is experiencing the dumping syndrome. You also know you need to eliminate other possible causes such as:

a. _____

b. _____

c. _____

d. _____

2. The nurse reviews Nancy's chart to see what medications she is receiving because she knows certain drugs increase the frequency of the syndrome in some patients. List several of these medications:

a. _____   d. _____

b. _____   e. _____

c. _____   f. _____

3. Because of the dumping syndrome, the physician reduces Nancy's current rate of infusion by 50%. The nurse should adjust the rate of the gastrostomy feeding to:

a. 8 ml/min.

b. 10 ml/min.

c. 12 ml/min.

d. 16 ml/min.

4. The nurse notes a residual gastric content of 50 ml. She should:

a. delay the feeding for 2 hours and reassess.

b. discard the 50 ml and administer the next feeding.

c. notify the physician.

d. return the solution through the tube and administer the next feeding.

36

Management of Patients With Gastric and Duodenal Disorders

Chapter Overview

Frequently gastric and duodenal disorders necessitate surgical intervention, which may result in removal of a significant segment of the stomach or duodenum. Because clinical manifestations can be diagnostic, the nurse assesses a patient's symptoms carefully. Again, assessment must include psychosocial aspects because several psychosomatic disorders are manifested by pathophysiologic changes in the gastrointestinal tract.

I. Knowledge-Based Questions

Deduction and Interpretation

Read each question carefully. Circle your answer.

1. Type B chronic gastritis can be distinguished from type A gastritis by its ability to:
   a. cause atrophy of parietal cells.
   b. affect only the antrum portion of the stomach.
   c. thin the lining of the stomach walls.
   d. decrease gastric secretions.

2. The most common site for peptic ulcer formation is the:
   a. duodenum.
   b. esophagus.
   c. pylorus.
   d. stomach.

3. A symptom that distinguishes a chronic gastric ulcer from a chronic duodenal ulcer is the:
   a. absence of any correlation between the presence of the ulcer and a malignancy.
   b. normal to below-normal secretion of acid.
   c. relief of pain after food ingestion.
   d. uncommon incidence of vomiting.

4. The blood group that seems most susceptible to peptic ulcer disease is group:
   a. A
   b. B.
   c. AB.
   d. O.

5. A goal of antacid therapy is to keep pepsin relatively inactive, which is possible when the pH exceeds:
   a. 2.0.
   b. 2.5.
   c. 3.0.
   d. 3.5.

6. The gastric phase of gastric secretion is stimulated by the release of:
   a. gastrin.
   b. secretin.
   c. pepsin.
   d. ptyalin.

7. A diagnostic clinical manifestation(s) of Zollinger-Ellison syndrome is(are):
  a. diarrhea.
  b. hypercalcemia.
  c. steatorrhea.
  d. all of the above.

8. A characteristic associated with peptic ulcer pain is a:
  a. burning sensation localized in the back or midepigastrium.
  b. feeling of emptiness that precedes meals from 1 to 3 hours.
  c. severe gnawing pain that increases in severity as the day progresses..
  d. combination of all of the above.

9. The best time to administer an antacid is:
  a. with the meal.
  b. 30 minutes before the meal.
  c. 1 to 3 hours after the meal.
  d. immediately after the meal.

10. The *most common* complication of peptic ulcer disease is:
  a. hemorrhage.
  b. intractable ulcer.
  c. perforation.
  d. pyloric obstruction.

11. Pyloric obstruction can occur when the area distal to the pyloric sphincter becomes stenosed by:
  a. edema.
  b. scar tissue.
  c. spasm.
  d. all of the above.

12. Symptoms associated with pyloric obstruction include all of the following *except:*
  a. anorexia.
  b. diarrhea.
  c. nausea and vomiting.
  d. weight loss.

13. A nursing intervention(s) associated with peptic ulcer is(are):
  a. checking the blood pressure and pulse rate every 15 to 20 minutes.
  b. frequently monitoring hemoglobin and hematocrit levels.
  c. observing stools and vomitus for color, consistency, and volume.
  d. all of the above.

14. If peptic ulcer hemorrhage were suspected, an immediate nursing action would be to:
  a. place the patient supine with his legs elevated.
  b. prepare a peripheral and central line for intravenous infusion.
  c. assess vital signs.
  d. accomplish all of the above.

15. *Morbid obesity* is a term applied to people who are more than:
  a. 20 lb above ideal body weight.
  b. 50 lb above ideal body weight.
  c. 75 to 80 lb above ideal body weight.
  d. 100 lb above ideal body weight.

16. A commonly used systemic antacid that can cause electrolyte imbalance is:
  a. aluminum hydroxide.
  b. magnesium hydroxide.
  c. milk of magnesia.
  d. sodium bicarbonate.

17. A Billroth I procedure is a surgical approach to ulcer management whereby:
  a. a partial gastrectomy is done with anastomosis of the stomach segment to the duodenum.
  b. a sectioned portion of the stomach is joined to the jejunum.
  c. the antral portion of the stomach is removed and a vagotomy is performed.
  d. the vagus nerve is cut and gastric drainage is established.

18. Anticholinergics are given to:
  a. block vagal stimulation of parietal cells.
  b. decrease gastric motor activity.
  c. reduce acid secretion.
  d. act by all of the above mechanisms.

170

19. Postoperative nursing care for a patient with a partial gastric resection would *not include:*

a. administering 30 ml of fluid through the naso-gastric tube every hour to maintain the patency of the tube and help prevent dehydration.

b. auscultating the abdomen for the presence of bowel sounds.

c. maintaining the patient in a modified Fowler's position to promote drainage from the stomach.

d. withholding fluids by mouth until peristalsis has returned.

20. Pulmonary complications frequently follow upper abdominal incisions because:

a. aspiration is a common occurrence associated with postoperative injury to the pyloric sphincter or the cardiac sphincter.

b. pneumothorax is a common complication of abdominal surgery when the chest cavity has been entered.

c. the patient tends to have shallow respirations in an attempt to minimize incisional pain.

d. all of the above are true.

21. Teaching points to help a total gastric resection patient avoid the dumping syndrome include all of the following except:

a. eating small, frequent meals.

b. increasing the carbohydrate content of the diet to supply needed calories for energy.

c. lying down after meals.

d. taking fluids between meals to decrease the total volume in the stomach at one time.

Read each statement carefully. Write the best response in the space provided.

1. List two measures used to treat the ingestion of corrosive acid.

1. _____

2. _____

2. Explain why patients with type A gastritis evidence malabsorption of vitamin B_{12}.

_____

_____

3. Name two conditions specifically related to peptic ulcer development.

_____

_____

4. List the bacillus that is commonly associated with gastric and possibly duodenal ulcers:

_____

5. List several findings characteristic of Zollinger-Ellison syndrome.

_____

_____

6. Describe those personality traits that are believed to predispose a person to peptic ulcer disease.

_____

_____

7. Define the term *stress ulcer.*

_____

8. Explain the current theory about diet modification for peptic ulcer disease.

_____

_____

9. Name the four major complications of a peptic ulcer.

1. _____   3. _____

2. _____

10. Describe the clinical manifestations associated with peptic ulcer perforation.

_____

_____

_____

11. Three current nonsurgical interventions that can be performed for hemorrhage are:

1. _____   3. _____

2. _____

12. Identify some of the early symptoms of gastric cancer.

_____

_____

II. Critical Analysis Questions

Generating Solutions: Clinical Problem Solving

Extracting Inferences

Examine Figure 36–1. Outline in detail the pathophysiology of peptic ulcer formation. Explain why specific sites are more common and what contributes to common inflammatory sites.

FIGURE 36–1 Peptic lesions may occur in the esophagus (esophagitis), stomach (gastritis), or duodenum (duodenitis). Note peptic ulcer sites and common inflammatory sites. Hydrochloric acid is formed by parietal cells in the fundus; gastrin is secreted by G cells in the antrum. The duodenal glands secrete an alkaline mucous solution.

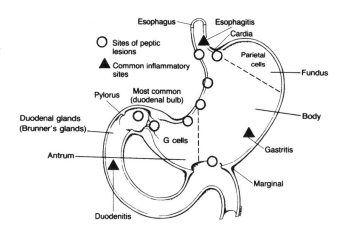

37

Management of Patients With Intestinal and Rectal Disorders

Chapter Overview

Intestinal disorders range from mild alterations in bowel function to the acute manifestations of peritonitis and the chronic problems associated with intestinal conduits subsequent to carcinoma. Nurses need to be alert to indicators of pathology, since prognosis can be influenced by early diagnosis and treatment. Covert physiologic symptoms can frequently be identified by analyzing psychosocial behavior. Nursing care plans need to address a person's total needs because the entire body is frequently adversely affected by localized gastrointestinal disorders.

I. Knowledge-Based Questions

Deduction and Interpretation

Read each question carefully. Circle your answer.

1. The pathophysiology of constipation may be related to interference with:
   a. myoelectric activity of the colon.
   b. mucosal transport.
   c. processes involved in defecation.
   d. all of the above mechanisms.

2. Nursing suggestions to help a person break the constipation habit include all of the following *except:*
   a. a fluid intake of 2 L/day; or more.
   b. a low-residue, bland diet.
   c. establishing a regular schedule of exercise.
   d. establishing a regular time for daily elimination.

3. The classification of *moderate* diarrhea refers to the quantity of daily unformed stools described as:
   a. more than two bowel movements a day.
   b. between two and four bowel movements daily.
   c. between three and six bowel movements daily.
   d. more than six bowel movements a day.

4. In assessing stool characteristics associated with diarrhea, the nurse knows that the presence of greasy stools suggests:
   a. disorders of the colon.
   b. inflammatory enteritis.
   c. intestinal malabsorption.
   d. small-bowel disorders.

5. Hypokalemia may occur rapidly in an elderly person who experiences diarrhea. The nurse should report a critical potassium level of _____ to the physician immediately.
   a. 3.0 mEq/L
   b. 4.0 mEq/L
   c. 4.5 mEq/L
   d. 5.0 mEq/L

6. A positive Rovsing's sign is indicative of appendicitis. The nurse knows to assess for this indicator by palpating the:
 a. right lower quadrant.
 b. left lower quadrant.
 c. right upper quadrant.
 d. left upper quadrant.

7. The most common site for diverticulitis is the:
 a. duodenum.
 b. ileum.
 c. jejunum.
 d. sigmoid.

8. Diverticulitis is clinically manifested by:
 a. a low-grade fever.
 b. a change in bowel habits.
 c. left lower quadrant pain.
 d. all of the above.

9. Common clinical manifestations of Crohn's disease are:
 a. abdominal pain and diarrhea.
 b. edema and weight gain.
 c. nausea and vomiting.
 d. obstruction and ileus.

10. A nurse suspects a diagnosis of regional enteritis when she assesses the symptom(s) of:
 a. abdominal distention and rebound tenderness.
 b. hyperactive bowel sounds in the right lower quadrant.
 c. intermittent pain associated with diarrhea.
 d. all of the above.

11. Nutritional management for regional enteritis consists of diet therapy that is:
 a. high in fats.
 b. high in fiber.
 c. low in protein.
 d. low in residue.

12. Remission of inflammation in ulcerative colitis is possible with:
 a. antidiarrheal medication.
 b. periods of rest after meals.
 c. steroid therapy.
 d. all of the above.

13. A problem unique to the patient with an ileostomy is that:
 a. regular bowel habits cannot be established.
 b. sexual activity is restricted.
 c. skin excoriation can occur.
 d. the collecting appliance is bulky and large.

14. Postoperative nursing management for a patient with a continent ileostomy includes all of the following *except:*
 a. checking to make certain that the rectal packing is in place.
 b. irrigating the ileostomy catheter every 3 hours.
 c. nasogastric tube feedings, 30 to 50 ml, every 4 to 6 hours.
 d. perineal irrigations after the dressings are removed.

15. Clinical manifestations associated with small bowel obstruction include all of the following *except:*
 a. dehydration.
 b. pain that is wavelike.
 c. the passage of blood-tinged stool.
 d. vomiting.

16. The mortality rate for cancer of the colon is:
 a. less than 20%.
 b. 25 to 35%.
 c. 40 to 50%.
 d. greater than 60%.

17. Preoperatively, intestinal antibiotics are given for colon surgery to:
 a. decrease the bulk of colon contents.
 b. reduce the bacteria content of the colon.
 c. soften the stool.
 d. do all of the above.

18. For colostomy irrigation, the enema catheter should be inserted into the stoma:
 a. 1 in.
 b. 2 to 3 in.
 c. 4 to 6 in.
 d. 8 in.

19. For colostomy irrigation, the patient should be directed to hold the enema can or bag at shoulder level approximately _____ above the stoma:
 a. 6 in.
 b. 8 to 16 in.
 c. 18 to 24 in.
 d. 30 in.

20. The total quantity of irrigating solution that can be instilled at one session is:

a. 1000 ml.

b. 1500 ml.

c. 2500 ml.

d. 3000 ml.

Match the physical complication listed in Column II with its associated medical condition listed in Column I. An answer may be used more than once.

Column I

1. _____ constipation

2. _____ appendicitis

3. _____ peritonitis

4. _____ diverticulitis

5. _____ abdominal hernia

6. _____ colostomies

Column II

a. megacolon

b. perforation

c. evisceration

d. intestinal obstruction

II. Critical Analysis Questions

Recognizing Contradictions

Rewrite each statement correctly. Underline the key concepts.

1. Diarrhea is a condition in which there is an increased frequency of bowel movements, more than six per day, associated with increased amount and consistency.

2. Peritonitis, the most common reason for emergency abdominal surgery, occurs in about 10% of the population.

3. The most serious complication of appendicitis is strangulation of adjacent bowel tissue which occurs in 5% of the cases.

4. The most common areas affected in Crohn's disease are the sigmoid colon and the cecum.

5. The most common presenting symptom of colon cancer is rectal bleeding.

Generating Solutions: Clinical Problem Solving

Read the following case studies. Fill in the blanks or circle the correct answer.

CASE STUDY: Appendicitis

Rory, an 18-year-old girl, is admitted to the hospital with a possible diagnosis of appendicitis. She had been symptomatic for several days before admission.

1. During assessment the nurse is looking for positive indicators of appendicitis, which include all of the following *except:*

a. a low-grade fever.

b. abdominal tenderness on palpation.

c. thrombocytopenia.

d. vomiting.

2. On physical examination the nurse should be looking for tenderness on palpation at McBurney's point, which is located in the:

a. left lower quadrant.

b. left upper quadrant.

c. right lower quadrant.

d. right upper quadrant.

3. A symptom or symptoms suggestive of acute appendicitis is(are):
   a. a positive Rovsing's sign.
   b. increased abdominal pain with coughing.
   c. tenderness around the umbilicus.
   d. all of the above.

4. Preparation for an appendectomy includes:
   a. an intravenous infusion.
   b. prophylactic antibiotic therapy.
   c. salicylates to lower an elevated temperature.
   d. all of the above.

CASE STUDY: Peritonitis

Sharon has peritonitis subsequent to ambulatory peritoneal dialysis. Her presenting symptoms are pain, abdominal tenderness, and nausea.

1. On assessment, the nurse should be looking for additional symptoms diagnostic of peritonitis, which include:
   a. abdominal rigidity.
   b. diminished peristalsis.
   c. leukocytosis.
   d. all of the above.

2. A central venous pressure (CVP) catheter is inserted to monitor fluid balance. The nurse's readings indicate low circulatory volume. The reading is probably between:
   a. 2 and 4 cm H_2O.
   b. 6 and 8 cm H_2O.
   c. 10 and 12 cm H_2O.
   d. 14 and 16 cm H_2O.

3. Given Sharon's CVP reading indicating hypovolemia, the nurse should assess for all of the following *except:*
   a. bradycardia.
   b. hypotension.
   c. oliguria.
   d. tachypnea.

4. With treatment, Sharon's peritonitis subsides. However, the nurse continues to assess for the common complication of:
   a. abscess formation.
   b. respiratory arrest owing to excessive pressure on the diaphragm.
   c. umbilical hernia.
   d. urinary tract infection.

Learner's Self-Evaluation Tool for End of Unit 8 Review

1. The most important concepts or facts I have learned from this unit are:

   1. _____

   2. _____

   3. _____

2. The most important reference page numbers for test review and clinical concepts are pages:

   _____   _____   _____

   _____   _____   _____

3. The concepts or facts that I do not fully understand are:

   _____

   _____

4. I will get the answer(s) to my questions by _____

_____

I will do this on _____ (date and time).

5. I believe my mastery of this unit to be:
    a.   100%   Great job! Good luck!
    b.   90%   2 hours of review recommended.
    c.   80%   4 hours of review recommended.
    d.   <80%   Make an appointment with your instructor.

UNIT 9
Metabolic and Endocrine Function

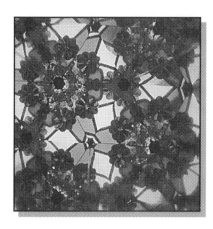

38

Assessment and Management of Patients With Hepatic and Biliary Disorders

Chapter Overview

The liver is vital to human survival. Among its functions are glucose, protein, and fat metabolism, drug metabolism, bile formation, and vitamin storage. The biliary system works synergistically with the hepatic system and plays a major role in digestion and absorption. Hepatic and biliary disorders always result in systemic as well as localized responses. Therefore, during assessment a nurse needs to be sensitive to covert as well as overt manifestations of organ and system pathophysiology that may result from hepatic or biliary dysfunction.

I. Knowledge-Based Questions

Deduction and Interpretation

Read each question carefully. Circle your answer.

1. Blood leaves the liver and enters the inferior vena cava through the:
   a. hepatic artery.
   b. hepatic vein.
   c. portal artery.
   d. portal vein.

2. The liver plays a major role in glucose metabolism by:
   a. producing ketone bodies.
   b. synthesizing albumin.
   c. participating in gluconeogenesis.
   d. doing all of the above.

3. The liver synthesizes prothrombin only if there is enough vitamin:
   a. A.
   b. B_{12}.
   c. D.
   d. K.

4. The substance necessary for the manufacture of bile salts by hepatocytes is:
   a. albumin.
   b. bilirubin.
   c. cholesterol.
   d. vitamin D.

5. The main function of bile salts is:
   a. albumin synthesis.
   b. fat emulsification in the intestines.
   c. lipid manufacture for the transport of proteins.
   d. urea synthesis from ammonia.

6. Hepatocellular dysfunction will result in all of the following *except:*
   a. decreased serum albumin.
   b. elevated serum bilirubin.
   c. increased blood ammonia levels.
   d. increased levels of urea.

7. Jaundice becomes evident when serum bilirubin levels exceed:
a. 0.5 mg/dl.
b. 1.0 mg/dl.
c. 1.5 mg/dl.
d. 2.5 mg/dl.

8. Negative sodium balance is important for a patient with ascites. An example of food permitted on a low-sodium diet is:
a. 1/4 cup of peanut butter.
b. 1 cup of powdered milk.
c. one frankfurter.
d. two slices of cold cuts.

9. A person who consumes contaminated shellfish would probably develop hepatitis:
a. A virus.
b. B virus.
c. non-A, non-B virus.
d. C virus.

10. The hepatitis virus that has the shortest average incubation period is hepatitis:
a. A virus.
b. B virus.
c. C virus.
d. D virus.

11. Immune serum globulin provides passive immunity to type A hepatitis if administered 2 to 7 days after exposure. Immunity is effective for about:
a. 1 month.
b. 2 months.
c. 3 months.
d. 4 months.

12. Choose the correct statement about hepatitis B vaccine.
a. All persons at risk should receive active immunization.
b. Evidence suggests that the HIV virus may be harbored in the vaccine.
c. It should be given only once because of its potency.
d. One dose in the dorsogluteal muscle is recommended.

13. Indications for postexposure vaccination with hepatitis B immune globulin include:
a. accidental exposure to HbsAg-positive blood.
b. perinatal exposure.
c. sexual contact with those who are positive for HbsAg.
d. all of the above exposures.

14. The chemical(s) *most commonly* implicated in toxic hepatitis is(are):
a. chloroform.
b. gold compounds.
c. phosphorus.
d. all of the above hepatoxins.

15. Fulminant hepatic failure may progress to hepatic encephalopathy _____ weeks after disease onset.
a. 2
b. 4
c. 6
d. 8

16. Late symptoms of hepatic cirrhosis include all of the following *except:*
a. edema.
b. hypoalbuminemia.
c. hypokalemia.
d. hyponatremia.

hypernatremic!

17. Cirrhosis results in shunting of the portal system blood into collateral blood vessels in the gastrointestinal tract. The most common site(s) is(are) the:
a. esophagus.
b. lower rectum.
c. stomach.
d. a combination of all of the above.

18. Signs of advanced liver disease include:
a. ascites.
b. jaundice.
c. portal hypertension.
d. all of the above.

19. The most common single cause of death in patients with cirrhosis is:
a. congestive heart failure.
b. hepatic encephalopathy.
c. hypovolemic shock.
d. ruptured esophageal varices.

20. The mortality rate from bleeding esophageal varices is about:
a. 10%.
b. 30%.
c. 50%.
d. 80%.

21. Indicator(s) of probable esophageal varices is(are):

a. hematemesis.

b. a positive guaiac test.

c. melena.

d. all of the above.

22. Bleeding esophageal varices result in a decrease in:

a. nitrogen load from bleeding.

b. renal perfusion.

c. serum ammonia.

d. all of the above.

23. Hepatic lobectomy for cancer can be successful when the primary site is localized. Because of the regenerative capacity of the liver, a surgeon can remove up to:

a. 25% of liver tissue.

b. 50% of liver tissue.

c. 75% of liver tissue.

d. 90% of liver tissue.

24. Statistics show that there is a greater incidence of gallbladder disease for women who are:

a. multiparous.

b. obese.

c. over 40 years of age.

d. characterized by all of the above.

25. Clinical manifestations of common bile duct obstruction include all of the following *except:*

a. amber-colored urine.

b. clay-colored feces.

c. pruritus.

d. jaundice.

26. The diagnostic test(s) used to distinguish hepatocellular jaundice from obstructive jaundice is(are):

a. intravenous cholecystography.

b. oral cholecystography.

c. percutaneous transhepatic cholangiography.

d. all of the above.

27. The most common side effect of extracorporeal shock-wave lithotripsy is:

a. bile duct obstruction.

b. cutaneous petechiae.

c. gross hematuria.

d. pancreatitis.

II. Critical Analysis Questions

Generating Solutions: Clinical Problem Solving

Read the following case studies. Circle the correct answer.

CASE STUDY: Liver Biopsy

Veronica is scheduled for a liver biopsy. The staff nurse assigned to care for Veronica is to accompany her to the treatment room.

1. Before a liver biopsy the nurse should check to see that:

a. a compatible donor blood is available.

b. hemostasis tests have been completed.

c. vital signs have been assessed.

d. all of the above have been done.

2. The nurse begins preparing Veronica for the biopsy by assisting her to the correct position, which is:

a. jackknife, with her entire back exposed.

b. recumbent, with her right upper abdomen exposed.

c. lying on her right side, with the left upper thoracic area exposed.

d. supine, with the left lateral chest wall exposed.

3. The nurse knows that the biopsy needle will be inserted into the liver between the:

a. third and fourth ribs.

b. fourth and fifth ribs.

c. sixth and seventh ribs.

d. eighth and ninth ribs.

4. Immediately before needle insertion, Veronica needs to be instructed to:

a. breathe slowly and deeply so that rib cage expansion will be minimized during needle insertion.

b. inhale and exhale deeply and then hold her breath at the end of expiration until the needle is inserted.

c. pant deeply and continue panting during needle insertion so pain perception will be minimized.

d. take a deep inspiration and not breathe for 30 to 40 seconds so that the area for needle insertion can be determined; she should then resume normal breathing for the remainder of the procedure.

5. After the biopsy the nurse assists Veronica to:
   a. high Fowler's position, in which she can effectively take deep breaths and cough.
   b. ambulate while splinting her incision.
   c. assume the Trendelenburg position to prevent postbiopsy shock.
   d. the right-side-lying position with a pillow placed under the right costal margin.

CASE STUDY: Paracentesis

Wendy is scheduled for a paracentesis for ascites formation subsequent to cirrhosis of the liver.

1. Before the procedure the nurse obtains several drainage bottles. She knows that the maximum amount of fluid to be aspirated at one time is:
   a. 1 L.
   b. 2 L.
   c. 3 L.
   d. 4 L.

2. The nurse helps Wendy to assume the proper position for a paracentesis, which is:
   a. recumbent so that the fluid will pool to the lower abdomen.
   b. lying on her left side so that fluid will not exert pressure on the liver.
   c. semi-Fowler's to avoid shock and provide the most comfort.
   d. upright with her feet resting on a support so that the puncture site will be readily visible.

3. After the paracentesis Wendy should be observed for signs of vascular collapse, which include all of the following *except:*
   a. bradycardia.
   b. hypotension.
   c. oliguria.
   d. pallor.

CASE STUDY: Laennec's Cirrhosis

Nathan, a 50-year-old physically disabled veteran, has lived alone for 30 years. He has maintained his independence despite chronic back pain resulting from a war injury. He has a long history of depression and limited food intake. He drinks six to ten bottles of beer daily. He was recently admitted to a veteran's hospital with a diagnosis of Laennec's cirrhosis. He was asymptomatic for ascites.

1. On assessment the nurse notes early clinical manifestations of Laennec's cirrhosis, which include all of the following *except:*
   a. pain caused by liver enlargement.
   b. a sharp edge to the periphery of the liver.
   c. a liver decreased in size and nodular. *Late*
   d. a firm liver.

2. An abnormal laboratory finding for Nathan is a:
   a. blood ammonia level of 35 mg/dl.
   b. serum albumin of 4.0 g/dl.
   c. total serum bilirubin of 0.9 mg/dl.
   d. total serum protein of 5.5 g/dl.

3. Nathan is 5 ft 10 in. tall and weighs 140 lb. The physician recommends 50 cal/kg for weight gain. Nathan's daily caloric intake would be approximately:
   a. 2200 cal.
   b. 2800 cal.
   c. 3200 cal.
   d. 3800 cal.

4. A recommended protein intake for Nathan to gain weight is:
   a. 31 to 44 g.
   b. 41 to 54 g.
   c. 51 to 64 g.
   d. 61 to 74 g.

5. The physician recommends a sodium-restricted diet. The nurse expects the suggested sodium intake to be approximately:
   a. 250 to 500 mg/24 hr.
   b. 500 to 1000 mg/24 hr.
   c. 2000 to 2500 mg/24 hr.
   d. 3000 to 3500 mg/24 hr.

CASE STUDY: Liver Transplant

Denise, a 54-year-old mother of three, is scheduled for a liver transplantation subsequent to an extensive hepatic malignancy.

1. Denise is hopeful that her surgery will be successful. She is aware that she has a(n) _____ % chance of a 1-year success rate.
   a. 10.
   b. 30.
   c. 50.
   d. 80.

2. Denise knows that a successful outcome to transplantation will be compromised by:
   a. fluid and electrolyte disturbances.
   b. malnutrition.
   c. massive ascites.
   d. all of the above.

3. The nurse is aware that, postoperatively, the leading cause of death is:
   a. bleeding.
   b. hypotension.
   c. infection.
   d. portal hypertension.

4. The nurse knows that a patient receiving cyclosporine to prevent rejection of the transplanted liver may develop a drug side effect of:
   a. nephrotoxicity.
   b. septicemia.
   c. thrombocytopenia.
   d. all of the above reactions.

CASE STUDY: Cholecystectomy

Brenda, a 33-year-old obese mother of four, is diagnosed as having acute gallbladder inflammation. She is 5 ft 4 in. tall and weighs 190 lb. The physician decides to delay surgical intervention until her acute symptoms subside.

1. Brenda's initial course of treatment would probably consist of:
   a. analgesics and antibiotics.
   b. intravenous fluids.
   c. nasogastric suction.
   d. all of the above.

2. After her acute attack, Brenda was limited to low-fat liquids. As foods are added to her diet, she needs to know that she should avoid:
   a. cooked fruits.
   b. eggs and cheese.
   c. lean meats.
   d. rice and tapioca.

3. Brenda is being medicated with chenodeoxycholic acid. The nurse needs to tell Brenda that the drug may not be effective if it is taken in conjunction with:
   a. dietary cholesterol.
   b. estrogens.
   c. oral contraceptives.
   d. all of the above.

Because Brenda's symptoms continue to recur, she is scheduled for gallbladder surgery.

1. Brenda has signed a consent form for removal of her gallbladder and ligation of the cystic duct and artery. She is scheduled to undergo a:
   a. cholecystectomy.
   b. cholecystostomy.
   c. choledochostomy.
   d. choledocholithotomy.

2. Postoperative nursing observation includes assessing for:
   a. indicators of infection.
   b. leakage of bile into the peritoneal cavity.
   c. obstruction of bile drainage.
   d. all of the above.

3. Brenda needs to know that fat restriction is usually lifted when the biliary ducts dilate to accommodate bile once held by the gallbladder. This takes about:
   a. 1 week.
   b. 2 to 3 weeks.
   c. 4 to 6 weeks.
   d. 2 months.

39

Assessment and Management of Patients With Diabetes Mellitus

Chapter Overview

Diabetes mellitus is an endocrine disorder associated with abnormalities in several major body systems. It is characterized by hyperglycemia, by insulin insufficiency, or by inadequate uptake of glucose in the peripheral tissues. Both acute and chronic manifestations are observed. The following questions and clinical situations refer to symptomatology and to nursing and medical management of patients who are diagnosed as having diabetes mellitus.

I. Knowledge-Based Questions

Deduction and Interpretation

Read each question carefully. Circle your answer.

1. A patient who is diagnosed with type I diabetes mellitus would be expected to:
  a. be restricted to an American Diabetic Association diet.
  b. have no damage to the islet cells of the pancreas.
  c. need exogenous insulin.
  d. need to receive daily doses of a hypoglycemic agent.

2. As a cause of death by disease in the United States, diabetes mellitus ranks:
  a. first.
  b. second.
  c. third.
  d. fourth.

3. A possible risk factor(s) associated with insulin-dependent diabetes mellitus (IDDM) is(are):
  a. an autoimmune susceptibility to diabetogenic viruses.
  b. premature onset of arteriosclerosis.
  c. the presence of human leukocyte antigen (HLA).
  d. all of the above.

4. Knowing that gluconeogenesis helps to maintain blood levels, a nurse should:
  a. document weight changes because of fatty acid mobilization.
  b. evaluate the patient's sensitivity to low room temperatures because of decreased adipose tissue insulation.
  c. protect the patient from sources of infection because of decreased cellular protein deposits.
  d. do all of the above.

5. Clinical manifestations associated with a diagnosis of IDDM include all of the following *except:*
a. hypoglycemia.
b. hyponatremia.
c. ketonuria.
d. polyphagia.

6. You are assigned to care for a patient who is suspected of having non–insulin-dependent diabetes mellitus (NIDDM). Clinical manifestations you should assess for include:
a. blurred or deteriorating vision.
b. fatigue and muscle cramping.
c. wounds that heal slowly or respond poorly to treatment.
d. all of the above.

7. You are asked to assess a patient for glucosuria. You would secure a specimen of:
a. blood.
b. sputum.
c. stool.
d. urine.

8. There seems to be a positive correlation between type II diabetes mellitus and:
a. hypotension.
b. kidney dysfunction.
c. obesity.
d. sex.

9. The fasting plasma glucose level suggestive of a diagnosis of diabetes is:
a. 110 mg/dl.
b. 120 mg/dl.
c. 130 mg/dl.
d. 140 mg/dl.

10. The most sensitive test for diabetes mellitus is the:
a. blood glucose test.
b. glucose tolerance test.
c. 2-hour postprandial test.
d. urine glucose test.

11. A diabetic who weighs 130 lb has an ideal body weight of 116 lb. For weight reduction, her daily caloric intake should be approximately:
a. 1000 cal.
b. 1200 cal.
c. 1500 cal.
d. 1800 cal.

12. The nurse should encourage exercise in the management of diabetes because it:
a. decreases total triglyceride levels.
b. improves insulin utilization.
c. lowers blood glucose.
d. accomplishes all of the above mechanisms.

13. Self-monitoring of blood glucose (SMBG) is recommended for patients with:
a. abnormal renal glucose thresholds.
b. hypoglycemia without warning symptoms.
c. unstable diabetes.
d. all of the above conditions.

14. An example of a commonly administered intermediate-acting insulin is:
a. NHP insulin.
b. PZI insulin.
c. regular insulin.
d. Ultralente insulin.

15. The nurse knows that an intermediate-acting insulin should reach its "peak" in:
a. 1 to 2 hours.
b. 4 to 6 hours.
c. 8 to 16 hours.
d. 18 to 20 hours.

16. The tissue area that provides the fastest absorption rate for regular insulin is believed to be the:
a. abdominal site.
b. anterior thigh.
c. deltoid site.
d. gluteal site.

17. Rotation sites for insulin injection should be separated from one another by 2.5 cm (1 in.) and should be used only once every:
a. third day.
b. week.
c. 2 to 3 weeks.
d. 2 to 4 weeks.

18. Current insulin pumps in use today:
a. can deliver a premeal dose (bolus) of insulin if the body signals such a need.
b. deliver a continuous basal rate of insulin throughout a 24-hour period.
c. estimate blood glucose measurements to determine variations in delivery.
d. are capable of doing all of the above.

19. A probable candidate for diabetic management with oral antidiabetic agents is one who is:
a. non–insulin-dependent.
b. stable and not prone to ketosis.
c. unable to be managed by diet alone.
d. characterized by all of the above.

20. The nurse should expect that insulin therapy will be temporarily substituted for oral antidiabetic therapy if the diabetic:
a. develops an infection with fever.
b. suffers trauma.
c. undergoes major surgery.
d. develops any or all of the above.

21. *Hypoglycemia,* an abnormally low blood glucose level, occurs with a glucose level:
a. below 50 mg/dl.
b. between 60 mg/dl and 75 mg/dl.
c. between 75 mg/dl and 85 mg/dl.
d. of 90 mg/dl.

22. A clinical feature that distinguishes a hypoglycemic reaction from a ketoacidosis reaction is:
a. blurred vision.
b. diaphoresing.
c. nausea.
d. weakness.

23. The nurse knows that treatment modalities for diabetic ketoacidosis should focus on management of:
a. acidosis.
b. dehydration.
c. electrolyte loss.
d. all of the above.

24. A patient exhibiting the *Somogyi effect* in contrast to the *dawn phenomenon* will evidence:
a. a progressive rise in blood glucose from bed-time to morning.
b. hypoglycemia at 2:00 to 3:00 AM after elevated glucose levels at bedtime.
c. normal glucose levels until 3:00 AM, when levels will begin to rise.
d. hyperglycemia in the early morning hours followed by an abrupt fall in glucose levels.

25. Mortality rates for patients with diabetes are positively correlated with atherosclerotic complications, especially in the coronary arteries, which account for about:
a. 10% of all deaths.
b. 30% of all deaths.
c. 40% of all deaths.
d. 60% of all deaths.

26. With nonproliferative retinopathy, examination of the retina may reveal:
a. leakage of fluid or serum (exudates).
b. microaneurysms.
c. weakened capillary walls.
d. all of the above pathologic changes.

27. A diagnostic manifestation of proliferative retinopathy is:
a. decreased capillary permeability.
b. microaneurysm formation.
c. neovascularization into the vitreous humor.
d. the leakage of capillary wall fragments into surrounding areas.

28. Clinical nursing assessment for a patient with microangiopathy who has manifested impaired peripheral arterial circulation includes all of the following *except:*
a. integumentary inspection for the presence of brown spots on the lower extremities.
b. observation for paleness of the lower extremities.
c. observation for blanching of the feet after the legs are elevated for 60 seconds.
d. palpation for increased pulse volume in the arteries of the lower extremities.

29. Nursing care for a diabetic with peripheral neuropathy includes:
a. assessing pain patterns to rule out peripheral vascular insufficiency.
b. inspecting the feet for breaks in skin integrity.
c. palpating the lower extremities for temperature variations.
d. all of the above.

30. With peripheral neuropathy a diabetic has limited sensitivity to:
a. heat.
b. pain.
c. pressure.
d. all of the above.

31. During surgery, glucose levels will rise because there is an increased secretion of:
a. cortisol.
b. epinephrine.
c. glucagon.
d. all of the above.

32. The nurse expects that a type I diabetic may receive _____ of his usual morning dose of insulin preoperatively.
   a. 10% to 20%.
   b. 25% to 40%.
   c. 50% to 60%.
   d. 85% to 90%.

For each of the clinical characteristics listed below, choose the associated classification of diabetes mellitus.

I refers to type I: *Insulin-dependent diabetes mellitus*

II refers to type II: *Non–insulin-dependent diabetes*

1. _II_ Etiology includes obesity

2. _II_ Ketosis is rare

3. _I_ Usually thin at diagnosis

4. _I_ Needs insulin to preserve life

5. _II_ Often has islet cell antibodies

6. _I_ No islet cell antibodies

7. _I_ Onset at any age

8. _II_ Usually is diagnosed after age 30

9. _II_ Hyperosmolar nonketotic syndrome is a complication

10. _II_ Little or no endogenous insulin

Match the physiologic change listed in Column II with its associated term listed in Column I.

Column I

1. _C_ gluconeogenesis

2. _A_ glucosuria

3. _B_ glycogenolysis

4. _E_ nephropathy

5. _D_ retinopathy

Column II

a. Filtered glucose that the kidney cannot absorb spills over into urine.

b. Glycogen breaks down in the liver through the action of glucagon.

c. New glucose is produced from amino acids.

d. Microvascular changes develop in the eyes.

e. Small vessel disease affects the kidneys.

II. Critical Analysis Questions

Generating Solutions: Clinical Problem Solving

Read the following case studies. Circle the correct answer.

CASE STUDY: IDDM

Albert, a 35-year-old insulin-dependent diabetic, is admitted to the hospital with a diagnosis of pneumonia. He has been febrile since admission. His daily insulin requirement is 24 units of NPH.

1. Every morning Albert is given NPH insulin at 7:30 AM. Meals are served at 8:30 AM, 12:30 PM, and 6:30 PM. The nurse expects that the NPH insulin will reach its maximum effect (peak) between the hours of:
   a. 11:30 AM and 1:30 PM.
   b. 1:30 PM and 7:30 PM.
   c. 3:30 PM and 9:30 PM.
   d. 5:30 PM and 11:30 PM.

2. A bedtime snack is provided for Albert. This is based on the knowledge that intermediate-acting insulins are effective for an approximate duration of:

a. 6 to 12 hours.

b. 12 to 18 hours.

c. 18 to 20 hours.

d. 24 to 28 hours.

3. Albert refuses his bedtime snack. This should alert the nurse to assess for:

a. an elevated serum bicarbonate and a decreased blood pH.

b. signs of hypoglycemia earlier than expected.

c. symptoms of hyperglycemia during the peak time of NPH insulin.

d. sugar in the urine.

CASE STUDY: Hypoglycemia

Betty, an 18-year-old insulin-dependent diabetic, is unconscious when admitted to the hospital. Her daily dose of insulin has been 32 units of NPH each morning.

1. Based on your knowledge of hypoglycemia, you would expect that Betty's serum glucose level, on admission, is approximately:

a. 50 mg/dl.

b. 70 mg/dl.

c. 90 mg/dl.

d. 110 mg/dl.

2. Betty is given 1 mg of glucagon hydrochloride, subcutaneously, in the emergency department. Your knowledge about the action of this drug alerts you to observe for latent symptoms associated with:

a. glucosuria.

b. hyperglycemia.

c. ketoacidosis.

d. rebound hypoglycemia.

3. After Betty is medically stabilized, she is admitted to the clinical area for observation and health teaching. The nurse should make sure that Betty is aware of warning symptoms associated with hypoglycemia, such as:

a. emotional changes.

b. slurred speech and double vision.

c. staggering gait and incoordination.

d. all of the above.

4. Betty should also be taught that hypoglycemia may be prevented by:

a. eating regularly scheduled meals.

b. eating snacks to cover the peak time of insulin.

c. increasing food intake when engaging in increased levels of physical exercise.

d. doing all of the above.

CASE STUDY: Diabetic Ketoacidosis

Christine, a 64-year-old woman, is admitted to the clinical area with a diagnosis of diabetic ketoacidosis. She is drowsy yet responsive on admission.

1. Nursing actions for a diagnosis of ketoacidosis include:

a. monitoring urinary output by means of an indwelling catheter.

b. evaluating serum electrolytes.

c. testing for glucosuria and acetonuria.

d. all of the above.

2. The nurse should expect that the rehydrating intravenous solution used will be:

a. 0.9% saline solution.

b. 5% dextrose in water.

c. 10% dextrose in water.

d. sterile water.

3. In evaluating the laboratory results, the nurse expects all of the following to indicate ketoacidosis *except* a(an):

a. decreased serum bicarbonate level.

b. elevated blood glucose.

c. increased blood urea.

d. increased blood pH.

4. The physician notes a change in Christine's respirations. Her breathing is described as Kussmaul respirations. The nurse knows that these respirations are:

a. deep.

b. labored.

c. rapid.

d. shallow.

5. Christine is started on low-dose intravenous insulin therapy. Nursing assessment includes all of the following *except* frequent:

a. blood pressure measurements to monitor the degree of hypotension.

b. estimates of serum potassium, since increased blood glucose levels are correlated with elevated potassium levels.

c. evaluation of blood glucose levels because glucose levels should decline as insulin levels increase.

d. elevation of serum ketones to monitor the course of ketosis.

6. As blood glucose levels approach normal, the nurse should assess for signs of electrolyte imbalance associated with:

a. hypernatremia.

b. hypercapnia.

c. hypocalcemia.

d. hypokalemia.

Identifying Patterns

Illustrate, in diagram format, the pathophysiologic sequence of changes that occur with type I diabetes.

40

Assessment and Management of Patients With Endocrine Disorders

Chapter Overview

The endocrine system is characterized by a feedback mechanism that functions interdependently with other systems to maintain homeostasis. Any imbalance in one area can quickly and adversely affect another area. Endocrine disorders are difficult to diagnose because of the multiplicity of nondescriptive symptoms associated with glandular dysfunction. Medical and nursing assessments need to be sensitive to the variety of clinical manifestations that may be present. Behavioral outcomes should be constantly monitored because even minor medical and nursing interventions may produce a change, necessitating a change in the approach to care.

I. Knowledge-Based Questions

Deduction and Interpretation

Read each question carefully. Circle your answer.

1. The pathophysiology of hypoparathyroidism is associated with all of the following *except* a(n):
   a. decrease in serum calcium.
   b. elevation of blood phosphate.
   c. increase in the renal excretion of phosphate.
   d. lowered renal excretion of calcium.

2. Nursing management for a hypoparathyroid patient *would not* include:
   a. maintaining a quiet, subdued environment.
   b. making certain that calcium gluconate is kept at the bedside.
   c. observing the patient for signs of tetany.
   d. supplementing the diet with milk and milk products.

3. A clinical manifestation not usually associated with hyperthyroidism is:
   a. a pulse rate below 90 beats per minute..
   b. an elevated systolic blood pressure.
   c. muscular fatigability.
   d. weight loss.

4. Patients with hyperthyroidism are characteristically:
   a. apathetic and anorexic.
   b. calm.
   c. emotionally stable.
   d. insensitive to heat.

5. The objective(s) of pharmacotherapy for hyperthyroidism is(are):
   a. inhibition of the activity of hormones formed before antithyroid drugs are administered.
   b. prevention of thyroid hormonal synthesis.
   c. suppression of the release of thyroid hormones formed before drug therapy.
   d. all of the above.

6. Iodine or iodide compounds are used for hyperthyroidism because they do all of the following *except:*
   a. decrease the basal metabolic rate.
   b. increase the vascularity of the gland.
   c. lessen the release of thyroid hormones.
   d. reduce the size of the gland.

7. After a single dose of radioactive iodine, the nurse should instruct the patient that symptoms of hyperthyroidism are expected to subside within:
   a. 24 to 48 hours.
   b. 1 to 2 weeks.
   c. 3 to 4 weeks.
   d. 2 to 6 months.

8. Signs of thyroid storm include all of the following *except:*
   a. bradycardia.
   b. delirium or somnolence.
   c. dyspnea and chest pain.
   d. hyperpyrexia.

9. Medical management for thyroid crisis includes:
   a. intravenous dextrose fluids.
   b. hypothermia measures.
   c. oxygen therapy.
   d. all of the above.

10. Pharmacotherapy for thyroid storm would *not* include the administration of:
   a. acetaminophen.
   b. iodine.
   c. propylthiouracil.
   d. synthetic levothyroxine.

11. A diagnosis of hyperparathyroidism can be established by all of the following signs *except:*
   a. a negative reading on a Sulkowitch test.
   b. a serum calcium level of 12 mg/dl.
   c. an elevated level of parathyroid hormone.
   d. bone demineralization seen on x-ray film.

12. A recommended breakfast for a hyperparathyroid patient would be:
   a. cereal with milk and bananas.
   b. fried eggs and bacon.
   c. orange juice and toast.
   d. pork sausage and canned fruit (pears and peaches).

13. A phoechromocytoma is an adrenal medulla tumor that causes arterial hypertension by increasing the level of circulating:
   a. catecholamines.
   b. enzymes.
   c. hormones.
   d. glucocorticoids.

14. A positive test for overactivity of the adrenal medulla is a total catecholamine value of:
   a. 50 pg/ml.
   b. 100 pg/ml.
   c. 100 to 300 pg/ml.
   d. 450 pg/ml.

15. Laboratory findings suggestive of Addison's disease include all of the following *except:*
   a. a relative lymphocytosis.
   b. hyperkalemia and hyponatremia.
   c. hypertension.
   d. hypoglycemia.

16. A positive diagnosis of Cushing's syndrome is associated with:
   a. the disappearance of lymphoid tissue.
   b. a reduction in circulating eosinophils.
   c. an elevated cortisol level.
   d. all of the above.

17. Clinical manifestations of Cushing's syndrome may be modified with a diet that is:
   a. high in protein.
   b. low in carbohydrates.
   c. low in sodium.
   d. all of the above.

18. The nurse needs to be aware that large-dose corticosteroid therapy is most effective when administered:
   a. at 8:00 AM.
   b. at 8:00 PM.
   c. between 4:00 AM and 5:00 AM.
   d. between 4:00 PM and 6:00 PM.

19. Nursing assessment for a patient who is receiving corticosteroid therapy includes observation for the unacceptable side effect of:
   a. glaucoma.
   b. facial mooning.
   c. potassium loss.
   d. weight gain.

20. A major symptom of pancreatitis is:
  a. severe abdominal pain.
  b. fever.
  c. jaundice.
  d. mental agitation.

21. The nurse should assess for an important early indicator of acute pancreatitis, which is an increased:
  a. serum amylase level.
  b. serum lipase level.
  c. white cell count.
  d. urine amylase level.

22. A nursing measure(s) for pain relief for acute pancreatitis include(s):
  a. encouraging bed rest to decrease the metabolic rate.
  b. teaching the patient about the correlation between alcohol intake and pain.
  c. withholding oral feedings to limit the release of secretin.
  d. all of the above.

23. With pancreatic carcinoma, insulin deficiency is suspected when the patient evidences:
  a. an abnormal glucose tolerance.
  b. glucosuria.
  c. hyperglycemia.
  d. all of the above.

24. A clinical manifestation(s) associated with a tumor of the head of the pancreas is(are):
  a. clay-colored stools.
  b. dark urine.
  c. jaundice.
  d. all of the above.

25. A nurse should monitor blood glucose levels for a patient who is diagnosed as having hyperinsulinism. A value inadequate to sustain normal brain function is:
  a. 30 mg/dl.
  b. 50 mg/dl.
  c. 70 mg/dl.
  d. 90 mg/dl.

Match the hormonal function listed in Column II with its corresponding hormone listed in Column I.

Column I

  1. _____ glucagon
  2. ___G___ aldosterone
  3. ___F___ oxytocin
  4. _____ somatotropin
  5. ___A___ vasopressin
  6. _____ thyrocalcitonin
  7. ___I___ prolactin
  8. _____ melatonin
  9. ___?___ parathormone
  10. ___B___ insulin

Column II

  a. controls excretion of water by the kidneys
  b. lowers blood sugar
  c. inhibits bone resorption
  d. influences metabolism that is essential for normal growth
  e. supports sexual maturation
  f. promotes the secretion of milk
  g. stimulates the reabsorption of sodium and the elimination of potassium
  h. promotes glycogenolysis
  i. increases the force of uterine contractions during parturition

II. Critical Analysis Questions

Generating Solutions: Clinical Problem Solving

Read the following case study. Circle the correct answer.

CASE STUDY: Primary Hypothyroidism

Connie had been hospitalized for 1 week for studies to confirm a diagnosis of primary hypothyroidism.

1. Several tests were used in Connie's assessment. All of the following results are consistent with her diagnosis of hypothyroidism *except* for a(n):
   a. elevated level of thyrotropin (TSH).
   b. low uptake of radioactive iodine (^{131}I).
   c. protein-bound iodine reading of 3 mg/dl.
   d. T_3 uptake value of 45%.

2. Nursing care for Connie includes assessing for clinical manifestations associated with hypothyroidism. A manifestation *not consistent* with her diagnosis is a:
   a. change in her menstrual pattern.
   b. pulse rate of 58 beats per minute.
   c. temperature of 95.8°F.
   d. weight loss of 10 lb over a 2-week period.

3. The principal objective of medical management is to:
   a. irradiate the gland in an attempt to stimulate hormonal secretion.
   b. replace the missing hormone.
   c. remove the diseased gland.
   d. withhold exogenous iodine to create a negative feedback response, which will force the gland to secrete hormones.

4. Nursing comfort measures for Connie should include:
   a. encouraging frequent periods of rest throughout the day.
   b. offering her additional blankets to help prevent chilling.
   c. using a cleansing lotion instead of soap for her skin.
   d. all of the above.

5. Health teaching for Connie includes making sure that she knows that iodine-based chemotherapy is:
   a. administered intravenously for 1 week so that her symptoms may be rapidly put into remission.
   b. needed for life.
   c. recommended for 1 to 3 months.
   d. used until her symptoms disappear.

CASE STUDY: Subtotal Thyroidectomy

Darrell, a 37-year-old father of two, has just returned to the clinical area from the recovery room. Darrell has had a subtotal thyroidectomy.

1. Postoperatively, Darrell is assisted from the stretcher to the bed. The most comfortable position for him to assume would be:
   a. high Fowler's with his neck supported by a soft collar.
   b. recumbent with his neck hyperextended and supported by a neck pillow.
   c. recumbent with sandbags preventing his neck from rotating.
   d. semi-Fowler's with his head supported by pillows.

2. Postoperative bleeding when the patient is in the dorsal position would probably be evidenced:
   a. anteriorly.
   b. laterally.
   c. posteriorly.
   d. in any of the above areas.

3. An indicator(s) of internal bleeding is(are):
   a. a sensation of fullness at the incision site.
   b. hypotension.
   c. tachycardia.
   d. all of the above.

4. The nurse should assess for the common manifestation of recurrent laryngeal nerve damage, which is:

   a. any voice change.

   b. the inability to speak.

   c. pain while speaking.

   d. pain while swallowing.

5. The nurse expects Darrell's postoperative diet to be:

   a. clear liquids, such as tea and carbonated beverages.

   b. high in calories.

   c. low in fat and protein.

   d. low in minerals, especially calcium.

6. The nurse should monitor serum calcium levels for hypocalcemia, which will occur with a serum calcium level of:

   a. 5 mg/dl.

   b. 9 mg/dl.

   c. 13 mg/dl.

   d. 17 mg/dl.

Learner's Self-Evaluation Tool for End of Unit 9 Review

1. The most important concepts or facts I have learned from this unit are:

   1. _____

   2. _____

   3. _____

2. The most important reference page numbers for test review and clinical concepts are pages:

   _____ _____ _____

   _____ _____ _____

3. The concepts or facts that I do not fully understand are:

   _____

   _____

4. I will get the answer(s) to my questions by _____

   _____

   I will do this on _____ (date and time).

5. I believe my mastery of this unit to be:

   a.   100%   Great job! Good luck!

   b.   90%   2 hours of review recommended.

   c.   80%   4 hours of review recommended.

   d.   <80%   Make an appointment with your instructor.

UNIT 10
Urinary
and Renal Function

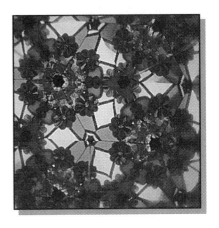

41

Assessment of Urinary and Renal Function

Chapter Overview

The urine is a valuable and readily accessible tool for indicating renal or urinary dysfunction. The nurse should always observe urine for abnormal characteristics and measure output in any patient suspected of having renal or urinary dysfunction. Patient education and preparation for invasive procedures used in diagnosing pathology should be part of any nursing care plan. Assessment includes observing for clinical manifestations of chronic as well as acute disorders in any patient suspected of having renal or urinary problems.

I. Knowledge-Based Questions

Deduction and Interpretation

Read each question carefully. Circle your answer.

1. An abnormal constituent of urine is:
   a. creatinine.
   b. glucose.
   c. potassium.
   d. urea.

2. The normal quantity of water ingested and excreted in the urine is approximately:
   a. 0.5 L/day.
   b. 1.5 L/day.
   c. 2.5 L/day.
   d. 4.0 L/day.

3. The normal amount of sodium ingested and excreted in the urine is approximately:
   a. 2 to 3 g/day.
   b. 4 to 5 g/day.
   c. 6 to 8 g/day.
   d. 9 to 10 g/day.

4. Increased blood osmolality will result in:
   a. antidiuretic hormone (ADH) stimulation.
   b. an increase in urine volume.
   c. diuresis.
   d. less reabsorption of water.

5. The nephrotic syndrome causes hypoalbuminemia, which results in:
   a. activation of the renin–angiotensin system.
   b. decreased oncotic pressure.
   c. edema.
   d. all of the above.

6. A major, sensitive indicator of kidney disease is the:
   a. blood urea nitrogen level.
   b. serum creatinine level.
   c. serum potassium level.
   d. uric acid level.

 Mary Jo Boyer: Study Guide to Accompany Brunner & Suddarth's Textbook of Medical-Surgical Nursing, 8th ed. © 1996 Lippincott-Raven Publishers

7. A major manifestation of uremia is:
   a. a decreased serum phosphorus level.
   b. hyperparathyroidism.
   c. hypocalcemia with bone changes.
   d. increased secretion of parathormone.

8. Oliguria is said to be present when urinary output is:
   a. less than 30 ml/hr.
   b. about 100 ml/hr.
   c. between 300 and 500 ml/hr.
   d. between 500 and 1000 ml/hr.

9. Significant nursing assessment data relevant to renal function should include information about:
   a. any voiding disorders.
   b. the patient's occupation.
   c. the presence of hypertension or diabetes mellitus.
   d. all of the above.

10. A 24-hour urine collection is scheduled to begin at 8:00 AM. The nurse should begin the procedure:
   a. after discarding the 8:00 AM specimen.
   b. at 8:00 AM, with or without a specimen.
   c. 6 hours after the urine is discarded.
   d. with the first specimen voided after 8:00 AM.

11. The nurse should inform a patient that preparation for intravenous pyelography includes:
   a. a liquid restriction for 8 to 10 hours before the test.
   b. clear liquids for 3 days before the test.
   c. enemas until clear.
   d. remaining NPO from midnight before the test.

12. Nursing responsibilities after renal angiography include:
   a. assessment of peripheral pulses.
   b. color and temperature comparisons between the involved and uninvolved extremities.
   c. examination of the puncture site for swelling and hematoma formation.
   d. all of the above.

13. A cystoscope allows visualization of the:
   a. bladder.
   b. ureteral orifices.
   c. urethra.
   d. above areas.

14. Nursing management after a renal biopsy includes:
   a. assessing for the clinical manifestations of hemorrhage.
   b. encouraging a fluid intake of 3 L every 24 hours.
   c. obtaining a sample of each voided urine to compare it with a prebiopsy specimen.
   d. all of the above.

Read each statement carefully and write the best response in the space provided.

   1. The functional unit of each kidney is the _____.

   2. The normal urine osmolality ranges between _____.

   3. The test that most accurately reflects glomerular filtration and renal excretory function is the _____ test.

   4. Water is reabsorbed, rather than excreted, under the control of _____.

   5. The most common, early manifestation of kidney disease is:

   _____.

II. Critical Analysis Questions

Identifying Patterns

Draw the sequence of pathophysiologic events that are triggered when the blood pressure decreases and the hormone renin is released from the cells in the kidneys.

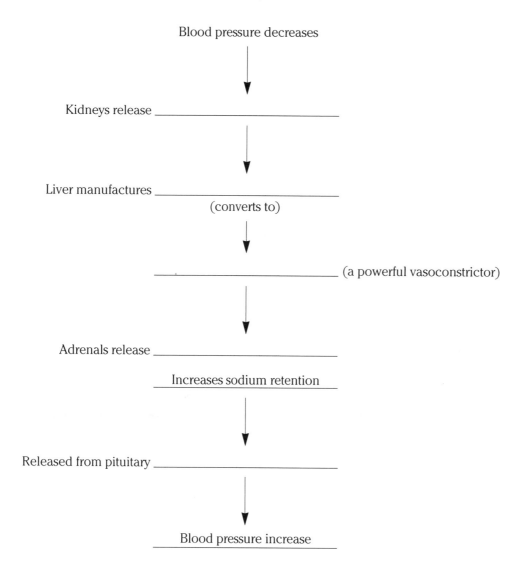

Blood pressure decreases

Kidneys release _____

Liver manufactures _____
(converts to)

_____ (a powerful vasoconstrictor)

Adrenals release _____
Increases sodium retention

Released from pituitary _____

Blood pressure increase

42

Management of Patients With Urinary and Renal Dysfunction

Chapter Overview

Renal and urinary dysfunctions range from discomfort related to urinary tract infections to toxemia and a life-threatening situation caused by renal failure. Without a renal transplant, a patient with end-stage renal disease needs to be dialyzed for the rest of his or her life.

Although dialysis can prolong life, the quality of that life can be severely compromised. A person must learn to deal with the psychosocial aspect of chronic illness and the emotional strain of dependence on a machine. Continuous ambulatory peritoneal dialysis (CAPD) allows a person to manage his or her care and have independence of movement. However, a renal transplantation is the ideal alternative for an acceptable candidate.

A major concern for patients with renal or urinary dysfunction is the multisystem alternations that result from the original pathology, in addition to the magnitude of psychosocial needs subsequent to the disorders. Other nursing concerns are nutrition, fluid and electrolyte imbalance, catheter management, medical and surgical asepsis, and infection.

I. Knowledge-Based Questions

Deduction and Interpretation

Read each question carefully. Circle your answer.

1. The most accurate indicator of fluid loss or gain in an acutely ill patient is:
   a. blood pressure.
   b. capillary refill.
   c. serum sodium levels.
   d. weight.

2. Urinary tract infections appear to be responsible for about _____ of all hospital-acquired infections.
   a. one-fifth
   b. one-quarter
   c. one-third
   d. one-half

3. A sign of a possible urinary tract infection is:
   a. a negative urine culture.
   b. an output of 200 to 900 ml with each voiding.
   c. cloudy urine.
   d. urine with a specific gravity of 1.005 to 1.022.

4. When managing a closed urinary drainage system, the nurse needs to remember *not to:*
   a. allow the drainage bag to touch the floor.
   b. disconnect the bag.
   c. raise the drainage bag above the level of the patient's bladder.
   d. do any of the above.

5. A female is taught to catheterize herself by inserting the catheter into the urethra:
   a. 1/2 to1 in.
   b. 2 in.
   c. 3 in.
   d. 5 in.

6. Nursing measures for a patient with a neurogenic bladder include:
   a. encouraging a liberal fluid intake.
   b. keeping the patient as mobile as possible.
   c. offering a diet low in calcium .
   d. all of the above.

7. The major complication of neurogenic bladder is:
   a. hypertrophy.
   b. infection.
   c. pain.
   d. spasm.

8. A spastic neurogenic bladder is associated with all of the following *except:*
   a. a loss of conscious sensation and cerebral motor control.
   b. a lower motor neuron lesion.
   c. hypertrophy of the bladder walls.
   d. reduced bladder capacity.

9. Choose the process that underlies/supports the procedure of hemodialysis.
   a. diffusion.
   b. osmosis.
   c. ultrafiltration.
   d. all of the processes.

10. An incomplete protein not recommended for the diet of a patient managed by long-term hemodialysis is that found in:
   a. eggs.
   b. fish.
   c. milk.
   d. nuts.

11. With peritoneal dialysis, urea and creatinine pass through the peritoneum by:
   a. active transport.
   b. diffusion.
   c. filtration.
   d. ultrafiltration.

12. The complete peritoneal dialysis process of removing toxic substances and body wastes takes approximately:
   a. 6 to 8 hours.
   b. 9 to 11 hours.
   c. 12 to 24 hours.
   d. 36 to 48 hours.

13. At the end of five peritoneal exchanges, the patient's fluid loss was 500 ml. This loss is equal to approximately:
   a. 0.5 lb.
   b. 1.0 lb.
   c. 1.5 lb.
   d. 2 lb.

14. The chief danger after renal surgery is:
   a. abdominal distention owing to reflex cessation of intestinal peristalsis.
   b. hypovolemic shock caused by hemorrhage.
   c. paralytic ileus caused by manipulation of the colon during surgery.
   d. pneumonia caused by shallow breathing because of severe incisional pain.

15. A nephrostomy tube is inserted to:
   a. conserve and restore tissue traumatized by obstruction.
   b. provide drainage from the kidney postoperatively.
   c. provide ureter drainage when there is an interruption of the normal drainage course.
   d. do all of the above.

Match the symptom listed in Column II with its associated fluid or electrolyte imbalance listed in Column I.

Column I

1. ___A B___ calcium deficit
2. ___b___ calcium excess
3. ___c___ fluid volume deficit
4. ___e___ fluid volume excess
5. ___D___ magnesium deficit
6. ___J___ potassium deficit
7. ___H___ potassium excess
8. _____ protein deficit
9. _____ sodium deficit G
10. _____ sodium excess

Column II

a. carpopedal spasm and tetany
b. muscle hypotonicity and flank pain
c. oliguria and weight loss
d. positive Chvostek's sign
e. crackles and dyspnea
f. chronic weight loss and fatigability
g. fingerprinting on the sternum
h. irritability and intestinal colic
i. rough, dry tongue and thirst
j. soft, flabby muscles, weakness

Read each statement carefully. Write your response in the space provided.

1. List four (4) reasons for catheterization:

1. _____
2. _____
3. _____
4. _____

2. List several pathogens responsible for catheter-associated urinary tract infections.

_____

_____

3. List several signs and symptoms associated with catheter-induced urinary tract infections.

_____

_____

4. List an "over-the-counter" antihistamine that is believed to cause urinary retention:

_____

5. The leading cause of death for patients undergoing chronic hemodialysis is:

_____

6. List seven potential complications of dialysis treatment:

1. _____   5. _____
2. _____   6. _____
3. _____   7. _____
4. _____

7. The most common and serious complication of CAPD is: _____.

8. List two complications of renal surgery that are believed to be caused by reflex paralysis of intestinal peristalsis.

_____   _____

II. Critical Analysis Questions

Recognizing Contradictions

Rewrite each statement correctly. Underline the key concept.

1. With a closed drainage system, only 10% of all patients experience bacteriuria.

2. About 2 million adults in the United States suffer from urinary incontinence.

3. Urinary incontinence afflicts about one third of all nursing home residents.

4. Hemodialysis can be used as a long-term management therapy that can reverse the progress of renal disease.

5. CAPD is a good choice for home management because the process needs to be completed only once a day.

Generating Solutions: Clinical Problem Solving

Read the following case study. Circle the correct answer.

CASE STUDY: CAPD

Edward, a 29-year-old diabetic, chose continuous ambulatory peritoneal dialysis (CAPD) as a way of managing his end-stage renal disease.

1. Edward chose CAPD because it helped him:
   a. avoid severe dietary restrictions.
   b. control his blood pressure.
   c. have control over his daily activities.
   d. do all of the above.

2. Using CAPD, Edward needs to dialyze himself:
   a. approximately three to six times a day with no night changes.
   b. every 3 hours while awake.
   c. every 4 hours around the clock.
   d. once in the morning and once in the evening every day.

3. Edward needs to be aware that toxic wastes are exchanged during the equilibration or dwell time, which usually lasts for:
   a. 10 minutes.
   b. 30 minutes.
   c. 1 hour.
   d. 2 to 3 hours.

4. Edward needs to be taught how to detect signs of the most serious and most common complication of CAPD, which is:
   a. an abdominal hernia.
   b. anorexia.
   c. edema.
   d. peritonitis.

5. Edward's diet should be modified to be:
   a. high in carbohydrates.
   b. high fats.
   c. high in protein.
   d. low in bran and fiber.

43

Management of Patients With Urinary and Renal Disorders

Chapter Overview

There are clinical manifestations common to renal and urinary disorders, as well as symptoms specific to the diagnosis (acute glomerulonephritis, cystitis, tuberculosis, urolithiasis). Nursing interventions must incorporate common approaches as well as individual adaptations.

A major renal disorder is acute renal failure (ARF), which has several causes, but one result: the sudden shutdown of renal function. ARF can be cured, or it can progress to chronic renal failure. Nursing care is directed toward managing renal dysfunction as well as those symptoms associated with the cause of the disorder.

Renal surgery (transplantation, diversion, conduit) demands expert preoperative and postoperative nursing management. Rehabilitative nursing care includes patient education about permanent catheters or collecting devices. Some communities offer support groups to patients with disorders that necessitate a major adjustment in body image and self-esteem. Nursing intervention in such circumstances includes referral and follow-up.

I. Knowledge-Based Questions

Deduction and Interpretation

Read each question carefully. Circle your answer.

1. The most common site of a urinary tract infection (UTI) is the:
   a. bladder.
   b. kidney.
   c. prostate.
   d. urethra.

2. There is an increased risk of urinary tract infections in the presence of:
   a. altered metabolic states.
   b. immunosuppression.
   c. urethral mucosa abrasion.
   d. all of the above.

3. The most common organism responsible for UTIs in the elderly is:
   a. *Klebsiella.*
   b. *Escherichia coli.*
   c. *Proteus.*
   d. *Pseudomonas.*

4. Health information for a female patient diagnosed as having cystitis includes all of the following *except:*
   a. cleanse around the perineum and urethral meatus (from front to back) after each bowel movement.
   b. drink liberal amounts of fluid.
   c. shower rather than bathe in a tub.
   d. void no more frequently than every 6 hours to allow urine to dilute the bacteria in the bladder.

5. Choose the *incorrect* statement about interstitial cystitis. It is:

a. associated with pain in the abdomen and perineum.

b. characterized by severe voiding symptoms.

c. seen in women between 40 and 50.

d. caused by *Escherichia coli*.

6. Complications of chronic pyelonephritis include:

a. end-stage renal disease.

b. hypertension.

c. kidney stone formation.

d. all of the above.

7. Tuberculosis of the lower genitourinary tract is always:

a. localized, rather than a systemic disease.

b. a primary infection.

c. secondary to renal tuberculosis.

d. subsequent to pulmonary tuberculosis.

8. *Acute glomerulonephritis* refers to a group of kidney diseases in which there is:

a. an inflammatory reaction.

b. an antigen–antibody reaction to streptococci that results in circulating molecular complexes.

c. cellular complexes that lodge in the glomeruli and injure the kidney.

d. a combination of all of the above.

9. In most cases, the major stimulus to acute glomerulonephritis is:

a. *Escherichia coli*.

b. group A streptococcal infection of the throat.

c. *Staphylococcus aureus*.

d. *Neisseria gonorrhoeae*.

10. Laboratory findings consistent with acute glomerulonephritis include all of the following *except:*

a. hematuria.

b. polyuria.

c. proteinuria.

d. white cell casts.

11. Chronic glomerulonephritis is manifested by:

a. anemia secondary to erythropoiesis.

b. hypercalcemia and decreased serum phosphorus.

c. hypokalemia and elevated bicarbonate.

d. metabolic alkalosis.

12. The major manifestation of nephrotic syndrome is:

a. hematuria.

b. hyperalbuminemia.

c. edema.

d. anemia.

13. Oliguria is a clinical sign of acute renal failure that refers to a daily urine output of:

a. 1.5 L.

b. 1.0 L.

c. less than 0.5 L.

d. less than 50 ml.

14. Hyperkalemia is a serious electrolyte imbalance that occurs in acute renal failure (ARF) and results from:

a. dietary intake.

b. electrolyte shifts in response to metabolic acidosis.

c. tissue breakdown.

d. all of the above.

15. A patient in ARF and negative nitrogen balance is expected to lose:

a. 0.5 kg/day.

b. 1.0 kg/day.

c. 1.5 kg/day.

d. 2 kg/day.

16. Potassium intake can be restricted by eliminating high-potassium foods, such as:

a. butter.

b. citrus fruits.

c. cooked white rice.

d. salad oils.

17. In chronic renal failure (end-stage renal disease), decreased glomerular filtration leads to:

a. increased pH.

b. decreased end products of protein catabolism.

c. increased serum phosphate levels.

d. all of the above.

18. Dietary intervention for renal deterioration includes limiting the intake of:

a. fluid.

b. protein.

c. sodium and potassium.

d. all of the above.

19. Recent research about the long-term toxicity of aluminum products had led physicians to recommend antacids that lower serum phosphorus such as:
a. calcium carbonate.
b. sodium bicarbonate.
c. magaldrate.
d. milk of magnesia.

20. Preoperative management for a patient who is to undergo kidney transplantation includes:
a. bringing the metabolic state to as normal a level as possible.
b. making certain that the patient is free of infection.
c. suppressing immunologic defense mechanisms.
d. all of the above.

21. Postoperative management for a recipient of a transplanted kidney includes:
a. aseptic technique to avoid infection.
b. hourly urinary outputs to estimate the degree of kidney function.
c. protective isolation while immunosuppressive drug therapy is at its maximum dosage.
d. all of the above.

22. A major clinical manifestation of renal stones is:
a. dysuria.
b. hematuria.
c. infection.
d. pain.

23. Patients with urolithiasis need to be encouraged to:
a. increase their fluid intake so they can excrete 3000 to 4000 ml every day, to prevent additional stone formation.
b. participate in strenuous exercises so that the tone of smooth muscle in the urinary tract can be strengthened to help propel calculi.
c. supplement their diet with calcium needed to replace losses to renal calculi.
d. limit their voiding to every 6 to 8 hours so that increased volume can increase hydrostatic pressure, which will help push stones along the urinary system.

24. A patient being managed on a diet moderately reduced in calcium and phosphorus should be taught to avoid:
a. citrus fruits.
b. milk.
c. pasta.
d. whole grain breads.

25. An early indicator of a renal tumor is:
a. a palpable mass.
b. painless hematuria.
c. localized tenderness.
d. renal colic.

26. The most common symptom of cancer of the bladder is:
a. back pain.
b. dysuria.
c. gross painless hematuria.
d. infection.

27. The most effective intravesical agent for recurrent bladder cancer is:
a. bacille Calmette-Guerin (BCG).
b. doxorubicin.
c. etoglucid.
d. thiotepa.

28. The urinary diversion whereby the patient will void from his rectum for the rest of his life is known as a:
a. cutaneous ureterostomy.
b. nephrostomy.
c. suprapubic cystotomy.
d. ureterosigmoidostomy.

Read each statement carefully. Write your response in the space provided.

1. Name the most common organism responsible for UTIs in women.

_____

2. Name common symptoms associated with UTI (cystitis).

_____

_____

3. List the six clinical manifestations of acute pyelonephritis.

1. _____ 4. _____

2. _____ 5. _____

3. _____ 6. _____

4. Describe the physical appearance of the urine early in the stage of acute glomerulonephritis.

_____

5. Name four physiologic disorders with which the nephrotic syndrome is associated.

_____

6. List five conditions that reduce blood flow to the kidneys and impair kidney function.

_____

_____

7. List several clinical manifestations seen in patients with chronic renal failure.

_____

_____

8. Name several signs or symptoms seen in patients with threatened kidney transplant rejection.

_____

_____

9. List three crystalline substances known to form stones in the urinary tract.

_____

_____

10. Identify seven complications that may occur following an ileal conduit.

_____

_____

II. Critical Analysis Questions

Generating Solutions: Clinical Problem Solving

Read the following case study. Circle the correct answer.

CASE STUDY: Acute Renal Failure

Fran is hospitalized with a diagnosis of acute renal failure (ARF). She had been taking gentamicin sulfate for a pseudomonal infection.

1. The nurse knows that the kidney is susceptible to damage by potent antimicrobials because it functions as a major excretory pathway and receives _____ of cardiac output at rest.
a. 5% c. 25%
b. 15% d. 45%

2. The nurse needs to assess for a symptom(s) consistent with pathology secondary to reduced renal blood flow. A symptom(s) would be:
a. reduced glomerular filtration. c. tubular damage.
b. renal ischemia. d. all of the above.

3. During the oliguric phase of ARF, Fran's protein intake for her 156 lb should be approximately:
   a. 35 g/24 hr.
   c. 120 g/24 hr.
   b. 70 g/24 hr.
   d. 156 g/24 hr.

4. While evaluating laboratory studies, the nurse expects that Fran's oliguric phase will be marked by all of the following *except:*
   a. blood urea nitrogen of 10 mg/dl.
   c. serum potassium of 6 mEq/L.
   b. serum creatinine of 0.8 mg/dl.
   d. urinary volume less than 600 ml/24 hr.

5. The nurse expects a period of diuresis to follow a period of oliguria in approximately:
   a. 24 to 48 hours.
   c. 10 days.
   b. 1 week.
   d. 3 to 6 weeks.

6. After the diuretic phase the nurse should recommend a:
   a. high-potassium diet.
   c. low-carbohydrate diet.
   b. high-protein diet.
   d. low-fat diet.

Learner's Self-Evaluation Tool for End of Unit 10 Review

1. The most important concepts or facts I have learned from this unit are:

   1. _____

   2. _____

   3. _____

2. The most important reference page numbers for test review and clinical concepts are pages:

   _____   _____   _____

   _____   _____   _____

3. The concepts or facts that I do not fully understand are:

   _____

   _____

4. I will get the answer(s) to my questions by _____

   _____

   I will do this on _____ (date and time).

5. I believe my mastery of this unit to be:
   a.   100%   Great job! Good luck!
   b.   90%   2 hours of review recommended.
   c.   80%   4 hours of review recommended.
   d.   <80%   Make an appointment with your instructor.

UNIT 11
Reproductive Function

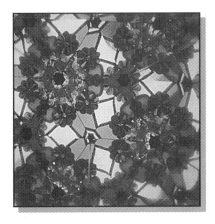

44

Assessment and Management of Patients With Problems Related to Female Physiologic Processes

Chapter Overview

Nursing intervention during the reproductive cycle includes patient education about individual promotion of health, impending signs of illness, self-examination of the breast, conception and birth control, prenatal care or pregnancy termination, nutrition for postmenopausal women, and hormonal pharmacotherapy.

A nurse should also support community efforts that encourage health care during the childbearing years by participating in seminars and functioning as a resource person.

I. Knowledge-Based Questions

Deduction and Interpretation

Read each question carefully. Circle your answer.

1. A neighbor tells you that she has had vaginal bleeding for the past several days. She is postmenopausal and has not had a menstrual period for the past 4 years. You tell her to:
   a. see her gynecologist or physician as soon as possible.
   b. mention the bleeding episode to her physician at her next appointment.
   c. disregard this bleeding episode because it is probably normal.
   d. use a birth control method because she may be fertile with her next ovulation.

2. The results of a patient's cytologic test for cancer (Pap test) were interpreted as class II. The nurse explains that a class II finding indicates:
   a. atypical cytology with no evidence of malignancy.
   b. malignancy.
   c. suggestive but not conclusive malignancy.
   d. the absence of atypical or abnormal cells.

3. Newer classifications are being used to describe the findings of the cytologic smear. For example, a *high-grade, squamous, intraepithelial lesion* corresponds to type:
   a. I.
   b. II.
   c. III.
   d. IV.

4. After a cervical biopsy the patient needs to be instructed to:
   a. leave the packing in place for 8 to 24 hours.
   b. report any excess bleeding.
   c. delay sexual intercourse for 1 week.
   d. do all of the above.

5. For vaginal irritations, the nozzle of the applicator should be inserted into the vagina for a distance of:
   a. 1.0 cm.
   b. 2.5 cm.
   c. 5.0 cm.
   d. 7.5 cm.

6. The secretion of progesterone and estrogen is highest during the phase of the menstrual cycle known as:
   a. follicular.
   b. luteal.
   c. ovulation.
   d. premenstrual.

7. In educating a patient with PMS (premenstrual syndrome) about changing her dietary practices, you would recommend that she increase her intake of:
   a. magnesium.
   b. vitamin D.
   c. iron.
   d. zinc.

8. Excessive bleeding at the time of the regular menstrual flow is referred to as:
   a. dysmenorrhea.
   b. amenorrhea.
   c. menorrhagia.
   d. metorrhagia.

9. A middle-aged woman experiencing dyspareunia can use _____ to diminish the discomfort.
   a. ibuprofen
   b. petroleum jelly
   c. K-Y jelly
   d. aspirin

10. A nutritional recommendation for postmenopausal women would be dietary increase in:
   a. calcium.
   b. iron.
   c. salt.
   d. vitamin K.

11. The most common side effect of the new implantable contraceptive (Norplant) is:
   a. breast cancer.
   b. irregular bleeding.
   c. thrombophlebitis.
   d. upper arm pain at insertion site.

12. Statistically, use of the calendar rhythm method as a means of contraception yields a pregnancy rate of:
   a. less than 10%.
   b. between 10% and 20%.
   c. about 40%.
   d. about 80%.

13. The most frequently occurring factor in infertility is:
   a. endometriosis.
   b. ovulatory failure.
   c. tubal damage.
   d. unexplained reasons.

14. In an ectopic pregnancy, the fallopian tube will rupture about _____ weeks after conception.
   a. 2 to 4
   b. 4 to 6
   c. 6 to 8
   d. 8 to 10

15. The incidence of recurrence of an ectopic pregnancy is:
   a. 5%.
   b. 10%.
   c. 20%.
   d. 40%.

Read each statement carefully. Write your response in the space provided.

1. List seven danger signals that any woman should report to a health care professional.

   1. _____   5. _____

   2. _____   6. _____

   3. _____   7. _____

   4. _____

2. The most accurate outpatient procedure for evaluating a woman for endometrial cancer is

_____

3. List eight major symptoms a woman with premenstrual syndrome (PMS) may experience:

1. _____   5. _____

2. _____   6. _____

3. _____   7. _____

4. _____   8. _____

4. Identify the normal range in years during which menopause usually begins.

_____

5. Describe the physiologic basis for "the pill" as a contraceptive.

_____

_____

6. Identify some risk factors that would absolutely contraindicate the use of oral contraceptives.

_____

_____

_____

7. Explain how the injection of Depo-Provera works.

_____

8. Name two investigational conception controls.

_____

9. Describe the use of laminaria tents in therapeutic abortions.

_____

_____

10. List four reproductive structures that are considered basic to infertility in women.

_____

11. Describe in vitro fertilization. _____

_____

_____

II. Critical Analysis Questions

Recognizing Contradictions

Rewrite each statement correctly. Underline the key concepts.

1. When conducting a health assessment, the nurse knows that about 10% of women have been victims of incest.

2. Women born to mothers who took diethylstilbestrol (DES) during their pregnancy have a higher than average chance of suffering miscarriage.

3. A cervical cone biopsy may be done without anesthesia because the cervix is less sensitive to pain.

4. Magnetic resonance imaging (MRI) exposes the patient to radiation and is more expensive than other pelvic diagnostic aids.

5. Estrogen prepares the uterus for implantation of the fertilized ovum.

6. Progesterone can cause painful cramps during ovulation because it causes myometrial contractility and arteriolar vasospasm.

7. More than 1 million yearly pregnancies in the United States are unintended.

8. An aborted fetus, not viable before the seventh month, usually weighs less than 500 g.

9. A bilateral vasectomy will interfere with the sexual potency of the male.

10. Infertility almost always follows an ectopic pregnancy.

45

Management of Patients With Disorders of the Female Reproductive System

Chapter Overview

Nursing management of patients with gynecologic disorders involves an awareness of the sensitivity of such patients. In the United States, society places such an exaggerated emphasis on female beauty and sexuality based on physical appearance that any threat to a woman's sexual image makes her anxious and fearful. Because sexual discussions are not considered proper in some cultures, nurses need to encourage patients to verbalize their fears and discomforts. Empathy, optimism, and a supportive attitude are needed in caring for patients with gynecologic disorders.

I. Knowledge-Based Questions

Deduction and Interpretation

Read each question carefully. Circle your answer.

1. Conditions that increase the chances of a woman developing candidiasis include:
   a. pregnancy.
   b. diabetes mellitus.
   c. antibiotic therapy.
   d. all of the above.

2. Metronidazole (Flagyl) is the recommended treatment for a vaginal infection caused by:
   a. *Candida albicans.*
   b. *Escherichia coli.*
   c. *Streptococcus.*
   d. *Trichomonas vaginalis.*

3. Nursing interventions for the relief of pain and discomfort for a woman with a vulvovaginal infection include:
   a. warm perineal irrigations.
   b. sitz baths.
   c. cornstarch for chafed inner thighs.
   d. all of the above.

4. To prevent the occurrence of toxic shock syndrome, women should be advised to do all of the following *except:*
   a. avoid the use of superabsorbent tampons.
   b. change tampons frequently.
   c. avoid the use of diaphragms.
   d. alternate the use of tampons with sanitary pads.

5. The bacterium responsible for mucopurulent cervicitis is:
   a. chlamydia.
   b. gonorrhea.
   c. staphylococcus.
   d. pseudomonas.

6. Mrs. Jakes has had a pessary inserted for long-term treatment of a prolapsed uterus. As part of your teaching plan, you would advise Mrs. Jakes to:
   a. see her gynecologist to remove and clean the pessary at regular intervals.
   b. keep the insertion site clean and dry.
   c. avoid sexual intercourse.
   d. avoid climbing stairs as much as possible.

7. Mrs. Schurman, who has been diagnosed as having endometriosis, asks for an explanation of the disease. The *best* response for the nurse is to explain that:
   a. she has developed an infection in the lining of her uterus.
   b. tissue from the lining of the uterus has implanted in areas outside the uterus.
   c. the lining of the uterus is thicker than usual, causing heavy bleeding and cramping.
   d. the lining of the uterus is too thin because endometrial tissue has implanted outside the uterus.

8. The highest frequency of endometriosis is found in the:
   a. cervix.
   b. cul-de-sac.
   c. ovaries.
   d. ureterovesical peritoneum.

9. Mrs. Schurman's treatment involves taking danazol (Danocrine), 200 mg po, for 9 months. Danazol is a(n):
   a. gonadotropin that decreases ovarian and pituitary stimulation.
   b. antigonadotropin that increases pituitary stimulation and decreases ovarian stimulation.
   c. gonadotropin that decreases pituitary stimulation and increases ovarian stimulation.
   d. antigonadotropin that decreases pituitary and ovarian stimulation.

10. A risk factor(s) commonly associated with cancer of the cervix is(are):
    a. early childbearing.
    b. exposure to DES in utero.
    c. multiple sexual partners.
    d. all of the above.

11. By incidence, cervical cancer is the _____ most common female reproductive cancer.
    a. first
    b. second
    c. third
    d. fourth

12. The two chief symptoms of early carcinoma of the cervix are:
    a. leukoplakia and metrorrhagia.
    b. dyspareunia and foul-smelling vaginal discharge.
    c. "strawberry" spots and menorrhagia.
    d. leukorrhea and irregular vaginal bleeding or spotting.

13. Using the International Classification of Carcinoma of the Uterine Cervix, a stage II Pap smear result indicates:
    a. cancer *in situ.*
    b. vaginal invasion.
    c. pelvic wall invasion.
    d. bladder extension.

14. A postmenopausal woman who has irregular uterine or vaginal bleeding should be encouraged by a nurse to:
    a. stop taking her Premarin (hormonal therapy).
    b. see her gynecologist as soon as possible.
    c. disregard this phenomenon because it is common during this life stage.
    d. mention it to her physician during her next annual examination.

15. Cancer of the uterus, the most common pelvic neoplasm in women, ranks _____ among cancer for women.
    a. first
    b. second
    c. third
    d. fourth

16. Women who experience postmenopausal bleeding have a _____ % chance of developing cancer of the uterus.
    a. 10
    b. 20
    c. 35
    d. 75

17. The most common symptom of cancer of the vulva is:
    a. a foul-smelling discharge.
    b. bleeding.
    c. pain.
    d. pruritus.

18. The primary treatment for vulvar malignancy is:
   a. chemotherapy creams.
   b. laser vaporization.
   c. radiation.
   d. wide excision.

19. Postoperative nursing care for a simple vulvectomy should include:
   a. cleansing the wound daily.
   b. offering a low-residue diet.
   c. positioning the patient with pillows.
   d. all of the above.

20. Ovarian cancer is the _____ most common cause of cancer deaths in women.
   a. second
   b. third
   c. fourth
   d. fifth

21. A diagnosis of ovarian cancer, stage III indicates that growth involves:
   a. only the ovaries.
   b. the ovaries with pelvic extension.
   c. metastases outside the pelvis.
   d. distant metastases.

22. Radiation therapy is the treatment of choice for:
   a. ovarian cancer.
   b. squamous cell carcinoma of the cervix.
   c. uterine carcinoma.
   d. vaginal wall cancer.

23. A medical measure(s) to modify possible side effects of external radiation beam therapy is(are):
   a. maintaining fluid intake to prevent cystitis and dysuria.
   b. restricting fiber and roughage to decrease the effects of a possible enteritis.
   c. using antispasmodic drugs.
   d. all of the above.

Complete the following scramblegram by circling the word(s) that answer each statement below. Terms may be written in any direction.

A	E	E	T	D	A	C	Y	C	L	O	V	I	R
H	L	B	K	E	M	O	M	C	M	U	R	S	C
C	E	D	H	R	A	L	Y	T	L	K	L	P	H
V	C	P	A	M	D	E	C	V	Y	L	M	R	A
P	O	A	L	O	N	G	O	S	G	B	E	O	D
B	T	P	U	I	M	D	S	C	A	R	N	L	S
Y	S	S	T	D	Y	L	T	N	L	I	O	A	M
M	Y	M	S	N	M	F	A	B	F	L	R	P	Y
O	C	E	I	R	A	C	T	G	O	T	R	S	T
T	R	A	F	O	S	F	I	Y	E	B	H	E	I
C	E	R	T	S	C	I	N	O	J	K	A	L	R
E	W	D	R	B	D	B	E	P	I	S	G	C	A
R	B	G	B	F	C	R	A	R	M	D	I	B	P
E	R	C	L	M	D	O	I	O	E	S	A	N	I
T	D	S	E	P	T	I	C	S	H	O	C	K	L
S	H	E	R	M	H	D	R	J	J	A	T	H	L
Y	B	A	G	A	C	S	Y	A	S	B	O	L	U
H	B	H	M	D	M	T	P	C	K	T	I	D	N

Definition of Terms

1. Intense burning and inflammation of the vulva.
2. A preferred treatment for candidiasis.
3. The recommended treatment for trichomoniasis.
4. The drug of choice for herpes genitalis.
5. A potential complication of toxic shock syndrome.
6. The downward displacement of the bladder toward the vaginal orifice.
7. This test is used for diagnosis of cervical cancer.
8. Term used to describe the surgical procedure where the uterus, cervix, and ovaries are removed.
9. A term to describe vaginal bleeding.
10. Another name for benign tumors of the uterus.
11. In utero exposure to this drug increases the incidence of vaginal cancer.
12. A risk factor for uterine cancer.
13. Exercises that strengthen the pelvic muscles.
14. An opening between two hollow organs.
15. Displacement of the uterus into the vaginal canal.
16. Cysts that arise from parts of the ovum.

II. Critical Analysis Questions

Generating Solutions: Clinical Problem Solving

Read the following case study. Circle the correct answer.

CASE STUDY: Vaginal Discharge

Maryanne, a 19-year-old college student, has recently noticed increased vaginal discharge.

1. After examination the nurse prepares a wet mount (vaginal smear). When potassium hydroxide solution is added to the smear, a fishy odor is noted. Maryanne probably has a nonspecific vaginitis known as:
   a. bacterial vaginosis.
   b. candidiasis.
   c. trichomoniasis.
   d. atropic vaginitis.

2. A characteristic symptom of bacterial vaginosis is:
   a. a scanty to minimal discharge.
   b. a fishlike odor.
   c. painful menstruation
   d. a greenish discharge between periods.

3. Metronidazole is prescribed, to be taken twice a day for 1 week. While taking this medication Maryanne should be instructed to:
   a. avoid dairy products.
   b. avoid sunlight.
   c. avoid alcohol.
   d. lie down flat for at least 30 minutes after inserting the medication.

4. If Maryanne's vaginal infection recurs, the nurse should recommend that:
   a. her sexual partner be tested and treated.
   b. she refrain from sexual intercourse.
   c. she avoid the use of tampons.
   d. she take only showers for a while, no tub baths.

5. An appropriate nursing diagnosis for Maryanne is:
   a. altered comfort: pain and discomfort related to burning or itching from the infectious process.
   b. self-care deficit related to inability to perform activities of daily living.
   c. altered comfort related to gardnerella-associated vaginitis.
   d. altered comfort related to candidiasis.

CASE STUDY: Toxic Shock Syndrome

Irene, a 23-year-old woman, is admitted to the emergency department in shock with an elevated temperature. She is diagnosed as having toxic shock syndrome (TSS).

1. The nurse knows that toxic shock syndrome is a bacterial infection associated with the use of tampons. The bacterial toxin is believed to be:
   a. *Escherichia coli.*
   b. *Haemophilus influenzae.*
   c. *Staphylococcus aureus.*
   d. *Pseudomonas aeruginosa.*

2. The onset of TSS is characterized by the sudden appearance of:
   a. an elevated fever (up to 102° F).
   b. a red, macular rash.
   c. myalgia and dizziness.
   d. uncontrolled hypotension.

3. Signs associated with toxic shock syndrome include all of the following *except:*
   a. an elevated blood urea nitrogen level.
   b. a decreased bilirubin level.
   c. leukocytosis.
   d. oliguria.

4. Diagnostic evaluation is made from examination of cultures from the:
   a. blood and urine.
   b. cervix.
   c. vagina.
   d. all of the above areas.

5. A priority of medical management is:
   a. alleviating respiratory distress.
   b. treating the shock.
   c. controlling the infection.
   d. managing the emotional distress.

CASE STUDY: Intracavitary Irradiation

Jill is 57 years old and is being treated with intracavitary irradiation. A nurse is assigned to care for Jill immediately after her "afterloading" of the radioactive material.

1. Jill asks how long the applicator will be in place. The nurse tells her that the application of radiation usually lasts for:
   a. 6 to 12 hours.
   b. 12 to 20 hours.
   c. 1 to 3 days.
   d. 1 week.

2. While caring for Jill, the nurse needs to remember that her total exposure to radiation must not exceed:
   a. 30 minutes.
   b. 60 minutes.
   c. 2 hours.
   d. 4 hours.

3. While in bed, Jill needs to be encouraged to:
   a. cough and breathe deeply.
   b. perform isometric exercises with her lower extremities.
   c. turn frequently from side to side.
   d. do all of the above.

46

Assessment and Management of Patients With Breast Disorders

Chapter Overview

Few things can be more traumatic to a woman than loss of a breast. Because society associates the breast with femininity and sexuality, loss of that tissue can be emotionally devastating. When developing a care plan for a patient who has had a mastectomy, the nurse needs to consider the woman's age, marital status, support systems, and mental attitude toward her breasts. These variables will significantly influence the direction of psychosocial care and nursing interventions.

I. Knowledge-Based Questions

Deduction and Interpretation

Read each question carefully. Circle your answer.

1. The optimal time for breast self-examination is usually beginning at the _____ day after menses.
   a. third
   b. fifth
   c. seventh
   d. tenth

2. The average percentage of women who perform self-breast examination is believed to be about:
   a. 15%.
   b. 25%.
   c. 40%.
   d. 80%.

3. Mammography can diagnose breast cancer before it is clinically palpable, meaning that the lump can be detected by x-ray when it is approximately:
   a. 1 cm in size.
   b. 1 mm in size.
   c. 2 cm in size.
   d. 1 m in size.

4. As part of health teaching, the nurse needs to alert patients that mammography can yield a false-negative result in _____ instances out of 100.
   a. 5 to 10
   b. 10 to 15
   c. 15 to 20
   d. 20 to 25

5. Mammography should be used to screen women annually:
   a. under age 35.
   b. between the ages of 35 and 40.
   c. from 40 to 50 years.
   d. over age 50.

 Mary Jo Boyer: Study Guide to Accompany Brunner & Suddarth's Textbook of Medical-Surgical Nursing, 8th ed. © 1996 Lippincott-Raven Publishers

6. Breast cancer is the leading cause of death for women:
 a. between 25 and 35.
 b. between 35 and 50.
 c. between 50 and 60.
 d. older than 60 years of age.

7. Characteristics of the lumps present in cystic disease of the breasts include all of the following *except:*
 a. a rapid increase and decrease in size.
 b. increased tenderness before menstruation.
 c. a painless or tender lump.
 d. skin dimpling and nipple retraction.

8. The risk of developing breast cancer is now one (1) woman out of _____.
 a. 8
 b. 20
 c. 35
 d. 50

9. The current 5-year survival rate is _____%.
 a. 50
 b. 70
 c. 85
 d. 93

10. The *strongest factor(s)* that influence the incidence of breast cancer is(are):
 a. chemical elements.
 b. environmental pollution.
 c. genetic predisposition.
 d. the number of menstrual cycles.

11. The chance of developing breast cancer doubles if:
 a. a woman has her first child after age 30.
 b. a woman's mother had breast cancer.
 c. the woman was exposed to radiation after puberty.
 d. all of the above are true.

12. The majority of breast cancers occur in the:
 a. upper, inner quadrant.
 b. lower, inner quadrant.
 c. upper, outer quadrant.
 d. lower, outer quadrant.

13. Early clinical manifestations of breast carcinoma include all of the following *except:*
 a. a nontender lump.
 b. asymmetry of the breasts.
 c. nipple retraction.
 d. pain in the breast tissue.

14. A noninvasive breast tumor between 2 cm and 5 cm is classified as a stage _____.
 a. I
 b. II
 c. III
 d. IV

15. Carcinoma of the breast results from a cell doubling. A cell that doubles every 60 days would become palpable after:
 a. 3 years.
 b. 5 years.
 c. 10 years.
 d. 15 years.

16. At diagnosis of breast carcinoma, the presence of metastasis is about:
 a. 25%.
 b. 45%.
 c. 65%.
 d. 85%.

17. The most common site of distant metastasis for breast carcinoma is the:
 a. adrenals.
 b. bone.
 c. lungs.
 d. liver.

18. A patient is scheduled for removal of her left breast and the axillary lymph nodes; the pectoralis minor muscle is to be left in place. This surgical intervention is called a(n):
 a. extended radical mastectomy.
 b. modified radical mastectomy.
 c. quadrantectomy.
 d. simple mastectomy.

19. The treatment of choice for cancer of the breast for lesions 4cm or smaller is:
 a. axillary node dissection.
 b. cobalt therapy to the remainder of the breast.
 c. lumpectomy.
 d. a combination of all three procedures.

20. The most common hormonal method of intervention is the use of:
   a. Cytodren.
   b. DES.
   c. Megace.
   d. Tamoxifen.

21. Suggested postoperative positioning of the affected arm following surgical intervention (mastectomy) is:
   a. abduction to promote incisional healing.
   b. adduction to minimize trauma to sensitive tissue.
   c. elevation to promote lumphatic drainage.
   d. extension to facilitate isometric exercises.

22. Postoperative arm exercises facilitate the development of collateral circulation, which decreases lymphedema. Collateral circulation is usually developed within:
   a. 1 month.
   b. 3 months.
   c. 5 months.
   d. 8 to 10 months.

23. A patient with lymphedema in an arm should be advised to avoid:
   a. blood pressure assessments in that arm.
   b. injections or needles in that arm.
   c. prolonged exposure of that arm to sunlight.
   d. all of the above.

24. The usual criterion used for selecting patients for breast reconstruction is:
   a. waiting for 6 months after a mastectomy or 2 to 5 years after completion of chemotherapy or radiotherapy.
   b. consideration of how much tissue was removed from the area during the mastectomy.
   c. the patient's age.
   d. the patient's potential for future development of breast cancer.

25. The most commonly encountered breast condition in the male is:
   a. breast cancer.
   b. mastitis.
   c. gynecomastia.
   d. cystic breast disease.

II. Critical Analysis Questions

Generating Solutions: Clinical Problem Solving

Read the following case study. Circle the correct answers.

CASE STUDY: Simple Mastectomy

Louise is 53 years old and single. The biopsy findings indicate that she has a malignancy in her breast. She is scheduled for a simple mastectomy.

1. Based on her knowledge about the cause of breast cancer, the nurse knows that the highest incidence of this type of cancer is found:
   a. among those who give birth to their first child after age 35.
   b. among those who have had multiple pregnancies.
   c. in the unmarried woman who has not had children.
   d. in the woman who has menopause after age 50.

2. On examination, Louise's tumor is found in the anatomic area where tumors usually develop, the:
   a. medial half of the breast.
   b. nipple area.
   c. posterior segment, inferior to the nipple.
   d. upper outer quadrant.

3. Louise is advised that if she chooses not to seek treatment, her life expectancy will be:
   a. less than 1 year.
   b. between 2 and 3 years.
   c. about 5 years.
   d. as long as 10 years.

4. The nurse can advise Louise that surgical management for her stage I cancer has a cure rate of:
   a. 30%.
   b. 50%.
   c. 80%.
   d. 100%.

Postoperatively, Louise returns to the clinical area and is alert and aware of her surroundings. She experiences moderate pain for the first 72 hours.

5. Postoperative care of the incision includes all of the following *except:*
   a. applying cocoa butter to increase elasticity.
   b. drying the area with slight friction to stimulate the circulation.
   c. gently bathing the area with a nonabrasive soap.
   d. massaging the area.

6. Louise's affected arm should be elevated on a pillow so that her:
   a. entire arm is in a horizontal plane.
   b. forearm is level with her heart.
   c. wrist is higher than her elbow, which should be higher than her shoulder.
   d. wrist is lower than her elbow so that circulation to her hand will not be decreased.

7. The nurse expects that Louise will be allowed out of bed in:
   a. 1 to 2 days.
   b. about 5 days.
   c. about 1 week.
   d. 1 to 2 weeks.

Identifying Patterns

Six figures of a woman performing breast self-examination follow. Start with the first figure and explain the activity associated with each step.

FIGURE 1

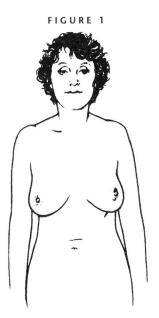

FIGURE 2

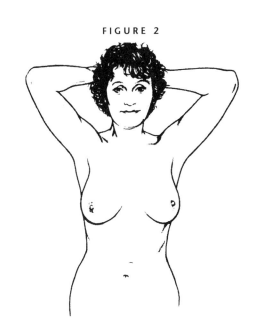

1. _____

2. _____

3. _____

1. _____

FIGURE 3

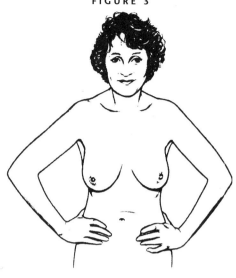

1. _____

FIGURE 4

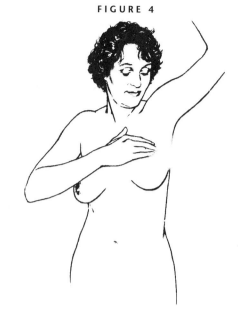

1. _____
2. _____
3. _____
4. _____
5. _____
6. _____

FIGURE 5

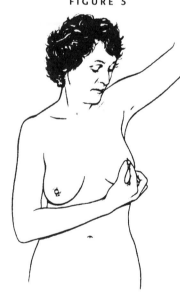

1. _____
2. _____

FIGURE 6

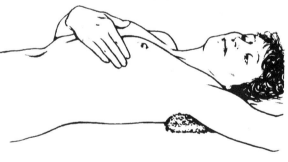

1. _____
2. _____
3. _____

47

Assessment and Management of Patients With Disorders of the Male Reproductive System

Chapter Overview

Nursing care for a male patient with a reproductive system disorder requires sensitivity to the patient's need for privacy and an awareness of society's tendency to correlate maleness with sexuality. Nursing care can be effective and positive if concern for body image and self-esteem is maintained.

Nurses need to be aware that sometimes the patient's psychosocial needs may have priority over his physiologic needs.

I. Knowledge-Based Questions

Deduction and Interpretation

Read each question carefully. Circle your answer.

1. Enlargement of the prostate gland, benign prostatic hyperplasia, is usually associated with:
   a. dysuria.
   b. dilation of the ureters.
   c. hydronephrosis.
   d. all of the above.

2. Health education for a patient with prostatitis includes all of the following *except:*
   a. avoiding drinks that increase prostatic secretions.
   b. forcing fluids to prevent urine from backing up and distending the bladder.
   c. taking several hot sitz baths daily.
   d. using antibiotic therapy for 10 to 14 days.

3. The closed procedure used for a prostatectomy is a(an) _____ approach.
   a. perineal
   b. suprapubic
   c. retropubic
   d. transurethral

4. The prostatectomy approach that is associated with a high incidence of impotency is:
   a. perineal.
   b. retropubic.
   c. suprapubic.
   d. transurethral.

5. Patients undergoing open surgical removal of the prostate seem to experience a high incidence of:
a. paralytic ileus.
b. pneumonia.
c. pulmonary embolism.
d. all of the above.

6. In most instances, patients can be advised that sexual activity can resume, postprostatectomy, in about:
a. 4 weeks.
b. 2 months.
c. 10 weeks.
d. after 4 months.

7. An expected postoperative outcome of prostatectomy is light pink urine within:
a. 24 hours.
b. 48 hours.
c. 3 days.
d. 1 week.

8. During the 2 months it take for the prostatic fossa to heal, the patient is advised not to:
a. engage in strenuous exercise.
b. perform the Valsalva maneuver.
c. take long automobile rides.
d. do all of the above.

9. As a cause of death in American men over age 55, cancer of the prostate ranks:
a. first.
b. second.
c. third.
d. fourth.

10. Prostatic cancer commonly metastasizes to the:
a. bone.
b. liver.
c. lungs.
d. brain.

11. The concentration of prostate-specific antigen (PSA) is proportional to the total prostatic mass. As a diagnostic tool, PSA would indicate all of the following *except:*
a. local progression of the disease.
b. patient responsiveness to cancer therapy.
c. recurrence of prostate cancer.
d. the presence of malignancy.

12. The life expectancy following a radical prostatectomy is about _____ years.
a. 3
b. 6
c. 10
d. > 15

13. In the 20- to 35-year-old age group, testicular cancer as a cause of death ranks:
a. first.
b. second.
c. third.
d. fourth.

14. Retroperitoneal lymphadenectomy after orchiectomy would probably lead to:
a. altered libido.
b. inability to have orgasm.
c. infertility.
d. all of the above.

15. One cause of infertility in men is a:
a. hydrocele.
b. varicocele.
c. paraphimosis.
d. phimosis.

16. Neonatal circumcision is an important protective measure against carcinoma of the:
a. penis.
b. testes.
c. scrotum.
d. urethra.

17. All of the following are true of priapism *except* that it:
a. is a urologic emergency.
b. may result in gangrene.
c. is painless.
d. may result in impotence.

Read each statement carefully. Write your response in the space provided.

1. Name two specific tests used to diagnose prostate cancer:

   _____   _____

2. List five symptoms associates with prostatis: _____,

   _____, _____,

   _____, _____.

3. List five symptoms found with benign prostatic hyperplasia (BPH):

   _____, _____,

   _____, _____,

   _____.

4. Explain why low-dose heparin is usually given to patients undergoing prostatectomy.

   _____

   _____

5. The most commonly used medication for estrogen therapy in the treatment of prostatic cancer is:

   _____.

6. Describe *epididymitis* and several of its common causes.

   _____

   _____

7. Define *priapism* and lists its major symptoms.

   _____

   _____

Learner's Self-Evaluation Tool for End of Unit 11 Review

1. The most important concepts or facts I have learned from this unit are:

   1. _____

   2. _____

   3. _____

2. The most important reference page numbers for test review and clinical concepts are pages:

   _____   _____   _____

   _____   _____   _____

3. The concepts or facts that I do not fully understand are:

   _____

   _____

4. I will get the answer(s) to my questions by _____

_____

I will do this on _____ (date and time).

5. I believe my mastery of this unit to be:
   a.   100%   Great job! Good luck!
   b.   90%   2 hours of review recommended.
   c.   80%   4 hours of review recommended.
   d.   <80%   Make an appointment with your instructor.

U N I T **12**
Immunologic Function

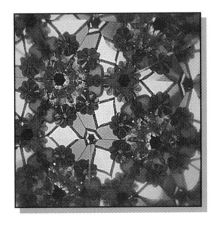

48

Assessment of Immune Function

Chapter Overview

Most people are familiar with the terms antigen, antibody, and interferon; however, understanding of these terms is frequently vague. Immunopathology is a complex field in which more is being learned every day. It involves understanding cellular activity that results in damage. Today, as the science and study of immunology advance, immunologic defects are being suggested as causative agents for acute disorders, such as acquired immune deficiency syndrome (AIDS), as well as for chronic illnesses, such as rheumatoid arthritis. As equipment becomes more sophisticated, we can expect to unravel many of the mysteries surrounding this science.

I. Knowledge-Based Questions

Deduction and Interpretation

Read each question carefully. Circle your answer.

1. The immune system is essentially composed of:
   a. bone marrow.
   b. lymphoid tissue.
   c. white blood cells.
   d. all of the above components.

2. An example(s) of a biologic response modifier that interferes with viruses is(are):
   a. bradykinin.
   b. eosinophils.
   c. granulocytes.
   d. interferon.

3. The body's first line of defense is the:
   a. antibody response.
   b. cellular immune response.
   c. phagocytic immune response.
   d. white blood cell response.

4. The primary cells responsible for recognition of foreign antigens are:
   a. leukocytes.
   b. lymphocytes.
   c. monocytes.
   d. reticulocytes.

5. Lymphocytes interfere with disease by picking up specific antigens from organisms to alter their function during the _____ stage of an immune response.
   a. effector
   b. proliferation
   c. recognition
   d. response

6. During the proliferation stage,
   a. antibody-producing plasma cells are produced.
   b. lymph nodes enlarge.
   c. lymphocytes rapidly increase.
   d. all of the above occur.

7. Cell-mediated immune responses are responsible for all of the following *except:*
   a. anaphylaxis.
   b. graft-versus-host reactions.
   c. transplant rejection.
   d. tumor destruction.

8. Antibodies are believed to be a type of:
   a. carbohydrate.
   b. fat.
   c. protein.
   d. sugar.

9. It is important to realize that cellular membrane damage results from all the following *except:*
   a. activation of complement.
   b. antibody–antigen coupling.
   c. arrival of killer T cells.
   d. attraction of macrophages.

10. Effector T cells destroy foreign organisms by:
   a. altering the antigen's cell membrane.
   b. causing cellular lysis.
   c. producing lymphokines, which destroy invading organisms.
   d. all of the above mechanisms.

11. Interferon is a lymphokine that exerts its effect by:
   a. increasing vascular permeability.
   b. inhibiting the growth of certain antigenic cells.
   c. stopping the spread of viral infections.
   d. suppressing the movement of macrophages.

12. Complement acts by:
   a. attracting phagocytes to an antigen.
   b. destroying cells through destruction of the antigen's membrane.
   c. rendering the antigen vulnerable to phagocytosis.
   d. a combination of all of the above mechanisms.

Read each statement carefully. Write your response in the space provided.

1. List four ways that disorders of the immune system occur:

   1. _____   3. _____

   2. _____   4. _____

2. Distinguish between natural, acquired and passively acquired immunity.

   Natural: _____

   Acquired: _____

   Passively acquired: _____

3. Explain what "complement" is and how it is formed.

   _____

4. Name the two ways biologic response modifiers affect the immune response:

   _____

   _____

5. Identify the trace elements that help the immune system function properly:

   _____

   _____

Match the immunoglobulin listed in Column II with its associated immunoglobulin activity listed in Column I. An answer may be used more than once.

Column I

1. _____ enhances phagocytosis

2. _____ appears in intravascular serum

3. _____ helps defend against parasites

4. _____ activates complement system

5. _____ protects against respiratory infections

6. _____ influences B-lymphocyte differentiation

7. _____ prevents absorption of antigens from food

Column II

a. IgA

b. IgD

c. IgE

d. IgG

e. IgM

49

Management of Patients With Immunodeficiency Disorders

Chapter Overview

Immunodeficiency disorders are challenging for their victim, the victim's family, and the medical–nursing health care team. The onset is frequently insidious, sometimes lying dormant for years. The symptoms are chronic and debilitating and the treatments palliative for the most part. Living with an immunodeficiency disorder is a daily juggling act, making certain that management is effective against current and future bacteria, viruses, and fungi. Vigilant attention to detail and compliance with life-long therapy are necessary for survival.

I. Knowledge-Based Questions

Deduction and Interpretation

Read each question carefully. Circle your answer.

1. Immunodeficiency disorders are caused by defects or deficiencies in:
   a. complement.
   b. B and T lymphocytes.
   c. phagocytic cells.
   d. all of the above.

2. The cardinal symptoms of immunodeficiency are:
   a. chronic diarrhea.
   b. chronic or recurrent severe infections.
   c. poor response to treatment of infections.
   d. inclusive of all the above.

3. The nitroblue tetrazolium reductase (NTB) test is used to diagnose immunodeficiency disorders related to:
   a. complement.
   b. B-cell lymphocytes.
   c. T-cell lymphocytes.
   d. phagocytic cells.

4. More than 50% of individuals with this disorder develop pernicious anemia:
   a. Bruton's disease.
   b. common variable immunodeficiency (CVID).
   c. DeGeorge's syndrome.
   d. Nezelaf's syndrome.

5. The primary cause of death for individuals with ataxia-telangiectasia is:
   a. acute renal failure.
   b. chronic lung disease.
   c. neurologic dysfunction.
   d. overwhelming infection.

6. Individuals with this disorder do not have a thymus gland:
   a. DeGeorge's.
   b. Job's.
   c. Nezelaf's.
   d. Burton's.

7. The most common *secondary* immunodeficiency disorder is:
- a. AIDS.
- b. DAF.
- c. CVID.
- d. SCID.

8. The recommended dose of IV gamma globulin for a 60 kg man is _____ given monthly.
- a. 15 g
- b. 30 g
- c. 45 g
- d. 60 g

9. When gamma globulin is infused intravenously, the rate should not exceed:
- a. 1.5 ml/min.
- b. 3 ml/min.
- c. 6 ml/min.
- d. 10 ml/min.

10. The nurse knows to stop an infusion of gamma globulin if the patient experiences:
- a. flank pain.
- b. shaking chills.
- c. tightness in the chest.
- d. any or all of the above.

II. Critical Analysis Questions

Identifying Patterns

For each group of clustered clues, write the corresponding immunodeficiency disorder.

1. Increased incidence of bacterial infections
Readily develops fungal infections from candida organism
Easily infected from herpes simplex
Afflicted with chronic eczematoid dermatitis

Disorder is: _____

2. Disappearance of germinal centers from lymphatic tissue
Complete lack of antibody production
Is associated with the *most common* immunodeficiency seen in childhood
Disease onset occurs most often in the second decade of life

Disorder is: _____

3. Lymphopenia is usually present
Failure of thymus gland to develop
Chronic mucocutaneous candidiasis is an associated disorder

Disorder is: _____

4. IgA deficiency is present in 40% of individuals
T-Cell deficiencies become more severe with age
Neurologic symptoms usually occur before age 5

Disorder is: _____

5. Usually occurs as a result of underlying disease processes
Frequently caused by certain autoimmune disorders
May be caused by certain viruses

Disorder is: _____

50

Acquired Immunodeficiency Syndrome

Chapter Overview

Acquired immunodeficiency syndrome (AIDS) is one of the newest (about 13 years ago in the United States) and most frightening infections that the United States and the world is struggling to conquer. Its virulence is directly proportional to its insidious onset, its confusing and myriad modes of transmission, its profound immunosuppression, life-threatening infections, rare malignancies, and devastating personal and social consequences. AIDS is a virus without a cure; a virus that has the potential of eliminating an entire generation of individuals, especially the young and innocent (sexually active young adults, newborns with HIV-infected mothers) who believe they are "invincible" or who are the victims of others' carelessness. Nursing's role encompasses patient education to prevent transmission, as well as the management and care of those who are infected and symptomatic. Cure may be possible only by eliminating transmission, since pharmacotherapy has been successful only in prolonging the manifestation of symptoms and the onset of active infection.

I. Knowledge-Based Questions

Deduction and Interpretation

Read each question carefully. Circle your answer.

1. The Centers for Disease Control and Prevention (CDC) officially "defined" AIDS after 100 cases were reported in:
   a. 1978.
   b. 1982.
   c. 1986.
   d. 1991.

2. Up to 65% of individuals infected with HIV will develop symptoms of AIDS within _____ years of infection.
   a. 3
   b. 6
   c. 10
   d. 15

3. The majority of AIDS cases in women occur in the _____ population(s).
   a. Caucasian
   b. black and Hispanic
   c. non-Hispanic white
   d. Asian

4. One of the fastest growing populations of women with AIDS are those:
   a. between the age of 18 and 35.
   b. who contracted the disease as children.
   c. who are in their 30s and 40s.
   d. who acquired the disease in adolescence.

5. HIV is transmitted only through:
- a. intimate sexual contact.
- b. parenteral exposure to infected blood or blood products.
- c. perinatal transmission: mother to neonate.
- d. all of the above routes.

6. The *most common* infection in persons with AIDS is:
- a. cytomegalovirus.
- b. legionnaire's disease.
- c. *Myocobacterium tuberculosis.*
- d. *Pneumocystis carinii.*

7. At least 90% of individuals with AIDS experience:
- a. anorexia.
- b. candidiasis.
- c. diarrhea.
- d. fungal infections.

8. The most common malignancy seen with HIV infection is:
- a. carcinoma of the skin.
- b. Kaposi's sarcoma.
- c. pancreatic cancer.
- d. stomach cancer.

9. Blood for transfusions was not checked for HIV contamination before:
- a. 1985.
- b. 1988.
- c. 1991.
- d. 1993.

10. An abnormal laboratory finding(s) seen with AIDS includes:
- a. decreased helper T cells.
- b. leukopenia.
- c. elevated serum globulin.
- d. all of the above.

11. Antibody formation, after HIV infection, may take as long as:
- a. 14 months.
- b. 2 years.
- c. 4 years.
- d. 10 years.

12. The minimum number of daily calories recommended for a 70-kg individual with AIDS-related "wasting syndrome" is:
- a. 1500.
- b. 2000.
- c. 2800.
- d. 4000.

13. The minimum number of daily protein calories for a 70-kg individual with AIDS-related "wasting syndrome" is:
- a. 20.
- b. 35.
- c. 45.
- d. 60.

Recognizing Contradictions

Rewrite each statement correctly. Underline the key concepts.

1. The HIV virus carries its genetic material in DNA.

2. Research data indicate that the increase in AIDS among the heterosexual population has dramatically increased on the West Coast, especially in California.

3. The percentage of AIDS infections in those over age 50 in the United States is less than 2%.

4. The current drug of choice for the treatment of *Pneumocystis carinii* pneumonia is pentamidine.

5. The most effective chemotherapy regimen for Kaposi's sarcoma is a combination of trimethoprim–sulfamethoxazole (Septra), pentamidine, and zidovudine (AZT).

Generating Solutions: Clinical Problem Solving

Read the following case study. Fill in the blanks or circle the correct answer.

CASE STUDY: AIDS

Brenden is a 39-year-old homosexual who has been recently diagnosed with AIDS.

1. On initial assessment, the nurse identifies two major potential risk factors associated with AIDS:

_____ and _____.

2. As part of her assessment, the nurse checks Brenden for candidiasis. To do this, she would inspect Brenden's:
  a. heart.
  b. lungs.
  c. oral cavity.
  d. skin.

3. Assessment data indicated dehydration as evidenced by:
  a. bradycardia.
  b. hypertension.
  c. urine specific gravity > 1.025.
  d. urine output > 70 ml/hr.

4. The assessment data indicates five possible collaborative problems; list two:

_____ and _____.

5. The nurse advises Brenden to avoid certain foods that are bowel irritants to prevent diarrhea. She advises him *not to eat:*
  a. bland foods.
  b. cooked cereal.
  c. jello and pudding.
  d. popcorn.

6. To improve Brenden's nutritional status, the nurse would:
  a. encourage him to rest before eating.
  b. limit fluids 1 hour before meals.
  c. serve five to six small meals per day.
  d. do all of the above.

51

Management of Patients With Allergic Disorders

Chapter Overview

Nursing assessment and management of a patient with an allergic disorder requires knowledge about the allergen that triggers the response, knowledge about expected symptoms and their anticipated severity, and knowledge about the usual protocol of therapy. Allergic responses range from mild erythema to anaphylactic shock. No reaction should be taken lightly because covert responses can be life-threatening. Some responses require prolonged hospitalization and complex nursing skills.

Patients with allergy disorders need expert medical and nursing management as well as an understanding attitude. They need to know that their discomfort is both perceived and appreciated.

I. Knowledge-Based Questions

Deduction and Interpretation

Read each question carefully. Circle your answer.

1. The body's first line of defense against potential invaders is the:
   a. gastrointestinal tract.
   b. respiratory tract.
   c. skin.
   d. combination of all the above.

2. Histamine acts on major organs by:
   a. contracting bronchial smooth muscle.
   b. dilating small venules.
   c. increasing gastric secretions.
   d. stimulating all of the above mechanisms.

3. Hypersensitivity reactions follow reexposure and are classified by type of reaction. An anaphylactic reaction is usually identified as type:
   a. I.
   b. II.
   c. III.
   d. IV.

4. Delayed hypersensitivity is said to have occurred when the inflammatory response to an allergen peaks within:
   a. 4 to 8 hours.
   b. 24 to 72 hours.
   c. 4 to 6 days.
   d. 1 to 2 weeks.

 Mary Jo Boyer: Study Guide to Accompany Brunner & Suddarth's Textbook of Medical-Surgical Nursing, 8th ed. © 1996 Lippincott-Raven Publishers

5. An atopic disorder(s) that results from an allergic response to an allergen is(are):

    a. allergic dermatoses.

    b. allergic rhinitis.

    c. bronchial asthma.

    d. all of the above.

6. The nurse monitors the patient's eosinophil level. She suspects a definite allergic disorder with a value of:

    a. 1% to 3% of total leukocyte count.

    b. 3% to 4% of total leukocyte count.

    c. 5% to 10% of total leukocyte count.

    d. 15% to 40% of total leukocyte count.

7. Pruritus and nasal congestion may be indicators of an impending anaphylactic reaction. If dysphagia is present, the reaction is classified as:

    a. initial.

    b. mild.

    c. moderate.

    d. severe.

8. Allergic rhinitis is induced by:

    a. airborne pollens or molds.

    b. ingested foods.

    c. parenteral medications.

    d. topical creams or ointments.

9. Patient who are sensitive to ragweed should be advised that weed pollen begins to appear in:

    a. early spring.

    b. early fall.

    c. summer.

    d. midwinter.

10. A major side effect of antihistamines that requires accurate patient education is:

    a. dryness of the mouth.

    b. anorexia.

    c. palpitations.

    d. sedation.

11. An area of nursing concern when administering a sympathomimetic drug is the drug's ability to:

    a. cause bronchodilation.

    b. constrict integumentary smooth muscle.

    c. dilate the muscular vasculature.

    d. do all of the above.

12. Injected allergens are used for "hyposensitization" and may produce systemic reactions that can be harmful. The medication that should be on hand for an adverse reaction is:

    a. Dramamine.

    b. epinephrine.

    c. Phenergan hydrochloride.

    d. Pyribenzamine.

13. The most serious manifestation of hereditary angioedema is:

    a. abdominal pain.

    b. conjunctivitis.

    c. larnygeal edema.

    d. urticaria.

14. For a 132-lb (60-kg) woman, who is experiencing anaphylaxis, the nurse should immediately administer a minimum of:

    a. 2 ml of Adrenalin, intramuscularly.

    b. 4 ml of Adrenalin, intramuscularly.

    c. 6 ml of Adrenalin, intramuscularly.

    d. 8 ml of Adrenalin, intramuscularly.

II. Critical Analysis Questions

Generating Solutions: Clinical Problem Solving

Read the following case study. Fill in the blanks or circle the correct answer.

CASE STUDY: Allergic Rhinitis

Chris is a 26-year-old contractor who specializes in finished basements. Because of his job, he is frequently working in environments where there are substances that stimulate an allergic reaction.

1. Based on assessment data, two likely nursing diagnoses would be:

    1. _____

    2. _____

2. Four probable patient goals would be:

1. _____   3. _____

2. _____   4. _____

3. The nurse advises Chris that his attacks may be preceded by the symptom(s) of:
a. breathing difficulty.   c. tingling sensations.
b. pruritus.   d. all of the above.

4. The nurse also advises him that other symptoms may be more alarming, such as:
a. hoarseness.   c. wheezing.
b. a rash or hives.   d. all of the above.

5. A teaching plan for Chris would include information about:
a. reducing exposure to allergens.   c. correct use of medications.
b. desensitization procedures.   d. all of the above.

6. The nurse tells Chris that if the physician recommends a series of inoculations for desensitization he should expect to receive injections every:
a. day for 30 days.   c. every 2 to 4 weeks.
b. week for 1 year.   d. monthly for 4 years.

52

Management of Patients With Rheumatic Disorders

Chapter Overview

Connective tissue disorders affect over 30 million persons in the United States and are indicative of some defect in the collagen and protein portions of connective tissue. Most of these diseases are characterized by exacerbations and remissions and are chronic. Many are debilitating and cause their victims to be handicapped.

Patient education needs to stress that when a disease is in remission, the person will feel as if he or she has been cured. Medications must still be taken and exercise programs continued. The patient needs to be aware that symptoms may reappear at any time.

I. Knowledge-Based Questions

Deduction and Interpretation

Read each question carefully. Circle your answer.

1. The most common symptom of rheumatoid arthritis that causes a patient to seek medical attention is:
   a. joint swelling.
   b. limited movement.
   c. fatigue.
   d. pain.

2. In rheumatoid arthritis joint swelling may be due to:
   a. bony overgrowth.
   b. fluid accumulation.
   c. hypertrophied synovium.
   d. all of the above.

3. Synovial fluid from an inflamed joint is:
   a. clear and pale.
   b. milky and cloudy.
   c. scanty in volume.
   d. straw-colored.

4. A serum study that is positive for the rheumatoid factor is:
   a. diagnostic for Sjögren's syndrome.
   b. diagnostic for systemic lupus erythematosus.
   c. specific for rheumatoid arthritis.
   d. suggestive of rheumatoid arthritis.

5. A disease-modifying agent that is successful in the treatment of rheumatoid arthritis yet has retinal eye changes as a side effect is:
   a. Butazolidin.
   b. Naprosyn.
   c. Plaquenil.
   d. Solganal.

6. Nonsteroidal anti-inflammatory agents include all of the following *except*:
- a. Clinoril.
- b. Cytoxan.
- c. Motrin.
- d. Tandearil.

7. In rheumatoid arthritis the cartilage is replaced with fibrous connective tissue during the stage of synovial joint destruction known as:
- a. cartilage erosion.
- b. increased phagocytic production.
- c. lymphocyte infiltration.
- d. pannus formation.

8. The most abundant type of connective tissue is known as:
- a. collagen.
- b. elastin.
- c. hematopoietic tissue.
- d. strong supporting tissue.

9. Complications of connective tissue disease include:
- a. leukopenia.
- b. thrombocytopenia.
- c. systemic infections.
- d. all of the above.

10. In rheumatoid arthritis (RA), the autoimmune reaction primarily occurs in the:
- a. joint tendons.
- b. cartilage.
- c. synovial tissue.
- d. interstitial space.

11. When a person with arthritis is temporarily confined to bed, the position recommended to prevent flexion deformities is:
- a. prone.
- b. semi-Fowler's.
- c. side-lying with pillows supporting the shoulders and legs.
- d. supine with pillows under the knees.

12. To immobilize an inflamed wrist, the nurse should splint the joint in a position of:
- a. slight dorsiflexion.
- b. extension.
- c. hyperextension.
- d. internal rotation.

13. The characteristic cutaneous lesion called the "butterfly rash" which appears across the bridge of the nose is found in:
- a. gout.
- b. rheumatoid arthritis.
- c. systemic sclerosis.
- d. systemic lupus erythematosus.

14. Clinical manifestations of systemic sclerosis include:
- a. decreased ventilation owing to lung scarring.
- b. dysphagia owing to hardening of the esophagus.
- c. dyspnea owing to fibrotic cardiac tissue.
- d. all of the above.

15. The single, most important medication for the treatment of systemic lupus erythematosus (SLE) is:
- a. immunosuppressants.
- b. corticosteroids.
- c. NSAIDs.
- d. salicylates.

16. The most common type of connective tissue disease in the United States is:
- a. carpal tunnel syndrome.
- b. degenerative joint disease.
- c. fibrositis.
- d. polymyositis.

17. Pathophysiologic changes seen with osteoarthritis include:
- a. joint cartilage degeneration.
- b. the formation of bony spurs at the edges of the joint surfaces.
- c. narrowing of the joint space.
- d. all of the above changes.

18. The nurse knows that a patient diagnosed with a spondyloarthropathy would *not have*:
- a. ankylosing spondylities.
- b. Raynaud's phenomenon.
- c. reactive arthritis.
- d. psoriatic arthritis.

19. With a diagnosis of gout, a nurse should expect to *find*:
- a. glucosuria.
- b. hyperuricemia.
- c. hypoproteinuria.
- d. ketonuria.

20. A purine-restricted diet is prescribed for a patient. The nurse should recommend:

    a. dairy products.

    b. organ meats.

    c. raw vegetables.

    d. shellfish.

II. Critical Analysis Questions

Generating Solutions: Clinical Problem Solving

Read the following case study. Fill in the blanks or circle the correct answer.

CASE STUDY: Rheumatoid Arthritis

Jane is a 33-year-old mother of two who is suspected of having rheumatoid arthritis. She went to her physician with concerns about joint pain and stiffness in her knees, decreased mobility (she is having discomfort playing tennis), and increased frequency of fatigue. She is unable to maintain her usual busy schedule and is depressed.

  1. The physician immediately suspects a diagnosis of rheumatoid arthritis, which she knows manifests itself primarily in the _____ decade of life.

    a. second

    b. third

    c. fourth

    d. fifth

  2. On initial examination the physician notes that Jane's knees are hot, swollen, and painful. She orders specific laboratory studies. The test result which is *not* significant for a diagnosis of rheumatoid arthritis is a(n):

    a. decreased red blood count.

    b. elevated C_4 complement component.

    c. elevated erythrocyte sedimentation rate.

    d. positive C-reactive protein.

  3. The nurse also assesses for the four systemic features found with rheumatoid arthritis:

    (1) _____ (2) _____,

    (3) _____, and (4) _____.

  4. Name the histocompatibility antigen whose presence is associated with a predisposition to rheumatoid arthritis: _____.

  5. Jane is scheduled for an arthrocentesis. The nurse advises her that her knee joint will be anesthetized locally and a fluid specimen obtained. There is no special preparation or precautions after the procedure. Jane is told that a positive finding would be joint fluid that:

    a. contains few inflammatory cells.

    b. does not contain leukocytes.

    c. is viscous and tan in color.

    d. will not form a mucin clot.

  6. A positive diagnosis of rheumatoid arthritis results in a multidisciplinary approach to treatment. Jane's pharmacotherapy regimen includes several drug classifications. A popular, nonsteroidal anti-inflammatory agent that is prescribed is:

    a. Aralen.

    b. Imuran.

    c. Motrin.

    d. Ridaura.

  7. A low-dose corticosteroid regimen is begun for a short period. The nurse advises Jane to be aware of certain drug-induced side effects, such as:

    a. elevated blood pressure.

    b. gastric upset.

    c. weight gain.

    d. all of the above.

Learner's Self-Evaluation Tool for End of Unit 12 Review

1. The most important concepts or facts I have learned from this unit are:

    1. _____

    2. _____

    3. _____

2. The most important reference page numbers for test review and clinical concepts are pages:

    _____   _____   _____

    _____   _____   _____

3. The concepts or facts that I do not fully understand are:

    _____

    _____

4. I will get the answer(s) to my questions by _____

    _____

    I will do this on _____ (date and time).

5. I believe my mastery of this unit to be:
    a. 100%   Great job! Good luck!
    b. 90%   2 hours of review recommended.
    c. 80%   4 hours of review recommended.
    d. <80%   Make an appointment with your instructor.

UNIT 13
Integumentary Function

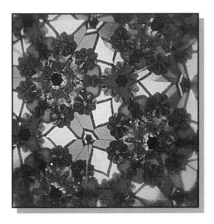

53

Assessment of Integumentary Function

Chapter Overview

If the eyes are the windows of the soul, then the skin is the doorway to the body—a door that can open slightly or all the way to let in helpful and destructive organisms. A door is characteristic of its owner and may be blank on the outside or covered with messages that help explain what is going on inside the body. Assessing the skin is as simple as it is complex because subtle messages can be overlooked or misinterpreted. This chapter will review the major types of skin lesions and describe the most accurate assessment techniques to distinguish types of lesions.

I. Knowledge-Based Questions

Deduction and Interpretation

Read each question carefully. Circle your answer.

1. For the average adult with a normal body temperature, a nurse needs to know that insensible water loss is approximately:
   a. 250 ml/day.
   b. 500 ml/day.
   c. 750 ml/day.
   d. 1000 ml/day.

2. When a nurse applies a cold towel to a patient's neck to reduce body heat, heat is reduced by:
   a. conduction.
   b. convection.
   c. evaporation.
   d. radiation.

3. Sweating, a process by which the body regulates heat loss, does not occur until the core body temperature exceeds the base level of:
   a. 24°C.
   b. 37°C.
   c. 43°C.
   d. 51°C.

4. In a dark-skinned person, color change that occurs in the presence of shock can be evidenced when the skin appears:
   a. ashen gray and dull.
   b. dusky blue.
   c. reddish pink.
   d. whitish pink.

5. Dark-skinned patients who have cherry red nail beds, lips, and oral mucosa may be exhibiting signs of:
   a. anemia.
   b. carbon monoxide poisoning.
   c. polycythemia.
   d. shock.

 Mary Jo Boyer: Study Guide to Accompany Brunner & Suddarth's Textbook of Medical-Surgical Nursing, 8th ed. © 1996 Lippincott-Raven Publishers

6. A clinical example of a primary skin lesion known as a macule is:

    a. hives.

    b. impetigo.

    c. port wine stains.

    d. psoriasis.

II. Critical Analysis Questions

Analyzing Comparisons

Read each analogy. Fill in the space provided with the best response.

1. Keratin: skin hardening :: melanin: _____.

2. Bluish skin color: insufficient oxygenation :: yellow-green skin:

_____.

3. Vitamin D deficiency: rickets :: vitamin C deficiency: _____.

4. Palpation: skin turgor :: _____: vesicle.

5. Acne: a pustule :: psoriasis: _____.

Identifying Patterns

Consider each of the systemic diseases listed in each grouping along with cutaneous manifestations of the disease. Cluster the data to identify the skin manifestation.

1. Seen in systemic lupus erythematosis
Characterized by red, spidery lines
Appear in placques on the nose and ears
Seen on scales on the cheek area

_____

2. Seen in syphilis
Appears as an ulcerated lesion
Is a painless chancre

_____

3. Seen in platelet disorders
Associated with vessel fragility
Characterized by purpura

_____

4. Occurs in infections
Seen with allergic reactions
Characteristic of drug reactions in infants

_____

5. Present as macules, papules, plaques, or nodules
Lesions are visually multiple
Lesions are characteristically blue-red or dark brown
Seen in AIDS

_____

54

Management of Patients With Dermatologic Problems

Chapter Overview

Dermatologic disorders can be physically unattractive and emotionally scarring, especially if the characteristics of the disorder are obvious to others. Age is also a consideration in understanding the impact of a skin disorder. A 14-year-old with pruritus of the hand will probably be more upset than a 40-year-old with the same condition. Considering the importance that society places on physical attractiveness, any dermatologic disorder needs to be treated as effectively as possible.

A major dermatologic disorder is skin cancer, which will eventually affect one in seven Americans if it continues to occur at its current rate. The incidence of skin cancer has been shown to be directly related to the amount of exposure one has to the sun. It is hoped that society will eventually place less importance on the tanned, "healthy" look since, in reality, the tanning process can be life-threatening.

A major implication for nursing is to educate people about the harmful effects of the sun. People need to be encouraged to use sun blockers, and mothers should use sunscreen on their children.

I. Knowledge-Based Questions

Deduction and Interpretation

Read each question carefully. Circle your answer.

1. Moisture-retentive dressings and commercially produced wet compresses are very efficient and may be able to stay in place up to:
   a. 3 hours.
   b. 6 hours.
   c. 12 hours.
   d. 18 hours.

2. The patient is advised to apply a lotion to a dermatosis site every 3 hours for a week. The nurse advised the patient to use:
   a. Bacitracin.
   b. Eucerin.
   c. Lubriderm.
   d. Vaseline petroleum jelly.

3. Occlusive dressings over topical medications:
   a. enhance the absorption of topical medications.
   b. improve hydration.
   c. increase the local skin temperature.
   d. do all of the above.

4. The nurse caring for a patient who has used occlusive dressings for some time knows to assess the skin daily for:
a. local skin atrophy.
b. striae.
c. telangiectasia.
d. all of the above.

5. Nurses should advise patients suffering with pruritus to avoid all of the following *except*:
a. drying soaps.
b. emollient lubricants.
c. vigorous towel drying.
d. warm to hot water.

6. An example of a cream commonly used as a topical medication is:
a. Bacitracin.
b. Dermassage.
c. Eucerin.
d. petroleum jelly.

7. The most common symptom of pruritus is:
a. a rash.
b. itching.
c. flaking.
d. pain.

8. The cause of acne vulgaris appears to be:
a. bacterial.
b. genetic.
c. hormonal.
d. an interplay of the above.

9. Management of follicular disorders includes all of the following *except*:
a. cleansing of the skin with an antibacterial soap to prevent spillage of bacteria to adjacent tissues.
b. rupture of the boil or pimple to release the pus.
c. systemic antibiotic therapy to treat the infection.
d. warm, moist compresses to increase resolution of the furuncle or carbuncle.

10. Herpes zoster (shingles) is:
a. a varicella–zoster viral infection related to chickenpox.
b. an inflammatory condition that produces vesicular eruptions along nerve pathways.
c. manifested by pain, itching, and tenderness.
d. characterized by all of the above.

11. The most common fungal infection that frequently affects young adults is:
a. tinea pedis.
b. tinea corporis.
c. tinea cruris.
d. tinea unguium.

12. Tinea capitis (ringworm of the scalp) can be identified by the presence of:
a. papules at the edges of inflamed patches.
b. circular areas of redness.
c. scaling and spots of baldness.
d. all of the above.

13. Patient education for the management of pediculosis capitis should include advising the patient to:
a. comb his hair with a fine-toothed comb dipped in vinegar to remove nits.
b. disinfect all combs and brushes.
c. wash his hair with a shampoo containing lindane (Kwell).
d. do all of the above.

14. A patient is complaining of severe itching that intensifies at night. The nurse decides to assess the skin using a magnifying glass and penlight to look for the "itch mite." The nurse suspects the skin condition known as:
a. contact dermatitis.
b. pediculosis.
c. scabies.
d. tinea corporis.

15. Psoriasis is an inflammatory dermatosis that results from:
a. a superficial infection with *Staphylococcus aureus*.
b. dermal abrasion.
c. epidermal proliferation.
d. excess deposition of subcutaneous fat.

16. The characteristic lesion of psoriasis is a:
a. circular patch covered with silver scales.
b. cluster of pustules.
c. group of raised vesicles.
d. pattern of bullae that rupture and form a scaly crust.

17. Exfoliate dermatitis is characterized by erythema and scaling and is associated with:
a. a loss of stratum corneum.
b. capillary leakage.
c. hypoproteinemia.
d. all of the above.

18. Nursing care for a patient with toxic epidermal necrolysis (TEN) should include:
a. inspection of the oral cavity.
b. assessment of urinary output.
c. application of topical skin agents.
d. all of the above actions.

19. The incidence of skin cancer in fair-skinned Americans is approximately:
a. 8%.
b. 12%.
c. 20%.
d. 35%.

20. The most common type of skin cancer is:
a. basal cell.
b. squamous cell.
c. malignant melanoma.
d. Kaposi's sarcoma.

21. The most lethal of all skin cancers is:
a. basal cell.
b. squamous cell.
c. malignant melanoma.
d. Kaposi's sarcoma.

22. Danger signals of melanoma include changes in a mole's:
a. color.
b. shape or outline.
c. size or surface.
d. appearance as included in all of the above.

23. The etiology of Kaposi's sarcoma is believed to be:
a. environmental.
b. genetic.
c. viral.
d. a combination of one or all of the above.

24. A living tissue transplant from the same person is known as a(n):
a. allograft.
b. alloplastic implant.
c. autograft.
d. xenograft.

25. For a graft to "take,"
a. the area must be free of infection.
b. the recipient bed must have an adequate blood supply.
c. immobilization must be ensured.
d. all of the above conditions must be present.

II. Critical Analysis Questions

Generating Solutions: Clinical Problem Solving

Read the following case study. Circle the correct answer.

Steve is a 26-year-old professional baseball player for a Florida farm team. He spent many hours in the sun practicing between 9:00 AM and 4:00 PM. His V-neck uniform left little protection to his chest. Steve had a mole on his chest for 5 years. One day last October he noticed that the margins of the mole were elevated and palpable and the color had become darker. Since his father had malignant melanoma when he was 32 years old, Steve decided to see a physician.

1. Steve knows that malignant melanoma currently causes 2% of all cancers. Based on statistical predictions, the number of deaths in 10 years will be approximately:
a. 2%.
b. 4%.
c. 5%.
d. 10%.

2. On examination, the physician noted a circular lesion with irregular outer edges and a pinkish hue in the center. The physician suspected the lesion to be a(n): _____ melanoma.
a. acral-lentiginous
b. lentigo-maligna
c. nodular
d. superficial spreading

3. The physician confirms the diagnosis by:
   a. complete blood count analysis.
   b. computed tomography.
   c. excisional biopsy.
   d. skin examination.

4. The lesion is >14 mm in thickness and growing vertically. The physician knows that:
   a. dermal invasion is likely.
   b. the prognosis is favorable.
   c. metastasis is probable.
   d. peripheral growth will occur next.

5. The physician considers immunotherapy with a biologic response modifier such as:
   a. interferon alfa.
   b. BCG vaccine.
   c. *Cornebacterium parvum.*
   d. levamisole

55

Management of Patients With Burn Injury

Chapter Overview

Nothing is more devastating than a burn. It is visually unattractive, heals slowly, may be disfiguring, and is frequently associated with months of rehabilitation and occupational therapy.

Nurses need to be knowledgeable about the pathophysiology as well as the treatment phase of burn management. The psychosocial aspects of burn care also need to be addressed. Burns of even 10% of the surface area can be accompanied by emotional responses that can hinder rehabilitation.

Burned patients are critically ill and in pain and have multiple biopsychosocial needs. Nursing patients with burns is a unique challenge. It requires a nurse who is a specialist in critical care procedures and who is able to work clinically in a burn unit or treatment center that is warm and has a high humidity. The nurse must also be able to deal with the emotional needs of a group of patients whose survival depends on accurate assessments and quick medical and nursing management decisions.

I. Knowledge-Based Questions

Deduction and Interpretation

Read each question carefully. Circle your answer.

1. Plasma seeps out into surrounding tissues after a burn. The greatest amount of fluid leaks out in:
   a. the first 2 hours.
   b. 4 to 8 hours.
   c. 12 hours.
   d. 24 to 36 hours.

2. As fluid is reabsorbed after injury, renal function maintains a diuresis for up to:
   a. 3 days.
   b. 1 week.
   c. 2 weeks.
   d. 1 month.

3. Fluid shifts during the first week of the acute phase of a burn injury cause electrolyte movements that result in:
   a. hypernatremia.
   b. hypokalemia.
   c. hyperkalemia.
   d. hypercalcemia.

4. Plasma leakage produces edema, which increases:
   a. circulating blood volume.
   b. the hematocrit level.
   c. systolic blood pressure.
   d. all of the above.

 Mary Jo Boyer: Study Guide to Accompany Brunner & Suddarth's Textbook of Medical-Surgical Nursing, 8th ed. © 1996 Lippincott-Raven Publishers

5. The leading cause of death in fire victims is believed to be:
a. cardiac arrest.
b. carbon monoxide intoxication.
c. hypovolemic shock.
d. septicemia.

6. A full-thickness burn is:
a. classified by the appearance of blisters.
b. identified by the destruction of the entire dermis.
c. not associated with edema formation.
d. usually very painful because of exposed nerve endings.

7. Generally, a burn wound has caused the most severe tissue injury in the inner layer where cellular death occurs. This inner layer is known as the zone of:
a. coagulation.
b. hyperemia.
c. necrosis.
d. stasis.

8. A child tips a pot of boiling water onto his bare legs. The mother should:
a. avoid touching the burned skin and take the child to the nearest emergency department.
b. cover the child's legs with ice cubes secured with a towel.
c. immerse the child's leg in cool water.
d. liberally apply butter or shortening to the burned area.

9. A man suffers leg burns from spilled charcoal lighter fluid. His son extinguishes the flames. While waiting for an ambulance the burn victim should:
a. have someone assist him into a bath of cool water, where he can wait for emergency personnel.
b. lie down, have someone cover him with a blanket, and cover his legs with petroleum jelly.
c. remove his burned pants so that the air can help cool the wound.
d. sit in a chair, elevate his legs, and have someone cut his pants off around the burned area.

10. As the first priority of care, a patient with a burn injury will initially need:
a. an airway established.
b. an indwelling catheter inserted.
c. fluids replaced.
d. pain medication administered.

11. Eyes that have been irritated or burned with a chemical should be flushed with cool, clean water:
a. immediately.
b. in 5 to 10 minutes.
c. after an eye examination.
d. after 24 hours.

12. Decreased urinary output during the first 48 hours of a major burn is secondary to all of the following *except*:
a. decreased adrenocortical activity.
b. hemolysis of red blood cells.
c. hypovolemia.
d. sodium retention.

13. Electrolyte changes in the first 48 hours of a major burn include:
a. base bicarbonate deficit.
b. hypernatremia.
c. hypokalemia.
d. all of the above.

14. The Evans formula for replacing fluid lost during the first 24 to 48 hours recommends the administration of:
a. colloids.
b. electrolytes.
c. glucose.
d. all of the above.

15. The most recent Consensus formula for fluid replacement recommends that a balanced salt solution be administered in the first 24 hours of a burn in the range of 2 ml/kg/% of burn. A 176-lb (80-kg) man with a 30% burn should receive:
a. 1200 ml in the first 8 hours.
b. 2400 ml in the first 8 hours.
c. 3600 ml in the first 8 hours.
d. 4800 ml in the first 8 hours.

16. One parameter of adequate fluid replacement is an hourly urinary output in the range of:
a. 10 to 30 ml.
b. 30 to 70 ml.
c. 80 to 120 ml.
d. 100 to 200 ml.

17. A serious gastrointestinal disturbance that frequently occurs with a major burn is:
a. diverticulitis.
b. hematemesis.
c. paralytic ileus.
d. ulcerative colitis.

18. Fluid remobilization usually begins:
a. within the first 24 hours, when massive amounts of fluid are being administered intravenously.
b. after 48 hours, when fluid is being reabsorbed from the interstitial tissue.
c. after 1 week, when capillary permeability has returned to normal.
d. after 1 month, when scar tissue covers the wound and prevents evaporative fluid loss.

19. An unexpected laboratory value during the fluid remobilization phase of a major burn is a:
a. hematocrit of 45%/dl.
b. pH, 7.20; PaO_2, 38 torr; bicarbonate, 15 mEq/L.
c. serum potassium of 3.2 mEq/L.
d. serum sodium of 140 mEq/L.

20. With partial-thickness (second-degree) burns, skin regeneration begins to take place:
a. within 7 days.
b. in 2 to 3 weeks.
c. after 2 months.
d. between the third and sixth month.

21. Wound cleansing and debridement usually begin when eschar begins to separate at:
a. 72 hours.
b. 1 week.
c. 1-1/2 to 2 weeks.
d. 1 month.

22. Leukopenia within 48 hours is a side effect associated with the topical antibacterial agent:
a. cerium nitrate solution.
b. gentamicin sulfate.
c. sulfadiazine, silver (Silvadene).
d. mafenide (Sulfamylon).

23. After an occlusive dressing is applied to a burned foot, the foot should be placed in the position of:
a. adduction.
b. dorsiflexion.
c. external rotation.
d. plantar flexion.

24. Biological dressings that use skin from living or recently deceased humans are known as:
a. autografts.
b. heterografts.
c. homografts.
d. xenografts.

25. The recommended route for administration of low-dose narcotics is:
a. intramuscular.
b. intravenous.
c. oral.
d. subcutaneous.

26. To meet his early nutritional demands for protein, a 198-lb (90-kg) burned patient will need to ingest a minimum of:
a. 90 g/day.
b. 110 g/day.
c. 180 g/day.
d. 270 g/day.

27. Early indicators of late-stage septic shock include all of the following *except*:
a. decreased pulse pressure.
b. a full bounding pulse.
c. pale cool skin.
d. renal failure.

II. Critical Analysis Questions

Recognizing Contradictions

Rewrite each statement correctly. Underline the key concepts.

1. The chances of survival are greatest for those who are very young and those between 40 and 50 years of age.

2. A localized burn response includes injury limited to 50% of a designated area.

3. All burn injuries greater than 25% of body surface area are associated with a pulmonary injury or some level of hypoxia.

4. During the acute phase of burn care the wound closes and cosmetic reconstruction begins.

5. Fluid replacement with colloids and crystalloids usually takes a week to restore normal plasma levels after a burn.

Generating Solutions: Clinical Problem Solving

Develop a nursing care plan for each of the following situations. Use the format below.

Nursing diagnosis:

Immediate goal(s):

Intermediate goal(s):

Long-term goal(s):

Nursing interventions   *Expected outcomes*

Suggested Situations

1. Aimee, 9 months old, climbed onto a stove where an electric range was on *high*. Her pajamas caught fire, and she was burned over 60% of her body (excluding her face and neck) with second- and third-degree burns. Her mother managed to extinguish the flames and immerse her in a sink of cool water before emergency help arrived. Aimee was transported to a burn treatment center. There are two other preschool children in her family.

2. Brad, 12 years old, sustained full-thickness burns on his upper chest, face, and neck when he was trying to start a charcoal fire to prepare dinner for his father. His father sprayed him with water from a hose and took him to a hospital emergency department 3 miles away. On arrival Brad was semiconscious and in extreme respiratory distress. He and his divorced father live together.

3. Claire is 27 years old and owns an arts and crafts store. During a recent demonstration of candle making, a container of hot liquid wax (230°F) spilled over her left forearm and hand. One of her students drove her to a nearby clinic. By the time Claire arrived at the clinic some of the wax had hardened and was falling off her arm, removing skin as it fell. She was in intense pain.

4. David, a 35-year-old single executive, was asleep when a fire began in his living room. A neighbor saw the flames and called the fire company. By the time David was rescued he was semiconscious and had suffered smoke inhalation. He was treated by emergency technicians and transported to an emergency d   rtment.

Learner's Self-Evaluation Tool for End of Unit 13 Review

1. The most important concepts or facts I have learned from this unit are:

    1. _____ _____
    2. _____
    3. _____

2. The most important reference page numbers for test review and clinical concepts are pages:

    _____   _____   _____

    _____   _____   _____

3. The concepts or facts that I do not fully understand are:

    _____

    _____

4. I will get the answer(s) to my questions by _____

    _____

    I will do this on _____ (date and time).

5. I believe my mastery of this unit to be:
    a.   100%   Great job! Good luck!
    b.   90%   2 hours of review recommended.
    c.   80%   4 hours of review recommended.
    d.   <80%   Make an appointment with your instructor.

UNIT 14
Sensorineural Function

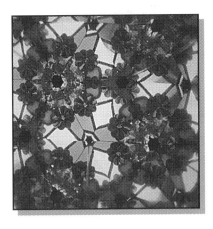

56

Assessment and Management of Patients With Vision Problems and Eye Disorders

Chapter Overview

Many bodily functions and activities of daily living require vision for successful performance. Patients with eye disorders need to be shown ways of altering their routines so that basic needs can be safely met.

Before developing a nursing care plan for a patient with a vision problem, the nurse should collect as much data as possible about such things as environment, hobbies, and interests. Goals and behavioral outcomes need to be realistic and attainable. The use of support services that offer volunteers to assist with transportation or help with meal preparation or that just offer companionship should be encouraged. Nurses should strive to assist handicapped patients to be as independent as possible.

I. Knowledge-Based Questions

Deduction and Interpretation

Read each question carefully. Circle your answer.

1. Vision becomes less efficient with age because aging is associated with:
   a. a decrease in pupil size.
   b. slowing of accommodation.
   c. an increase in lens opaqueness.
   d. a change in all of the above.

2. The physician prescribed a mydriatic to dilate the patient's pupil. The nurse expects her to order the most commonly used mydriatic:
   a. Adrenalin.
   b. Glaucon.
   c. Neo-Synephrine.
   d. Paredrine.

3. An example of a parasympathomimetic drug that is used as a miotic is:
   a. atropine sulfate.
   b. lidocaine hydrochloride.
   c. phenylephrine hydrochloride.
   d. pilocarpine hydrochloride.

4. A patient interested in contact lenses wants the type that will last for more than 10 years. The nurse recommends:
   a. extended-wear lenses.
   b. hard contact lenses.
   c. gas-permeable lenses.
   d. soft contact lenses.

5. During a routine eye examination, a patient complains that she is unable to read road signs at a distance when driving her car. The physician knows to check for:
   a. an astigmatism.
   b. anisometropia.
   c. myopia.
   d. presbyopia.

6. The most common neoplasm of the eyelids is:
   a. basal cell carcinoma.
   b. a chalazion.
   c. xanthelasmas.
   d. squamous cell carcinoma.

7. Acute conjunctivitis is associated with:
   a. blurred vision.
   b. elevated intraocular pressure.
   c. moderate to copious ocular discharge.
   d. severe pain.

8. After cataract surgery a patient is encouraged to:
   a. maintain bed rest for 1 week.
   b. lie on his stomach while sleeping.
   c. avoid bending his head below the waist.
   d. life weights to increase muscle strength.

9. Increased ocular pressure is indicated by a reading of:
   a. 0 to 5 mm Hg.
   b. 6 to 10 mm Hg.
   c. 11 to 20 mm Hg.
   d. 23 to 30 mm Hg.

10. A diagnostic clinical manifestation of glaucoma is:
    a. a significant loss of central vision.
    b. diminished acuity.
    c. pain associated with a purulent discharge.
    d. the presence of halos around lights.

11. When assessing acute glaucoma, you would expect to find a:
    a. clear cornea.
    b. constricted pupil.
    c. marked blurring of vision.
    d. watery ocular discharge.

12. Pharmacotherapy for primary glaucoma that increases the outflow of aqueous humor would include all of the following *except*:
    a. anticholinesterase drugs.
    b. carbonic anhydrase inhibitors.
    c. epinephrine drops.
    d. miotics.

13. A clinical symptom(s) of a detached retina is(are):
    a. a sensation of floating particles.
    b. a definite area of blank vision.
    c. momentary flashes of light.
    d. all of the above.

14. Macular degeneration is characterized by:
    a. purulent periorbital drainage.
    b. pupil dilation.
    c. loss of central vision.
    d. ptosis.

15. The success rate of surgical repair for retinal detachments is about:
    a. 35%.
    b. 60%.
    c. 75%.
    d. 90%.

16. One of the most significant symptoms associated with corneal abrasions is:
    a. blurred vision.
    b. photophobia.
    c. serous drainage.
    d. intense pain.

17. Chemical burns of the eye are treated with:
    a. local anesthetics and antibacterial drops for 24 to 36 hours.
    b. hot compresses applied at 15-minute intervals.
    c. flushing of the lids, conjunctiva, and cornea.
    d. cleansing of the conjunctiva with a small cotton-tipped applicator.

18. Postoperatively the patient who has had eye surgery should be placed:

a. flat on his back with pillows supporting both sides of his head to prevent unnecessary movement.

b. in high Fowler's position with his neck supported with a neck collar to prevent unnecessary jarring and to minimize eye movement.

c. on the side opposite his surgery to eliminate pressure near the surgical area.

d. supine with a small pillow under his head.

19. Legal blindness refers to visual acuity that is _____ or worse.

a. 20/50

b. 20/100

c. 20/150

d. 20/200

Match the characteristic or function of the eye listed in Column II with its associated structure listed in Column I.

Column I

1. _____ choroid

2. _____ lens

3. _____ pupil

4. _____ retina

5. _____ vitreous humor

6. _____ cornea

7. _____ sclera

8. _____ iris

9. _____ uvea

10. _____ limbus

Column II

a. maintains the form of the eyeball

b. area where most of the blood vessels for the eye are located

c. degree of convexity modified by contraction and relaxation of the ciliary muscles

d. contractile membrane between the cornea and lens

e. transparent part of the fibrous coat of the eyeball

f. accommodates to the intensity of light by dilating or contracting

g. white part of the eye

h. the pigmented, vascular coating of the eye

i. the edge of the cornea where it joins the sclera

j. contains nerve endings that transmit visual impulses to the brain

Complete the following crossword puzzle using common ophthalmologic terms.

Down

1. Excessive production of tears
2. Another term for an external hordeolum
3. The term *oculus dexter* refers to the _____ eye.
4. A term used to describe an inflammatory condition of the uveal tract
7. Another term for nearsightedness
8. An inflammatory condition affecting the iris
9. People who are photosensitive function better outdoors during this time of day.
10. Inflammation of the cornea
13. A loss of cornea substance or tissue as a result of inflammation

Across

5. Abnormal sensitivity to light
6. The term *oculus sinister* refers to the _____ eye.
9. Absence of the lens
11. Uneven curvature of the cornea
12. Drooping of the upper eyelid
14. A tear in the eye tissue
15. A condition in which one eye deviates from the object at which the person is looking

II. Critical Analysis Questions

Identifying Patterns

Analyze the following clusters of information about disorders of the eyes and identify the specific disorder.

1. A chronic inflammation of the eyelid margins
   Formation of scales and granulations on the eye lashes
   White eyelashes may result from this condition
   Staphylococcus aureus may be a primary infecting organism

   _____

2. A superficial infection of the glands of the eyelids
   Pain and swelling of the eyelids are characteristic signs
   Warm, moist compresses on the eyelids facilitate healing
   Topical sulfonamides may be prescribed

   _____

3. Symptoms include hyperemia and edema of conjunctiva
   Etiology may be bacterial, fungal, viral, or allergic
   Lay person's term for condition is "pink-eye"

   _____

4. Corneal edema is a common sign in this disorder
   Ulceration and infection are associated with this disorder
   Cycloplegics and mydriatics may be prescribed
   Etiology is usually associated with trauma or compromise
   Systemic or local defense mechanisms

   _____

5. Characterized by an opacification of the lens
   Usually associated with the aging process
   Vision is clouded because light to the retina is blocked
   Associated with compromised night vision

   _____

Generating Solutions: Clinical Problem Solving

Develop a nursing care plan for Elise, who is 65 years old and needs to have cataract surgery on her right eye. Elise lives with her daughter in a three-story house and has rheumatoid arthritis. She needs a cane to walk. Her daughter has a Down's syndrome child at home who requires constant care. Share your nursing care plan with your instructor for comments.

   Nursing diagnosis:

   Immediate goal(s):

Intermediate goal(s):

Long-term goal(s):

Nursing interventions   *Expected outcomes*

57

Assessment and Management of Patients With Hearing Problems and Ear Disorders

Chapter Overview

Hearing disorders can limit a person's normal activities of daily living, depending on the patient's age, occupation, degree of impairment, and attitude toward the handicap. The capability of a person with impaired hearing to live a normal life has improved over the past 25 years because of increased public awareness of the disorder, the ability of those with hearing problems to communicate with sign language, and the positive performance of hearing-impaired people on the job and in sports.

Even with recent improvements in society's attitude, major adjustments need to be made by the patient and his or her family. Nursing care plans need to be all-inclusive, and the nurse needs to take an active role in patient education and consumer awareness.

I. Knowledge-Based Questions

Deduction and Interpretation

Read each question carefully. Circle your answer.

1. The organ of hearing is known as the:
a. cochlea.
b. eardrum.
c. semicircular canal.
d. stapes.

2. A sensorineural (perceptive) hearing loss results from impairment of the:
a. eighth cranial nerve.
b. middle ear.
c. outer ear.
d. seventh cranial nerve.

3. Those who are born with normal hearing but lose their hearing because of illness or accident are classified as:
a. adventitiously deaf.
b. congenitally deaf.
c. deaf.
d. hard of hearing.

4. A hearing loss that is a manifestation of an emotional disturbance is known as a _____ hearing loss.
a. conductive.
b. functional.
c. mixed.
d. sensorineural.

 Mary Jo Boyer: Study Guide to Accompany Brunner & Suddarth's Textbook of Medical-Surgical Nursing, 8th ed. © 1996 Lippincott-Raven Publishers

5. Noise-induced hearing loss can result from noise at a minimum decibel (dB) level of:
   a. 35 to 40 dB
   b. 60 dB
   c. 70 dB
   d. 85 to 90 dB

6. To straighten the ear canal for examination, the nurse would grasp the auricle and pull it:
   a. backward.
   b. upward.
   c. slightly outward.
   d. in all of these directions.

7. Changes in the ear that occur with aging may include:
   a. atrophy of the tympanic membrane.
   b. increased hardness of the cerumen.
   c. degeneration of cells at the base of the cochlea.
   d. all of the above.

8. The critical level of loudness that most people (without a hearing loss) are comfortable with is a decibel reading of:
   a. 15 dB.
   b. 30 dB.
   c. 45 dB.
   d. 60 dB.

9. The most common fungus associated with ear infections is:
   a. *Staphylococcus albus.*
   b. *Staphylococcus aureus.*
   c. *Aspergillus.*
   d. *Pseudomonas.*

10. Nursing instructions for a patient suffering from external otitis should include the:
   a. application of heat to the auricle.
   b. avoidance of swimming.
   c. ingestion of over-the-counter analgesics such as aspirin.
   d. information included in all of the above.

11. Solutions for ear irrigations should be at a temperature of:
   a. 98° to 103°F
   b. 105° to 110°F
   c. 110° to 120°F
   d. 120° to 125°F

12. Choose the symptom *not usually* found with acute otitis media.
   a. Aural tenderness
   b. Rhinitis
   c. Otalgia
   d. Otorrhea

13. An incident of otitis media is usually associated with:
   a. ear canal swelling.
   b. discharge.
   c. intense ear pain.
   d. prominent localized tenderness.

14. A myringotomy is performed primarily to:
   a. drain purulent fluid.
   b. identify the infecting organism.
   c. relieve tympanic membrane pressure.
   d. accomplish all of the above.

15. A tympanoplasty is surgically performed to:
   a. close a perforation.
   b. prevent recurrent infection.
   c. reestablish middle ear function.
   d. accomplish all of the above.

16. Postoperative nursing assessment for a patient who has had a mastoidectomy should include observing for facial paralysis, which might indicate damage to the _____ cranial nerve.
   a. first
   b. fourth
   c. seventh
   d. tenth

17. A diet for Ménière's disease would include avoiding:
   a. bread.
   b. cheese.
   c. eggs.
   d. milk.

II. Critical Analysis Questions

Generating Solutions: Clinical Problem Solving

Read the following case study. Fill in the blanks or circle the correct answer.

CASE STUDY: Mastoid Surgery

Amber is a 73-year-old grandmother who is scheduled for mastoid surgery to remove a cholesteatoma, a cystlike sac filled with keratin debris, which was large enough to occlude the ear canal.

1. Preoperatively, the physician reviews the results of the audiogram and assesses for the presence of associated ear problems such as: _____

   _____

   _____

2. Identify four major nursing goals for the patient, preoperatively:

   1. _____   3. _____

   2. _____   4. _____

3. Postoperatively, it is common for the patient to experience: _____

   _____

4. The patient is advised that the postauricular incision should be kept dry for:
   a. 7 days.   c. 3 weeks.
   b. 2 weeks.   d. 1 month.

5. Two important signs of infection are: _____ and

   _____.

6. Manipulation of the semicircular canals during surgery may result in the symptom of:
   a. sharp, shooting pain.   c. purulent drainage.
   b. inner ear fullness.   d. vertigo.

7. The patient is advised that it is normal to hear popping and crackling sounds in the affected ear for about:
   a. 3 days.   c. 3 to 5 weeks.
   b. 1 week.   d. 2 to 4 months.

8. The patient is advised to prevent activities that increase intracranial pressure, such as:

   _____

   _____

Learner's Self-Evaluation Tool for End of Unit 14 Review

1. The most important concepts or facts that I have learned from this unit are:

   1. _____

   2. _____

   3. _____

2. The most important reference page numbers for test review and clinical concepts are pages:

_____   _____   _____

_____   _____   _____

3. The concepts or facts that I do not fully understand are:

_____

_____

4. I will get the answer(s) to my questions by _____

_____

I will do this on _____ (date and time).

5. I believe my mastery of this unit to be:
   a.   100%   Great job! Good luck!
   b.   90%   2 hours of review recommended.
   c.   80%   4 hours of review recommended.
   d.   <80%   Make and appointment with your instructor.

UNIT 15
Neurologic Function

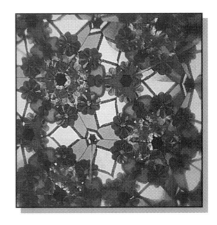

58

Assessment of Neurologic Function

Chapter Overview

The central and autonomic nervous systems are complex and interrelated. Assessment of neurologic function requires an expert knowledge of the brain, the spinal cord, and the actions of each nerve. Nurses need to be knowledgeable about the norm and acutely sensitive to any deviations.

Because of the complexity of neurologic function, sophisticated technology is used for diagnostic studies. Nurses need to assist patients undergoing these procedures by making sure they understand what will be involved in the procedure and why.

I. Knowledge-Based Questions

Deduction and Interpretation

Read each question carefully. Circle your answer.

1. The normal adult produces 500 ml of cerebrospinal fluid daily from the:
   a. arachnoid.
   b. dura mater.
   c. circle of Willis.
   d. corpus callosum.

2. A person's personality and judgment are controlled by that area of the brain known as the _____ lobe.
   a. frontal
   b. occipital
   c. parietal
   d. temporal

3. The lobe of the cerebral cortex that influences sensation is the _____ lobe.
   a. frontal
   b. occipital
   c. parietal
   d. temporal

4. Voluntary muscle control is governed by a vertical band of "motor cortex" located in the _____ lobe.
   a. frontal
   b. occipital
   c. parietal
   d. temporal

5. The sleep regulator and the site of the hunger center is known as the:
   a. hypothalamus.
   b. medulla oblongata.
   c. pituitary gland.
   d. thalamus.

6. The "master gland" is also known as the _____ gland.
   a. adrenal
   b. thyroid
   c. pineal
   d. pituitary

7. Motor axons form pyramidal tracts that cross to the opposite side. This crossed pyramidal tract occurs in the brain in the area of the:
   a. frontal cerebrum.
   b. lateral portion of the cerebellum.
   c. medulla oblongata.
   d. pons.

8. The spinal cord tapers off to a fine thread of tissue at the level of the:
   a. coccygeal nerve.
   b. cerebral cortex.
   c. lateral ventricle.
   d. medulla oblongata.

9. The brain center responsible for balancing and coordination is the:
   a. cerebellum.
   b. second lumbar vertebra.
   c. first sacral nerve.
   d. sacrum.

10. The major receiving and communication center for afferent sensory nerves is the:
    a. medulla oblongata.
    b. pineal body.
    c. pituitary gland.
    d. thalamus.

11. The overall supervision of the autonomic nervous system is the function of the:
    a. cerebellum.
    b. hypothalamus.
    c. pons.
    d. temporal lobe of the cerebral cortex.

12. Parasympathetic impulses are mediated by the secretion of:
    a. acetylcholine.
    b. epinephrine.
    c. norepinephrine.
    d. all of the above.

13. The preganglionic fibers of the sympathetic neurons are located in those segments of the spinal cord identified as:
    a. C1–T1.
    b. C3–L1.
    c. C8–L3.
    d. T1–S5.

14. Myelography with an oil-based medium requires the patient to lie _____ for 12 to 24 hours to reduce CSF leakage.
    a. in high Fowler's position
    b. in semi-Fowler's position
    c. prone
    d. recumbent

15. Patient preparation for electroencephalography includes omitting, for 24 hours before the test, all of the following *except*:
    a. coffee and tea.
    b. solid foods.
    c. stimulants.
    d. tranquilizers.

16. For a lumbar puncture the nurse should assist the patient to flex his head and thighs while lying on his side so that the needle can be inserted between the:
    a. fourth and fifth cervical vertebrae.
    b. fifth and sixth thoracic vertebrae.
    c. third and fourth lumbar vertebrae.
    d. first and second sacral vertebrae.

II. Critical Analysis Questions

Generating Solutions: Clinical Problem Solving

Write the effects produced by the parasympathetic and sympathetic nervous systems on each organ or tissue listed in Column I. Use the terms provided, and document in the space below.

Terms to be used:	acceleration	inhibition
	constriction	increased motility
	dilation	secretion

Organ or Tissue	Parasympathetic Effect	Sympathetic Effect
a. bronchi (sample)	constriction	dilation
b. cerebral vessels		
c. coronary vessels		
d. heart		
e. iris of the eye		
f. salivary glands		
g. smooth muscle of		
(1) bladder wall		
(2) large intestine		
(3) small intestine		

Next to each cranial nerve listed by number, write the appropriate corresponding terminology in Column I and a major associated function in Column II.

Nerve No.	Column I	Column II
1 (sample)	olfactory	smell
2		
3		
4		
5		
6		
7		
8		
9		
10		
11		
12		

59

Management of Patients With Neurologic Dysfunction

Chapter Overview

Patients with neurologic dysfunction represent a challenge to nursing care because of the complexity of their symptoms, the frequent involvement of other systems, and their prolonged rehabilitative course. Recovery is usually slow, with small increments in progress noted. Nurses need to be supportive and to encourage patients to have positive attitudes toward improvement, no matter how minor the gains.

I. Knowledge-Based Questions

Deduction and Interpretation

Read each question carefully. Circle your answer.

1. An indicator of compromised respiratory status significant enough to require mechanical ventilation for an average-weight adult patient with a neurologic dysfunction would be:
   a. expiratory reserve volume of 1300 ml.
   b. inspiratory capacity of 3000 ml.
   c. residual volume of 1400 ml.
   d. vital capacity of 1000 ml.

2. Intracranial pressure can be increased by a:
   a. decrease in venous outflow.
   b. dilation of the cerebral blood vessels.
   c. rise in $PaCO_2$.
   d. change in all of the above.

3. Initial compensatory vital sign changes with increased intracranial pressure include all of the following *except* a(an):
   a. decreased pulse rate.
   b. increased systemic blood pressure.
   c. decreased temperature.
   d. slowed respiratory rate with irregularities.

4. The normal range of intracranial fluid pressure (ICP) is:
   a. 60 to 100 mm H_2O.
   b. 110 to 140 mm H_2O.
   c. 150 to 180 mm H_2O.
   d. 180 to 210 mm H_2O.

5. The earliest sign of increasing ICP is:
   a. a bounding pulse.
   b. bradycardia.
   c. hypertension.
   d. lethargy.

6. The nurses assess the patient's level of consciousness using the Glasgow Coma Scale. Her score of _____ indicates severe impairment of neurologic function.
a. 3
b. 6
c. 9
d. 12

7. Nursing care activities for a patient with increased intracranial pressure *would not* include:
a. assisting him with isometric exercises.
b. avoiding activities that interfere with venous drainage of blood from the head.
c. use of a cervical collar.
d. teaching him to exhale when being turned (to avoid the Valsalva maneuver).

8. As ICP rises, the nurse knows that she may be asked to give _____, a commonly used osmotic diuretic.
a. glycerin
b. isosorbide
c. mannitol
d. urea

9. Unconsciousness may have a _____ origin.
a. neurologic
b. metabolic
c. toxicologic
d. multisystem involvement

10. The initial mortality rate for a stroke is as high as:
a. 10%.
b. 20%.
c. 35%.
d. 50%.

11. The most common cause of cerebrovascular accident is cerebral:
a. arteriosclerosis.
b. hemorrhage.
c. ischemia.
d. thrombosis.

12. Risk factors associated with cerebrovascular accident include:
a. high-normal hematocrit level.
b. hypertension.
c. preexisting cardiovascular disease.
d. all of the above.

13. Aphasia resulting from injury or disease of the brain centers is primarily a disturbance in:
a. memory.
b. swallowing.
c. language.
d. vision.

14. It is expected that _____ % of stroke patients develop aphasia.
a. 10
b. 20
c. 50
d. 80

15. Postcraniotomy cerebral edema is maximum _____ after brain surgery.
a. 6 hours
b. 12 to 20 hours
c. 24 to 36 hours
d. 48 hours

16. A neurosurgical approach(es) to pain relief would be:
a. stimulation procedures.
b. administration of intraspinal opiates.
c. interruption of nerve tracts that conduct pain.
d. all of the above mechanisms.

Match the need interference found with neurologic dysfunction in Column II with its associated nursing intervention(s) found in Column I. An answer may be used more than once.

Column I

1. _____ assist with daily active or passive range of motion.

2. _____ elevate the head of the bed 30°.

3. _____ institute a bowel-training program.

4. _____ maintain dorsiflexion to affected area.

5. _____ place patient in a lateral position.

Column II

a. footdrop

b. incontinence

c. impaired cough reflex

d. keratitis

e. paralyzed diaphragm

f. paralyzed extremity

II. Critical Analysis Questions

Generating Solutions: Clinical Problem Solving

1. Develop a plan of care for Miss Potter, a 32-year-old, single circus performer who has been unconscious since she was admitted to the hospital 1 week ago after falling from a high wire. Her family must leave the area to travel with the circus and is expected to return in 2 months.

Nursing interventions   *Rationale*

Immediate goal(s)

Intermediate goal(s)

Long-term goal(s)

Nursing interventions   *Expected outcomes*

2. Construct a nursing care plan for Mrs. Coe, who recently sustained a cerebrovascular accident. Mrs. Coe is 41 years old and lives with her husband and three sons. Emphasize the rehabilitative phase, which should have begun with her diagnosis, and stress the retraining of her flaccid right upper and lower extremities. She also needs to be taught how to sit, stand, and walk with balance and how to use a wheelchair.

Nursing interventions   *Rationale*

Immediate goal(s)

Intermediate goal(s)

Long-term goal(s)

Nursing interventions   *Expected outcomes*

60

Management of Patients With Neurologic Disorders

Chapter Overview

Nursing care for patients with neurologic disorders demands a multiplicity of resources and skills, since neurologic disorders are not isolated problems. Any neurologic disorder affects other systems and involves psychosocial adjustment to changes in one's self-image and self-esteem.

The specifics of care will depend on the diagnosis. Generally, there are some common denominators to be considered by nurses when developing a care plan, including alterations in mobility, bowel and bladder elimination, comfort, health maintenance, nutrition, sexual functioning, and family processes.

The sequelae of neurologic damage can be heartbreaking, especially when the victim is young or has many dependents. Patient education should be realistic and optimistic because continued research has brought society closer to some cures and has improved rehabilitative measures.

I. Knowledge-Based Questions

Deduction and Interpretation

Read each question carefully. Circle your answer.

1. The most common drug used for the prevention of a migraine headache is:
   a. Cafergot.
   b. Inderal.
   c. Sansert.
   d. Seconal.

2. The most frequently seen brain neoplasm is a(an):
   a. acoustic neuroma.
   b. angioma.
   c. glioma.
   d. meningioma.

3. Choose the common tumor type(s) seen in the elderly:
   a. Cerebral metastases.
   b. Glioblastomas.
   c. Meningiomas.
   d. All of the above.

4. The majority of brain tumors are treated by:
   a. neurosurgery.
   b. chemotherapy.
   c. radioisotope implants.
   d. all of the above measures.

5. The most significant form of meningitis is:
   a. bacterial.
   b. aseptic.
   c. septic.
   d. viral.

6. Bacterial meningitis alters intracranial physiology, causing:
   a. cerebral edema.
   b. increased permeability of the blood–brain barrier.
   c. raised intracranial pressure.
   d. all of the above changes.

7. A brain abscess is a collection of pus within the substance of the brain and is caused by:
   a. direct invasion of the brain.
   b. spread of infection from nearby sites.
   c. spread of infection by other organs.
   d. all of the above mechanisms.

8. The clinical manifestations of Parkinson's disease (bradykinesia, rigidity, and tremors) is directly related to a decreased level of:
   a. acetylcholine.
   b. dopamine.
   c. seratonin.
   d. phenylalanine.

9. The most effective pharmacologic agent for the treatment of Parkinson's disease is:
   a. Levadopa.
   b. Permax.
   c. Selegilene.
   d. Symmetrel.

10. A clinical manifestation(s) of Huntington's disease is(are):
   a. abnormal involuntary movements (chorea).
   b. emotional disturbances.
   c. intellectual decline.
   d. all of the above.

11. A surgical intervention that can cause substantial remission of myasthenia gravis is:
   a. esophagostomy.
   b. myomectomy.
   c. thymectomy.
   d. spleenectomy.

12. The normal life expectancy for 50% of patients with amyotropic lateral sclerosis (ALS) is:
   a. 3 years.
   b. 5 years.
   c. 10 years.
   d. 20 years.

13. Nursing care for a patient who is experiencing a convulsive seizure includes all of the following *except*:
   a. loosening constrictive clothing.
   b. opening the patient's jaw and inserting a mouth gag.
   c. positioning the patient on his side with head flexed forward.
   d. providing for privacy.

14. A seizure characterized by loss of consciousness and tonic spasms of the trunk and extremities, rapidly followed by repetitive generalized clonic jerking, is classified as a:
   a. focal seizure.
   b. generalized seizure.
   c. jacksonian seizure.
   d. partial seizure.

15. Choose the *incorrect statement* about the occurrence of head injuries:
   a. Almost 70% of all victims are below 30 years of age.
   b. An estimated 100,000 persons die annually from these injuries.
   c. Detectable blood alcohol levels are present in more than 50% of the victims.
   d. The majority of injuries occur in females.

16. A cerebral hemorrhage located under the dura mater is classified as a(n):
   a. epidural hematoma.
   b. extradural hematoma.
   c. intracerebral hematoma.
   d. subdural hematoma.

17. Most victims of spinal cord injury are:
   a. 30 years of age or younger.
   b. 30 to 40 years of age.
   c. 40 to 50 years of age.
   d. 50 years of age or older.

18. In the United States the number of new spinal cord injuries each year averages approximately:
   a. 5,000 cases.
   b. 10,000 cases.
   c. 15,000 cases.
   d. 25,000 cases.

19. Respiratory difficulty and paralysis of all four extremities occur with spinal cord injury:
   a. above C4.
   b. at C6.
   c. at C7.
   d. around C8.

20. A common complication of immobility in a spinal cord injury is:
   a. pressure ulcers.
   b. deep vein thrombosis.
   c. urinary tract infections.
   d. pneumonia.

21. The majority of lumbar disk herniations occur at the level of:
   a. L1–L2.
   b. L3–L4.
   c. L4–L5.
   d. S1–S2.

22. Tic douloureux is a(n) _____ cranial nerve disorder characterized by paroxysms of pain and burning sensations.
   a. third
   b. fifth
   c. seventh
   d. eighth

23. Bell's palsy is a _____ cranial nerve disorder characterized by weakness or paralysis of the facial muscles.
   a. third
   b. fifth
   c. seventh
   d. eighth

II. Critical Analysis Questions

Generating Solutions: Clinical Problem Solving

Read the following case studies. Circle the correct answer.

CASE STUDY: Multiple Sclerosis

Toni, a 32-year-old mother of two, has had multiple sclerosis for 5 years. She is currently enrolled in a school of nursing. Her husband is supportive and helps with the care of their preschool sons. Toni has been admitted to the clinical area for diagnostic studies related to symptoms of visual disturbances.

1. The nurse is aware that multiple sclerosis is a progressive disease of the central nervous system characterized by:
   a. axon degeneration.
   b. demyelination of the brain and the spinal cord.
   c. sclerosed patches of neural tissue.
   d. all of the above.

2. During the physical assessment the nurse recalls that the areas most frequently affected by multiple sclerosis are the:
   a. lateral, third, and fourth ventricles.
   b. optic nerve and chiasm.
   c. pons, medulla, and cerebellar peduncles.
   d. above areas.

3. During the nursing interview Toni minimizes her visual problems, talks about remaining in school to attempt advanced degrees, requests information about full-time jobs in nursing, and mentions her desire to have several more children. The nurse recognizes her emotional responses as being:
   a. an example of inappropriate euphoria characteristic of the disease process.
   b. a reflection of coping mechanisms used to deal with the exacerbation of her illness.
   c. indicative of the remission phase of her chronic illness.
   d. realistic for her current level of physical functioning.

4. Toni's disease process involves a sacral plexus. Assessment should include:
   a. bladder problems or urinary tract infections.
   b. bowel management.
   c. sexual activity.
   d. all of the above.

CASE STUDY: Parkinson's Disease

Charles is a 76-year-old retired professional golfer. He has recently been diagnosed as having Parkinson's disease.

1. The nurse knows that Parkinson's disease, a progressive neurologic disorder, is characterized by:
   a. bradykinesia.
   b. muscle rigidity.
   c. tremor.
   d. all of the above.

2. The nurse assesses for the characteristic movement of Parkinson's disease, which is a(n):
   a. exaggerated muscle flaccidity that leads to frequent falls.
   b. hyperextension of the back and neck that alters normal movements.
   c. pronation–supination of the hand and forearm that interferes with normal hand activities.
   d. combination of all of the above.

3. Charles is started on chemotherapy, which is aimed at restoring dopaminergic activities. An example of such a drug is:
   a. Artane.
   b. Benadryl.
   c. Elavil.
   d. Dopar.

4. Nutritional considerations as part of the nursing care plan would include all of the following *except* that:
   a. the diet should be semisolid to facilitate the passage of food.
   b. calcium should be avoided.
   c. the patient should be sitting in an upright position during feeding.
   d. thick fluids should be encouraged to provide additional calories.

Develop nursing care plans for three case studies.

CASE STUDY: Huntington's Disease

Develop a nursing care plan for *Mike,* a 49-year-old television producer who has been diagnosed as having Huntington's disease. He lives alone in a penthouse apartment and is extremely busy and successful in his business. He has no living relatives. He is experiencing uncontrollable movements and difficulties feeding himself. He recently started chemotherapy with haloperidol (Haldol). Share your care plan with your instructor for comments.

Nursing Diagnosis: Potential for accidental injury related to abnormal involuntary movements.

Immediate goal(s):

Intermediate goal(s):

Long-term goal(s):

Nursing interventions   *Expected outcomes*

CASE STUDY: Cervical Spine Injury

Develop a nursing care plan for *Katie,* an 11-year-old who suffered a cervical spine injury after diving into a swimming pool. Katie is in traction applied by Crutchfield tongs and is on a Stryker frame. She is the oldest of three children and has never been hospitalized before. Complete your care plan and share it with your instructor for comments. Use the format below.

Nursing diagnosis:

Immediate goal(s):

Intermediate goal(s):

Long-term goal(s):

Nursing interventions   *Expected outcomes*

CASE STUDY: Paraplegia

Develop a nursing care plan for *Matthew,* a 29-year-old Navy pilot who was recently injured in a training maneuver. Matthew is a paraplegic. He has been hospitalized for 1 week. He was recently married, and his wife is expecting their first child in 2 months. Emphasize the following areas in your nursing care plan: psychological support, weight-bearing activities, muscle exercises, mobilization, and sexual needs. Share your work with your clinical instructor. Use the suggested format below.

Nursing diagnosis:

Immediate goal(s):

Intermediate goal(s):

Long-term goal(s):

Nursing interventions   *Expected outcomes*

Learner's Self-Evaluation Tool for End of Unit 15 Review

1. The most important concepts or facts I have learned from this unit are:

1. _____

2. _____

3. _____

2. The most important reference page numbers for test review and clinical concepts are pages:

_____   _____   _____

_____   _____   _____

3. The concepts or facts that I do not fully understand are:

_____

_____

4. I will get the answer(s) to my questions by _____

_____

   I will do this on _____ (date and time).

5. I believe my mastery of this unit to be:
   a.   100%   Great job! Good luck!
   b.   90%   2 hours of review recommended.
   c.   80%   4 hours of review recommended.
   d.   <80%   Make an appointment with your instructor.

UNIT 16
Musculoskeletal Function

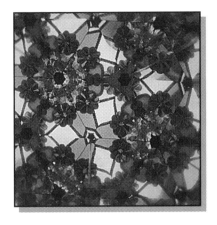

61

Assessment of Musculoskeletal Function

Chapter Overview

The synergistic interplay between muscles and bones provides a person with freedom of movement to perform his or her daily tasks and to participate in exercise activities. The interaction between muscles and bones can be influenced by one's genetic makeup, age, nutrition, environment, occupation, and activity levels.

When assessing musculoskeletal function, a nurse needs to be aware of the normal range of motor function and should be able to correlate symptoms of pathology to other data to diagnose and plan care.

I. Knowledge-Based Questions

Deduction and Interpretation

Read each question carefully. Circle your answer.

1. The vertebrae can be classified as a type of _____ bone(s).
   a. flat
   b. irregular
   c. long
   d. short

2. The sternum, a bone that is a site for hematopoiesis, is classified as a _____ bone.
   a. flat
   b. irregular
   c. long
   d. short

3. The basic cells responsible only for the formation of bone matrix are:
   a. osteoblasts.
   b. osteoclasts.
   c. osteocytes.
   d. all of the above.

4. About 3 weeks postfracture, an internal bridge of fibrous material, cartilage, and immature bone join bone fragments so that ossification can occur. The building of a "fracture bridge" occurs during the stage of bone healing known as:
   a. inflammation.
   b. cellular proliferation.
   c. callus formation.
   d. ossification.

5. The hip and shoulder are examples of articular joints that are classified as:
   a. ball-and-socket types.
   b. hinge joints.
   c. pivot joints.
   d. saddle joints.

6. The primary energy source for muscle cells is:
   a. adenosine triphosphate (ATP).
   b. creatine phosphate.
   c. glucose.
   d. glycogen.

 Mary Jo Boyer: Study Guide to Accompany Brunner & Suddarth's Textbook of Medical-Surgical Nursing, 8th ed. © 1996 Lippincott-Raven Publishers

7. Isometric contraction of the vastus lateralis is part of the exercises known as:
   a. biceps-tightening exercises.
   b. triceps-resisting exercises.
   c. gluteal-setting exercises.
   d. quadriceps exercises. *(circled)*

8. Patient education for musculoskeletal conditions for the aging is based on the understanding that bone mass peaks at age _____ after which there is a gradual loss of bone.
   a. 20
   b. 35 *(circled)*
   c. 40
   d. 50

9. By age 75, the average woman has lost about _____ % of cancellous bone and is susceptible to bone fractures.
   a. 15
   b. 40 *(circled)*
   c. 60
   d. 75

10. The removal of synovial fluid from a joint is called:
   a. arthrectomy.
   b. arthrocentesis. *(circled)*
   c. arthrography.
   d. arthroscopy.

Match the range-of-motion term listed in Column II with its associated description listed in Column I.

Column I

1. __H__ pulling down toward the midline of the body
2. __I__ the act of turning the foot inward
3. __B__ the opposite movement of flexion
4. __J__ turning around on an axis
5. __G__ turning the palms down
6. __E__ pulling the jaw forward
7. __D__ moving away from the midline
8. __C__ conelike circular movement
9. __A__ turning the palm up
10. __F__ turning the foot outward

Column II

a. supination
b. extension
c. circumduction
d. abduction
e. protraction
f. eversion
g. pronation
h. adduction
i. inversion
j. rotation

Read each statement carefully and write the best response in the space provided.

1. List several general functions of the musculoskeletal system.

_____

_____

2. The approximate percentage of total body calcium present in the bones is _____ %.

3. In the human body there are __206__ bones.

4. Name the major bones in which red bone marrow is located.

_____   _____

_____   _____

5. Explain how vitamin D helps to regulate the balance between bone formation and resorption.

_____

_____

6. The major hormonal regulators of calcium homeostasis are _____

_____.

Unscramble the letters to answer each statement.

1. The fibrous membrane that covers the bone:

E O P T R M E S U I

2. These connect muscles to muscles:

A N S I G M L T E

3. The contractile unit of skeletal muscle:

O E S E A R M R C

4. These attach muscles to bone:

N T S O E D N   *tendons*

5. Loss of bone mass common in postmenopausal women:

I S S T P O O R E O O S   *osteoporosis*

6. A lateral curving deviation of the spine:

L S O S O S I I C   *scoliosis*

62

Management Modalities for Patients With Musculoskeletal Dysfunction

Chapter Overview

Assistive orthopedic devices are used to treat musculoskeletal dysfunctions. Nurses need to be familiar with the various devices to make sure that they are performing their intended function. Nurses need to assure patients that the devices are necessary for recovery, seldom cause pain, can be uncomfortable, and will be removed when recovery is complete. Some joint replacements are permanent and may initially cause pain, but the patient should eventually be pain-free.

Nursing care plans must include the maintenance of any orthopedic device, since proper functioning is vital to the healing process.

I. Knowledge-Based Questions

Deduction and Interpretation

Read each question carefully. Circle your answer.

1. The nurse who assesses bone fracture pain expects the patient to describe the pain as:
   a. a dull, deep, boring ache.
   b. sharp and piercing.
   c. similar to "muscle cramps."
   d. sore and aching.

2. The nurse suspects "compartment syndrome" for a casted extremity. She would assess for characteristic symptoms such as:
   a. decreased sensory function.
   b. excruciating pain.
   c. loss of motion.
   d. all of the above.

3. A common pressure problem area for a long leg cast is the:
   a. dorsalis pedis.
   b. peroneal nerve.
   c. popliteal artery.
   d. posterior tibialis.

4. Choose the *incorrect* statement about a plaster cast. After a plaster cast has been set, it:
   a. will take 1 to 3 days to dry.
   b. may be dented with pressure from the fingers of the hands when being moved.
   c. should be covered with a blanket to promote quick drying.
   d. will not have maximum strength until it is dry.

Mary Jo Boyer: Study Guide to Accompany Brunner & Suddarth's Textbook of Medical-Surgical Nursing, 8th ed. © 1996 Lippincott-Raven Publishers   **291**

5. After removal of a cast, the patient needs to be instructed to do all of the following *except*:
    a. apply an emollient lotion to soften the skin.
    b. control swelling with elastic bandages, as directed.
    c. gradually resume activities and exercise.
    d. use friction to remove dead surface skin by rubbing the area with a towel.

6. A patient with an arm cast complains of pain. The nurse should do all of the following *except*:
    a. assess the fingers for color and temperature.
    b. administer a prescribed analgesic to promote comfort and allay anxiety.
    c. suspect that the patient may have a pressure sore.
    d. determine the exact site of the pain.

7. The nurse assesses for peroneal nerve injury by checking the patient's casted leg for the primary symptom(s) of:
    a. burning.
    b. numbness.
    c. tingling.
    d. all three indicators.

8. The nurse is very concerned about the potential debilitating complication of peroneal nerve injury which is:
    a. permanent paresthesis.
    b. footdrop.
    c. deep vein thrombosis.
    d. infection.

9. Choose the *incorrect* statement about turning a patient in a hip spica cast.
    a. A minimum of three persons are needed so that the cast can be adequately supported by their palms.
    b. Points over body pressure areas need to be supported to prevent the cast from cracking.
    c. The abduction bar should be used to ensure that the lower extremity can be moved as a unit.
    d. The patient should be encouraged to use the trapeze or side rail during repositioning.

10. Nursing assessment of a patient in traction should include:
    a. lung sounds and bowel sounds.
    b. circulation, sensation, and motion of the extremities in traction.
    c. his level of anxiety and apprehension.
    d. all of the above interventions.

11. A patient in pelvic traction needs his circulatory status assessed. The nurse should check for a positive (+) Homans' sign by asking the patient to:
    a. extend both hands while she compares the volume of both radial pulses.
    b. extend each leg and dorsiflex each foot to determine if pain or tenderness is present in the lower leg.
    c. plantar flex both feet while she performs the blanch test on all his toes.
    d. squeeze her hands with his hands to evaluate any difference in strength.

12. Skin traction is usually limited to a weight between:
    a. 1 and 3 lbs.
    b. 4 and 7 lbs.
    c. 8 and 10 lbs.
    d. 11 and 13 lbs.

13. The nurse expects that up to _____ lbs of weight can be used for a patient in skeletal traction:
    a. 10
    b. 25
    c. 40
    d. 60

14. When a patient is in continuous skeletal leg traction, it is important for the nurse to remember to do all of the following *except*:
    a. encourage the patient to use the trapeze bar.
    b. maintain adequate countertraction.
    c. remove the weights when pulling the patient up in bed to prevent unnecessary pulling on the fracture site.
    d. use a fracture bedpan to prevent soiling and to maintain patient comfort.

15. The surgical procedure in which damaged knee joint fibrocartilage is excised is called:
    a. arthroplasty.
    b. fasciectomy.
    c. meniscectomy.
    d. open reduction.

16. Preoperative nursing measures that are appropriate for an orthopedic patient should include:
    a. encouraging fluids to prevent a urinary tract infection.
    b. teaching isometric exercises and encouraging active range of motion.
    c. discouraging smoking to improve respiratory function.
    d. all of the above interventions.

17. Postoperative nursing concerns when caring for an orthopedic patient should include:
    a. determining that his pain is controlled by administering prescribed analgesics.
    b. observing for signs of shock, such as hypotension and tachycardia.
    c. preventing infection by using aseptic technique when giving wound care.
    d. all of the above interventions.

18. One of the most dangerous of all postoperative complications is:
    a. atelectasis.
    b. hypovolemia.
    c. pulmonary embolism.
    d. urinary tract infection.

19. A diet for a skeletal traction patient who must remain in bed would *not* be high in:
    a. calcium.
    b. iron.
    c. protein.
    d. vitamin C.

20. Fusion of a bone to eliminate a joint is called:
    a. an osteotomy.
    b. arthrodesis.
    c. cup arthroplasty.
    d. tenorrhaphy.

21. An artificial joint for total hip replacement involves an implant that consists of:
    a. an acetabular socket.
    b. a femoral shaft.
    c. a spherical ball.
    d. all of the above.

22. The recommended leg position to prevent prosthesis dislocation after a total hip replacement is:
    a. abduction.
    b. adduction.
    c. flexion.
    d. internal rotation.

23. Postoperatively a patient with a total hip replacement is allowed to turn:
    a. 45 degrees onto his unoperated side if he keeps his affected hip abducted.
    b. from the prone to the supine position only, and he must keep his affected hip extended and abducted.
    c. to any comfortable position as long as the affected leg is extended.
    d. to his operative side if his affected hip remains extended.

24. After a total hip replacement, stair climbing and stooping are to be avoided for:
    a. 1 month.
    b. 3 months.
    c. 5 months.
    d. 8 months.

25. After a total hip replacement, the patient is usually able to resume daily activities after:
    a. 3 months.
    b. 6 months.
    c. 9 months.
    d. 1 year.

Read each statement carefully. Write your response in the space provided.

1. List four reasons or purposes for applying a cast.

   (1) _____   (3) _____

   (2) _____   (4) _____

2. The typical plaster of paris cast is impregnated with a powdered chemical called

   _____

3. Describe suggested methods of vascular assessment to determine circulatory constriction in a casted extremity.

_____

_____

4. List the danger signs of possible circulatory constriction in a casted extremity.

_____

_____

5. Name at least four purposes of traction application.

_____   _____

_____   _____

6. List two examples of straight or running traction.

_____

7. The most common cause of postoperative mortality in musculoskeletal patients is:

_____

_____

8. Name several indicators of hip prosthesis dislocation.

_____

_____

II. Critical Analysis Questions

Generating Solutions: Clinical Problem Solving

Read the following case study. Fill in the blanks or circle the correct answer.

CASE STUDY: Buck's Traction

Bernadette is a 32-year-old bank secretary who was admitted to the hospital for unilateral Buck's extension traction to the left leg following a hip injury. Bernadette is the single parent of three children under age 12.

1. Based on her knowledge of running traction, the nurse knows to expect that:
   a. the patient's leg will be flat on the bed to allow for a straight pulling force.
   b. the patient's leg will be flexed at the knee to allow for mobility without disruption of the pulling force.
   c. the traction will be applied directly to the bony skeleton to maintain a constant pulling force.
   d. the traction will allow the patient's leg to be suspended off the bed so no further damage can occur to the hip.

2. The nurse knows that countertraction must be considered whenever traction is applied with Buck's traction, countertraction is provided by:

   (a) _____ and (b) _____

3. In preparing the patient's skin for Buck's traction application the nurse knows that it is necessary to:

_____

_____

4. The nurse makes certain that the weights applied will not exceed _____ kg.
   a. 0.5
   b. 1
   c. 2
   d. 3

5. The nurse consistently assesses neurovascular status when traction is in place. List the seven indicators that the nurse would evaluate.

_____   _____

_____   _____

_____   _____

_____

6. On assessment, the nurse notes a positive Homans' sign. Explain what this means.

_____

_____

63

Management of Patients With Musculoskeletal Disorders

Chapter Overview

Two major nursing considerations for patients with musculoskeletal disorders are the chronicity of symptoms and the course of progressive deterioration that tends to characterize such conditions. Nurses need to address these two areas to help patients have a positive attitude toward acceptable levels of functioning. When dealing with musculoskeletal disorders, the nurse needs to call on her knowledge of pharmacotherapy, nutrition, and physical medicine to implement and evaluate planned care.

I. Knowledge-Based Questions

Deduction and Interpretation

Read each question carefully. Circle your answer.

1. The intervertebral disks that are subject to the greatest mechanical stress and greatest degenerative changes are:
   a. C3 and C4.
   b. L1 and L2.
   c. L4 and L5.
   d. S1 and L5.

2. Back pain is classified as "chronic" when the pain lasts longer than:
   a. 4 weeks.
   b. 2 months.
   c. 6 months.
   d. 1 year.

3. The best position to ease low back pain is:
   a. high Fowler's to allow for maximum hip flexion.
   b. supine with the knees slightly flexed and the head of the bed elevated 30°.
   c. prone with a pillow under the shoulders.
   d. supine with the bed flat and a firm mattress in place.

4. Pelvic traction for low back pain promotes:
   a. lumbar flexion.
   b. lumbar lordosis.
   c. sacral extension.
   d. sacral lordosis.

 Mary Jo Boyer: Study Guide to Accompany Brunner & Suddarth's Textbook of Medical-Surgical Nursing, 8th ed. © 1996 Lippincott-Raven Publishers

5. When lifting objects, patients with low back pain should be encouraged to maximize the use of the:
a. gastrocnemius.
b. latissimus dorsi.
c. quadriceps.
d. rectus adominis.

6. The nurse should encourage a patient with low back pain to do all of the following *except*:
a. lie prone with legs slightly elevated.
b. strengthen abdominal muscles.
c. avoid prolonged sitting or walking.
d. maintain appropriate weight.

7. Bone formation is enhanced by:
a. calcium intake.
b. muscular activity.
c. weight-bearing.
d. all of the above.

8. The most common symptoms of osteomalacia are:
a. bone fractures and kyphosis.
b. bone pain and tenderness.
c. muscle weakness and spasms.
d. softened and compressed vertebrae.

9. Most cases of osteomyelitis are caused by:
à. *Proteus.*
b. *Pseudomonas.*
c. *Salmonella.*
d. *Staphylococcus aureus.*

10. Signs and symptoms of osteomyelitis may include all of the following *except*:
a. pain, erythema, and fever.
b. leukopenia, swelling, and purulent drainage.
c. elevated erythocyte sedimentation rate and increased white blood cell count.
d. positive wound cultures and localized discomfort.

11. The specific treatment for chronic osteomyelitis would probably be:
a. antibiotic therapy.
b. drainage of localized foci of infection.
c. immobilization.
d. surgical removal of the sequestrum.

12. The most common benign bone tumor is a(n):
a. enchondroma.
b. giant cell tumor.
c. osteochondroma.
d. osteoid osteoma.

13. Appropriate nursing actions when caring for a patient with a primary malignant bone tumor would include all of the following *except*:
a. allowing the patient to independently plan his daily routine.
b. estimating the size and location of the mass daily by vigorously palpating the affected area.
c. assuring the patient receiving chemotherapy that alopecia, if it occurs, it temporary.
d. encouraging range-of-motion exercises to prevent atrophy of unaffected muscles.

14. The multiple myeloma tumor has its origin and principal location in the:
a. bone marrow.
b. liver.
c. lymph nodes.
d. spleen.

II. Critical Analysis Questions

Generating Solutions: Clinical Problem Solving

Read the following case study. Fill in the blanks or circle the correct answer.

CASE STUDY: Osteoporosis

Emily is a 49-year-old administrative assistant at a community college who has just been diagnosed with osteoporosis. The physician has asked you to answer some of her questions and explain his directions for her level of activity and her nutritional needs.

1. Emily asks the nurse to explain why she is losing her bone mass. The nurse's explanation is based on the physiologic rationale that bone mass loss occurs when

_____

2. What two reasons could the nurse use to explain why women develop osteoporosis more frequently than men.

   _____ Estrogen loss _____   _____

3. The nurse advises Emily that about _____ % of women over age 45 have some degree of osteoporosis.
   a. 10
   b. 25
   c. 50
   d. 80

4. The nurse advises Emily that the development of osteoporosis is significantly dependent on:
   a. decreased estrogen, which inhibits bone breakdown.
   b. increased calcitonin, which enhances bone re-sorption.
   c. increased vitamin D use, which interferes with calcium use.
   d. increased parathyroid hormone, which de-creases with aging.

5. Part of Emily's teaching plan includes nutritional information about dietary calcium and vitamin D. The nurse advised Emily that she needs _____ mg of calcium a day.
   a. 500
   b. 1000
   c. 1500
   d. 2000

6. Emily is told that her x-ray results indicated bone radiolucency. The nurse knows that Emily has probably al-ready exhibited _____ % of demineralization.
   a. 5
   b. 10
   c. 20
   d. 30

64

Management of Patients With Musculoskeletal Trauma

Chapter Overview

Any break in bone integrity causes pain, dysfunction, and frequently loss of motion. The pain and blood loss associated with a fracture can be so overwhelming that a person may experience shock and die. All fractures are considered serious because fracture complications, such as thromboembolism, may cause death or disability.

Another type of musculoskeletal trauma is amputation. Whether amputation is therapeutic or traumatic, it causes many physiologic and psychosocial adjustments.

Nursing care for patients who are suffering musculoskeletal trauma must address priority patient needs, such as pain relief, rehabilitation to achieve a functional level of activity and locomotion, and assistance to adjust to an altered body image.

I. Knowledge-Based Questions

Deduction and Interpretation

Read each question carefully. Circle your answer.

1. A muscle tear that is microscopic and due to overuse is called a:
   a. contusion.
   b. dislocation.
   c. sprain.
   d. strain.

2. The acute inflammatory stage of a strain or sprain usually lasts:
   a. less than 24 hours.
   b. between 24 and 48 hours.
   c. about 72 hours.
   d. at least 1 week.

3. After arthroscopy a patient can usually resume some activity in:
   a. 24 to 48 hours.
   b. 2 to 3 days.
   c. 1 week.
   d. all of the above.

4. Patients who have a surgically repaired Achilles tendon need to know that normal activities can usually be resumed after:
   a. 1 month.
   b. 8 weeks.
   c. 3 months.
   d. 6 months.

5. Emergency management of a fracture should include:
   a. covering the area with a clean dressing, if the fracture is open.
   b. immobilizing the affected site.
   c. splinting the injured limb.
   d. all of the above nursing interventions.

6. The longest immobilization time necessary for fracture union occurs with a fracture of the:
   a. intratrochanteric area of the femur.
   b. midshaft of the humerus.
   c. pelvis.
   d. tibial shaft.

7. The most serious complication of an open fracture is:
   a. infection.
   b. muscle atrophy caused by loss of supporting bone structure.
   c. necrosis of adjacent soft tissue caused by blood loss.
   d. nerve damage.

8. Shock, as an immediate complication of fractures, is usually classified as:
   a. cardiogenic.
   b. hypovolemic.
   c. neurogenic.
   d. septicemic.

9. Fat emboli, as a complication of fractures,
   a. represents the major cause of death in fracture patients.
   b. result in symptoms of decreased mental alertness.
   c. may compromise the patient's respiratory status, necessitating ventilator support.
   d. are characterized by all of the above.

10. Patients who experience a fracture of the humeral neck are advised that healing will take an average of _____ weeks with restricted vigorous activity for an additional _____ weeks.
   a. 6; 2
   b. 10; 4
   c. 10; 6
   d. 16; 2

11. After an arm fracture, pendulum exercises are begun:
   a. as soon as tolerated.
   b. in 2 to 3 weeks, when callus ossification prevents easy movements of bony fragments.
   c. in about 4 to 5 weeks, after new bone is well established.
   d. in 2 to 3 months, after normal activities are resumed.

12. Nursing assessment for a pelvic fracture includes:
   a. checking the urine for hematuria.
   b. palpating peripheral pulses in both lower extremities.
   c. testing the stool for occult blood.
   d. all of the above.

13. The two most serious complications of pelvic fractures are:
   a. paresthesias and ischemia.
   b. hemorrhage and shock.
   c. paralytic ileus and a lacerated urethra.
   d. thrombophlebitis and infection.

14. An intracapsular fracture of the femur involves the:
   a. neck of the femur.
   b. shaft of the femur.
   c. supracondylar area of the femur.
   d. trochanteric region of the femur.

15. The femur fracture that commonly leads to aseptic necrosis or nonunion because of an abundant supply of blood vessels in the area is a fracture of the:
   a. condylar area.
   b. neck.
   c. shaft.
   d. trochanteric region.

16. The most common complication of a hip fracture in the elderly is:
   a. avascular necrosis.
   b. infection.
   c. nonunion.
   d. thromboembolism.

17. An immediate nursing concern for a patient who has suffered a femoral shaft fracture is assessment for:
   a. hypovolemic shock.
   b. infection.
   c. knee and hip dislocation.
   d. pain resulting from muscle spasm.

18. The major indicator of lower extremity amputation is:
   a. congenital deformity.
   b. malignant tumor.
   c. peripheral vascular disease.
   d. trauma.

19. A complication(s) of an upper extremity amputation would be:
   a. contact dermatitis.
   b. infection and necrosis.
   c. phantom sensations.
   d. all of the above.

20. A nurse can foster a positive self-image in a patient who has had an amputation by all of the following *except*:
   a. encouraging the patient to care for the residual limb.
   b. allowing the expression of grief.
   c. introducing the patient to local amputee support groups.
   d. encouraging family and friends to refrain from visiting temporarily because this may increase the patient's embarrassment.

Matching Items

Match the type of fracture in Column II with its descriptive terminology listed in Column I.

Part I

Column I

1. _____C_____ A break occurs across the entire section of the bone.

2. _____A_____ A fragment of the bone is pulled off by a ligament or tendon.

3. _____B_____ Bone is splintered into several fragments.

4. _____E_____ One side of a bone is broken and the other side is bent.

Column II

a. avulsion

b. comminuted

c. complete

d. epiphyseal

e. greenstick

Part II

Column I

1. _____C_____ A fracture occurs at an angle across the bone.

2. _____B_____ Fragments are driven inward.

3. _____A_____ The fractured bone is compressed by another bone.

4. _____D_____ The fracture extends through the skin.

Column II

a. compressed

b. depressed

c. oblique

d. open

e. pathologic

II. Critical Analysis Questions

Generating Solutions: Clinical Problem Solving

Read the following case study. Circle the correct answers.

CASE STUDY: Above-the-Knee Amputation

William, a 70-year-old Catholic priest, lives in a center city rectory. He is scheduled to have an above-the-knee amputation of his left leg because of peripheral vascular disease.

1. Preoperatively the nurse knows that the circulatory status of the affected limb should be evaluated by assessing for:
   a. color and temperature.
   b. palpable pulses.
   c. positioning responses.
   d. all of the above.

2. The level of William's amputation was determined after assessing:
   a. the circulatory status of the affected limb.
   b. the type of prosthesis to be used.
   c. William's ability to understand and use the prosthetic device.
   d. all of the above.

3. Preoperatively the nurse needs to assist William in exercising the muscles needed for crutch walking. The major muscle to be strengthened is the:
   a. pectoralis major.
   b. gastrocnemius.
   c. quadriceps femoris.
   d. triceps brachii.

4. Postoperatively William experiences phantom limb sensations. The most appropriate nursing response is to:
   a. agree with his statements, recognizing that he is expressing a psychological need.
   b. consistently stress the absence of the lower leg.
   c. disagree with him and reorient him to reality.
   d. keep him as active as possible and encourage self-expression.

5. William's amputation is treated with a soft compression dressing. Nursing care would include all of the following *except*:
   a. keeping the residual limb slightly elevated on a pillow to decrease edema.
   b. monitoring vital signs to detect any indication of bleeding.
   c. placing the residual limb in an extended position, with brief periods of elevation.
   d. keeping a tourniquet nearby in case of hemorrhage.

6. Preprosthetic nursing care should attempt to avoid any problem that can delay prosthetic fitting, such as:
   a. abduction deformities of the hip.
   b. flexion deformities.
   c. nonshrinkage of the residual limb.
   d. all of the above.

7. The nurse who is preparing to apply a bandage to William's residual limb knows that she should:
   a. anchor the bandage on the posterior surface of the residual limb.
   b. begin the vertical turns on the anterior surface of the residual limb.
   c. maintain the residual limb in a position of flexion while bandaging.
   d. use circular turns that run in a horizontal plane from the proximal to the distal segment.

8. The nurse teaches William to massage his residual limb to:
   a. decrease local tenderness.
   b. improve vascularity.
   c. mobilize the scar.
   d. accomplish all of the above.

Learner's Self-Evaluation Tool for End of Unit 16 Review

1. The most important concepts or facts that I have learned from this unit are:

   1. _____

   2. _____

   3. _____

2. The most important reference page numbers for test review and clinical concepts are pages:

   _____ _____ _____

   _____ _____ _____

3. The concepts or facts that I do not fully understand are:

   _____

   _____

4. I will get the answer(s) to my questions by _____

   _____

   I will do this on _____ (date and time).

5. I believe my mastery of this unit to be:
   a.   100%   Great job! Good luck!
   b.   90%   2 hours of review recommended.
   c.   80%   4 hours of review recommended.
   d.   <80%   Make an appointment with your instructor.

UNIT 17
Other Acute Problems

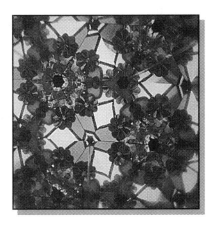

65

Management of Patients With Infectious Diseases

Chapter Overview

Diseases of an infectious nature are potentially life-threatening and are managed with chemotherapy or isolation measures, or both. Nurses should be aware of the mechanisms of disease incubation and transmission and follow expected protocols of disease control. The patient needs to understand the severity of his or her disease and its potential for harm. In addition, the nurse should assure the patient that he or she is not "dirty" and that isolation measures are used to protect the patient and others from the disease, not to isolate or ignore him or her.

When a new infectious disease surfaces and knowledge about the organism is insufficient to determine medical management (*e.g.*, AIDS), protective isolation measures are instituted. Again, nursing interventions are directed toward meeting the psychosocial needs associated with strict isolation procedures and helping family members deal with their fears and anxieties.

FACTS:

- *The CDC 24-hour telephone hotline for information about pediatric or adult vaccine advice is 1-404-332-4553.*

- *The 24-hour Traveler's Hotline for communicable disease while traveling abroad is 1-404-332-4559.*

- *Chickenpox vaccine was approved in spring, 1995, with an immunization schedule, by the American Academy of Pediatrics.*

I. Knowledge-Based Questions

Deduction and Interpretation

Read each question carefully. Circle your answer.

1. The single most important means of preventing the spread of infection is:
   a. antibiotic therapy.
   b. gowning and gloving.
   c. handwashing.
   d. isolation measures.

2. The blood-borne pathogen of greatest concern for occupational transmission in the 1990s is:
   a. hepatitis B virus (HBV)
   b. hepatitis C virus (HCV)
   c. human immunodeficiency virus (HIV)
   d. all three are of major concern.

 Mary Jo Boyer: Study Guide to Accompany Brunner & Suddarth's Textbook of Medical-Surgical Nursing, 8th ed. © 1996 Lippincott-Raven Publishers

3. The most important potential source of pathogens such as HIV, HBV, and HCV is:
a. blood.
b. cerebrospinal fluid.
c. peritoneal fluid.
d. semen and vaginal secretions.

4. A fluid not associated with the risk of blood-borne transmission is:
a. amniotic fluid.
b. pericardial fluid.
c. synovial fluid.
d. urine.

5. Each year nosocomial infections affect about _____ patients.
a. 250,000
b. 1/2 million
c. 1 million
d. 2 million

6. A gram-positive organism that is less virulent than a gram-negative organism is:
a. *Escherichia coli.*
b. *Pseudomonas aeruginosa.*
c. *Proteus.*
d. *Staphylococcus aureus.*

7. The nurse should know that the mortality rate associated with nosocomial pneumonia is about:
a. 10%.
b. 25%.
c. 50%.
d. 80%.

8. MRSA is a common nosocomial infection caused by _____, the most frequently occurring pathogen identified with this disorder.
a. *Escherichia coli.*
b. *Proteus.*
c. *Pseudomonas aeruginosa.*
d. *Staphylococcus aureus.*

9. Gonorrhea is a sexually transmitted infection that involves the mucosal surface of the:
a. genitourinary tract.
b. pharynx.
c. rectum.
d. areas mentioned above.

10. Acquired immunodeficiency syndrome (AIDS) is a:
a. condition of unknown cause.
b. disorder of immunoregulation.
c. syndrome associated with high mortality.
d. condition consistent with all of the above.

11. Late syphilitic lesions may appear _____ after early manifestations disappear.
a. 2 to 3 months.
b. 3 to 6 months.
c. 1 to 2 years.
d. about 4 years.

12. The primary site for gonorrhea in women is the:
a. urethra.
b. kidney.
c. vagina.
d. uterine cervix.

13. Characteristics of the tuberculosis mycobacterium include all of the following *except* that it:
a. can be transmitted only by droplet nuclei.
b. is able to lie dormant within the body for years.
c. is acid-fast.
d. survives in anaerobic conditions.

14. For the tubercle bacillus to multiply and initiate a tissue reaction in the lungs, it must be deposited in:
a. the alveoli.
b. the bronchi.
c. the trachea.
d. all of the above tissues.

15. Patients with hepatitis B infection are considered infectious for at least:
a. 6 months.
b. 12 months.
c. 2 years.
d. 4 years.

16. Hepatitis C is primarily transmitted:
a. parenterally.
b. perinatally.
c. sexually.
d. by contaminated food.

17. Gas gangrene is caused by a species of gram-positive *Clostridium* that can be treated by:
a. chemotherapy.
b. hyperbaric oxygenation.
c. surgery.
d. all of the above.

II. Critical Analysis Questions

Recognizing Contradictions

Read each statement correctly. Underline the key concepts.

1. The purpose of the Occupational Safety and Health Administration (OSHA) agency is the investigation and prevention of communicable disease.

2. The underlying premise of Universal Precautions is that barrier precautions be taken for patients who are believed to be infected.

3. Used needles should be recapped so they do not puncture someone by mistake.

4. Gonorrhea and syphilis are different strains of the same microorganism.

5. Hepatitis B is transmitted primarily by the fecal–oral route.

6. Most cases of Rocky Mountain spotted fever occur in the Rockies.

7. There are currently ten vaccines licensed in the United States, for example, measles, mumps, rubella.

8. Mumps is also referred to as rubeola.

66

Emergency Nursing

Chapter Overview

Emergency management for injuries and trauma requires a collaborative effort of the physician, nurse, and emergency team. Nursing care depends on constant assessment of a patient's changing status.

Specifics of nursing interventions will depend on the injury. Nursing care should be provided in a calm, efficient manner, and the patient and his or her family should be kept informed with concise, simple statements. Explanations may need to be given repeatedly because of the high level of anxiety that emergency departments tend to create.

I. Knowledge-Based Questions

Deduction and Interpretation

Read each question carefully. Circle your answer.

1. The elderly, who are major consumers of emergency health care, account for about _____ of visits to the emergency room.
   a. 50%.
   b. 15%.
   c. 25%.
   d. 45%.

2. John, 16 years old, is brought to the emergency department after a vehicular accident. He is pronounced dead on arrival (DOA). When his parents arrive at the hospital, the nurse should:
   a. ask them to sit in the waiting room until she can spend time alone with them.
   b. speak to both parents together and encourage them to support each other and express their emotions freely.
   c. speak to one parent at a time in a private setting so that each can ventilate feelings of loss without upsetting the other.
   d. ask the emergency physician to medicate the parents so that they can handle their son's unexpected death quietly and without hysteria.

3. An oropharyngeal airway should be inserted:
   a. at an angle of 90 degrees.
   b. upside down and then rotated 180 degrees.
   c. with the concave portion touching the posterior pharynx.
   d. with the convex portion facing upward.

4. A clinical indicator(s) for emergency endotracheal intubation is(are):
   a. airway obstruction.
   b. respiratory arrest.
   c. respiratory insufficiency.
   d. all of the above.

5. Drowning is the fourth leading cause of accidental death with about _____ occurring to children under 4 years of age.
   a. 10%
   b. 25%
   c. 40%
   d. 75%

6. The initial nursing measure for the control of hemorrhage caused by trauma is to:
   a. apply a tourniquet.
   b. apply firm pressure over the involved area or artery.
   c. elevate the injured part.
   d. immobilize the area to control blood loss.

7. Indicators of hypovolemic shock associated with internal bleeding include all of the following *except*:
   a. bradycardia.
   b. cool, moist skin.
   c. hypotension.
   d. thirst.

8. The most common cause of shock in emergency situations is:
   a. cardiac failure.
   b. decreased arterial resistance.
   c. hypovolemia.
   d. septicemia.

9. Nursing management for a crushing lower extremity wound includes:
   a. applying a clean dressing to protect the wound.
   b. elevating the site to limit the accumulation of fluid in the interstitial spaces.
   c. splinting the wound in a position of rest to prevent motion.
   d. all of the above measures.

10. A nursing measure(s) for a penetrating abdominal injury would include:
   a. assessing for manifestations of hemorrhage.
   b. covering any protruding viscera with sterile dressings soaked in normal saline solution.
   c. looking for any associated chest injuries.
   d. all of the above actions.

11. Identify the sequence of medical or nursing management for a patient who experiences multiple injuries.
   a. Assess for head injuries, control hemorrhage, establish an airway, prevent hypovolemic shock.
   b. Control hemorrhage, prevent hypovolemic shock, establish an airway, assess for head injuries.
   c. Establish an airway, control hemorrhage, prevent hypovolemic shock, assess for head injuries.
   d. Prevent hypovolemic shock, assess for head injuries, establish an airway, control hemorrhage.

12. A nursing measure(s) for an extremity fracture would include:
   a. assessing for manifestations of shock.
   b. immobilizing the fracture site.
   c. palpating peripheral pulses.
   d. all of the above actions.

13. Progressive deterioration of body systems occurs when hypothermia lowers the body temperature to:
   a. 98°F.
   b. 97°F.
   c. 96°F.
   d. 95°F.

14. Rose, a 19-year-old student, has been sexually assaulted. When assisting with the physical examination, the nurse should do all of the following *except*:
   a. have the patient shower or wash the perineal area before the examination.
   b. assess and document any bruises and lacerations.
   c. record a history of the event, using the patient's own words.
   d. label all torn or bloody clothes and place each item in a separate brown bag so that any evidence can be given to the police.

II. Critical Analysis Questions

Generating Solutions: Clinical Problem Solvin

For each of the following situations, identify a nursing action with supporting rationale.

1. Condition   **Action**   **Rationale**

Heimlich maneuver for standing or   1. _____   _____
sitting conscious patient   2. _____   _____
                                       3. _____   _____

Heimlich maneuver with patient lying   1. _____   _____
unconscious   2. _____   _____
                                       3. _____   _____

Finger sweep   1. _____   _____
                                       2. _____   _____
                                       3. _____   _____

Chest thrusts with conscious patient   1. _____   _____
standing or sitting   2. _____   _____
                                       3. _____   _____

Chest thrusts with patient lying   1. _____   _____
(unconscious)   2. _____   _____
                                       3. _____   _____

For each of the following situations, supply nursing diagnosis, nursing interventions and supporting rationales for intervention.

2. Consider a patient who has experienced blunt, abdominal trauma. Formulate nursing diagnoses and nursing interventions for the patient in the emergency department. Cite a rationale for each nursing action. List interventions in order of priority.

Nursing Diagnosis   **Nursing Interventions**   **Rationale**

3. List the emergency nursing measures you would carry out if you were present when someone experienced an anaphylactic reaction to a bee sting. Formulate nursing diagnoses, list nursing interventions, and cite supporting rationales for your actions.

Nursing Diagnosis   **Nursing Interventions**   **Rationale**

4. Ann is admitted to the emergency department because she ingested approximately 30 diet capsules 1 hour before admission. The nurse is to assist with gastric lavage. State nursing diagnoses, with nursing interventions and supporting rationale for each action.

Nursing Diagnosis   *Nursing Interventions*   *Rationale*

5. List specific nursing interventions that can be used for drug abuse with each of the following drugs. It is assumed that the patient is presenting to the emergency department for treatment.

Drug   *Nursing Interventions*

Cocaine

Dexedrine

Valium

Aspirin

6. Compare nursing actions for psychiatric emergencies in dealing with the following patients.

Psychiatric Patients   *Nursing Actions*

An overactive patient

A violent patient

A depressed patient

A suicidal patient

Learner's Self-Evaluation Tool for End of Unit 17 Review

1. The most important concepts or facts that I have learned from this unit are:

1. _____

2. _____

3. _____

2. The most important reference page numbers for test review and clinical concepts are pages:

_____   _____   _____

_____   _____   _____

3. The concepts or facts that I do not fully understand are:

_____

_____

4. I will get the answer(s) to my questions by _____

_____

I will do this on _____ (date and time).

5. I believe my mastery of this unit to be:
    a.   100%   Great job! Good luck!
    b.   90%   2 hours of review recommended.
    c.   80%   4 hours of review recommended.
    d.   <80%   Make an appointment with your instructor.

Chapter Summaries

Chapter 1 **Health Care Delivery and Nursing Practice**

- During the past several decades, major changes in the health care delivery system have occurred as a result of societal, technological, economic, political, and demographic changes. Emphasis has shifted from disease cure and prevention to health maintenance and promotion.

- The spiraling costs of health care have led to cost-containment measures, managed health care systems, and renewed national interest in and demand for health care reform.

- Care that was once provided primarily in hospitals is now being redirected to outpatient settings, the community, and the home.

- Nursing has been significantly affected by the changes in the delivery of health care. The profession and its practitioners are challenged by increased acuity of patients in hospitals, shortened hospital stays, increased utilization of outpatient services, and the increasing trend toward care in the home and community.

- Nursing is meeting these challenges through measures directed toward maintaining quality of care and services while at the same time promoting continuity of care, effective utilization of services, and cost containment.

- Primary nursing, case management, advanced practice roles, and multidisciplinary collaboration are being utilized to promote health care that will effectively and efficiently meet the needs of patients in a variety of settings.

Chapter 2 **Community-Based Nursing Practice**

- Changes in the health care system have increased the needs for medical-surgical nurses to practice in community-based settings.

- Nurses working in community settings face different conditions from those who work in hospitals. Nurses making home visits are essentially guests in the patient's home.

- Discharge planning and collaboration with other health care providers are an important aspect of community-based care.

- Community-based nurses work in a variety of ambulatory health care settings and provide nursing care based on the needs of the patients they serve.

- A systematic process is involved in preparing for and conducting a home visit.

Chapter 3 **Critical Thinking and the Nursing Process**

- Critical thinking skills that involve analysis, synthesis, interpretation, and decision making are required in all encounters that the nurse has with the patient. They are used in all phases of the nursing process.

- The nursing process is a deliberate, problem-identification, and problem-solving approach to meeting the health care and nursing needs of patients.

- The cyclic and recurrent steps of the nursing process are assessment, diagnosis, planning, implementation, and evaluation. Each step is ongoing and is related to all other steps.

Chapter 4 **Health Education and Health Promotion**

- The goal of health education is to teach people to strive toward achievement of their maximum health potentials.

- The teaching–learning process is an integral part of the nursing process and consists of the same recurrent steps: assessment, diagnosis, planning, implementation, and evaluation. Each step is ongoing and is related to all other steps.

- Continuous evaluation provides the means for maintaining the effectiveness of the entire teaching–learning process and for demonstrating accountability for the quality of the teaching provided.

- Health promotion is an active process, the purpose of which is to focus on the person's potential for wellness and to encourage a change in personal habits, life-style, and environment in ways that will enhance health and well-being.

- Health promotion involves the principles of self-responsibility, nutritional awareness, stress reduction and management, and physical fitness.

- Health promotion is not limited to any particular age group but extends throughout the life span for people of both sexes and all socioeconomic and cultural backgrounds, and it applies both to those who have no health problems and to those with chronic illnesses and disabilities.

- Nurses are assuming vital roles in health promotion. They are involved in developing programs and in leading interdisciplinary teams in providing health promotion services.

- The promotion of positive health attitudes and behaviors has become an integral component of nursing care in all practice settings.

Chapter 5 **Ethical Issues in Medical-Surgical Nursing**

- Ethics refers to formal theory, rules, principles or codes of conduct to determine the right course of action.

- Morality refers to the individual's values that incorporate a sense of right and wrong.

- Moral dilemmas involve a clear conflict between two or more moral claims.

- Applied ethics utilizes ethical discussion to arrive at a morally correct decision in a specific discipline.

- Ethical terms help clarify the realm of moral philosophy. From a broad perspective, there are different approaches to the study of ethical issues. When one is attempting to answer questions regarding a specific course of action, one is engaging in normative ethics.

- Historically there are two common types of ethical theory: teleological (or utilitarianism), which is predominantly concerned with the consequences of the action, and deontological (or formalism), which is concerned with adherence to moral principles. Within these two frameworks there are a variety of perspectives espoused by different philosophers.

- In practice, many people use a combination of these two approaches. Combining these methods is called ethical pluralism. With a pluralistic framework, individuals incorporate the universal moral principles in the moral reasoning process, but they will also take into consideration various virtues or behaviors as well as the ethos of the profession as they attempt to answer the normative question, "What should I do in this situation?"

- Nursing ethical behavior is described in ANA's code of ethics.

- Common ethical principles include autonomy, beneficence, confidentiality, double effect, fidelity, justice, nonmaleficence, paternalism, respect for persons, sanctity of life and veracity.

- Ethical decision making involves analyzing the ethical situation, identifying and validating all pertinent information, identifying alternative courses of action, and choosing an action based on a determinant of what appears to be morally correct.

Chapter 6   Clinical Interviewing: The Health History

- The process of eliciting a health history is a complex one that requires knowledge and understanding, clinical experience, and reinforcement in the practice setting. There is no one way to approach a patient or to elicit a health history.

- The nurse is encouraged to develop a style of interviewing that is personally comfortable and to use a health history format that is flexible to accommodate the practice setting and the person's needs. The health history format and interviewing techniques outlined in this chapter are presented as guidelines for acquiring the initial components of the data base.

- The health history is conducted to obtain information about the person's health problem; functional status; medical history; psychosocial, ethnic, and cultural factors; life-style; health-related behaviors; family and interpersonal relationships; and a general patient profile.

- The health history should be conducted in an open manner that informs the person being interviewed of the purpose of the interview and the manner in which the information gathered will be used.

- The interview should be conducted in such a way as to reduce anxiety, encourage communication, provide for a flexible approach to collect the information, avoid personal biases, promote understanding, and consider cultural factors.

- The history database covers such pertinent information as biographical data, past and present health problems, family history, diagnostic tests, patient profile, and a possible review of body systems or functional state.

- The health history of an elderly person should include questions related to any subtle changes in functioning and a complete history of medications taken. If necessary, a family member can be present to provide additional information.

Chapter 7   Physical Assessment and Nutritional Assessment

- Inspection, palpation, percussion, and auscultation are assessment skills that can be mastered with practice and experience. These skills provide valuable information that is useful to follow up and confirm information obtained through the health history.

- Inspection provides an opportunity to gain information about general appearance, posture, stature, body movements, nutrition, speech patterns, and temperature.

- Palpation elicits information through the sense of touch. Sounds such as murmurs, thrills, and tactile fremitus may be detected with this technique.

- Percussion involves striking the finger of one hand with the finger of the other hand to produce sound that reflects the density of the underlying structure.

- Auscultation detects specific body sounds such as bowel sounds and heart sounds, which are amplified by a stethoscope.

- Assessment of a person's nutritional status provides information about the person's previous dietary intake, understanding of the principles of good nutrition, and the availability of resources for purchase and consumption of an adequate diet.

- Nutritional assessment may identify those who are poorly nourished and at risk for complications of illness and hospitalization because of poor nutrition. Early detection of these risks enables the nurse to intervene to prevent such occurrences or minimize their severity.

Chapter 8   Homeostasis and Pathophysiologic Processes

- The natural protective mechanisms that sustain life include adaptive and homeostatic processes that maintain the constancy or steady state of the internal environment so that changes in temperature, fluid and electrolyte balance, acid–base balance, and so on are compensated for and balance is maintained within a narrow range. These processes occur rapidly and go on constantly. Adaptive responses, when repeated over time, cause changes in structures and functions.

- When homeostatic and adaptive responses fail, disease sets in and the structure and function of cells, tissues, and organs are altered. Pathologic changes in structure and pathophysiologic mechanisms become operative. If not halted, death will ensue.

- Injury to the cell has many causes, including physical, chemical, and infectious agents; problems of immunity; genetic defects; hypoxia; nutritional imbalance; and psychogenic factors.

- Inflammation is a defensive response to injury and results in the following five signs: redness, heat, swelling, pain, and loss of function. Inflammation may be acute, chronic, or subacute.

- Repair and healing take place through regeneration or replacement.

- Physiologic and pathophysiologic mechanisms have characteristic signs and symptoms. The optimal point of intervention to promote health and prevent disease is when the person's own compensatory mechanisms are working. When assessing clients, nurses can detect variations from normal and plan interventions to support compensation and reduce further disordered function.

Chapter 9   Stress and Adaptation

- Stressors create a change in a person's dynamic balance or equilibrium. The amount of stress that results will be influenced by the number of stressors that occur simultaneously, previous experience with the stressors, the individual's appraisal of the stressors, the organ or system of the body affected, and the magnitude and duration of the stressors.

- Each person has a range within which he or she is capable of adapting to change and the stress that results. Changes occurring within this range produce demands that fall within the individual's existing coping ability. Changes falling outside this range lead to imbalance and require readjustment; such readjustment may lead to a new adaptation level, increasing the person's repertoire of adaptive responses.

- The body's physiologic response to a stressor is an adaptive mechanism directed toward maintaining equilibrium. The initial components of this physiologic response, the sympathetic response and the sympathetic-adrenal-medullary response, occur in almost all stressful situations. The observable behaviors (*e.g.,* changes in blood pressure and pulse rate) may vary, but the essential neuroendocrine response is the same.

- With the onset of the more chronic phase of the physiologic response there is great variability. The hypothalamic-pituitary-adrenal-cortical response will be activated in most cases, but the total pattern of the endocrine response will vary with the nature, duration, and severity of the chronic stressor. With continued exposure to the same stressor, the response will be attenuated.

- People perceive and react to situations and change differently depending on personal characteristics, abilities, experiences, external support systems, and the characteristics of the stressor itself. The stress response produced may be elicited by real, potential, or imagined threats. Individuals who can mobilize their energy resources to cope with the stressor will experience adaptive outcomes.

- In the health care setting, it is the nurse's role to appraise and diagnose the individual's health state (including life-style, self-care activities, health promotion activities, coping behaviors, and resources) and to support and instruct the person in stress reduction or coping enhancement techniques.

- Strategies available to help reduce stress include common relaxation techniques, education, support groups, therapy groups, and health-promoting life-style practices.

Chapter 10   Human Response to Illness

- Illness is an unpredictable event that has an impact on one's homeostasis and sense of well-being. Moving from health to illness is a process to which each individual adapts in stages based on past coping behaviors.

- To facilitate the patient's adaptation to illness or injury, the nurse must use effective communication. Communication is an essential mechanism by which the nurse can assess and intervene to meet mutually established goals.

- Caring for the dying patient involves examining one's own feelings about death and at the same time utilizing the entire scope of nursing knowledge and judgment to provide physical and emotional care and comfort.

Chapter 11   Transcultural Perspectives in Nursing

- Transcultural nursing refers to a formal area of study and practice that focuses on the cultural care values, beliefs, and practices of individuals and groups from a particular culture. Its focus is to provide culture-specific and culture-universal care that promotes well-being or health for individuals, families, groups, communities, and/or institutions.

- Subcultures may be based on ethnicity, religion, occupation, age, gender, sexual orientation, or geographic location.

- Minority refers to a group of people who may be isolated or treated differently from others in a society because of certain physical or cultural characteristics.

- In order to provide culturally congruent care, the nurse must practice cultural or culturologic assessment—a systematic appraisal or examination of individuals, families, groups, and communities in terms of their cultural beliefs, values, and practices.

- When communicating cross-culturally, the nurse should note the following signals of a lack of effective communication: efforts to change the subject; absence of questions; inappropriate laughter; and nonverbal cues.

- Space and distance, eye contact, time, touch, observance of holidays, and diet are key areas in which the nurse must be aware of the potential for vast differences in cultural actions and attitudes.

- Three major views that attempt to explain causes of disease or illness are the biomedical/scientific, the naturalistic/holistic, and the magico/religious.

- Some cultures may turn to a folk or indigenous healer to treat disease or sickness.

Chapter 12   Health Care of the Older Adult

- The population over age 65 is growing in numbers and in average age. Health problems, particularly those associated with chronic illness, increase with age. To proide optimal health care to elderly persons, nurses must work cooperatively with other health professionals. Emphasis of care must be on promotion of health and maximizing independence.

- Ageism and negative false beliefs are common in the United States. Older people know these beliefs, and many unconsciously adjust their behavior to correspond to them. Adaptation and life patterns continue across a lifetime. The older adult will most likely achieve a successful life adjustment by retaining a connection with the past.

- Normal changes of aging occur universally and negatively affect body system functions. However, many age-related symptoms can be delayed or minimized if the person practices preventive health measures and avoids known health risks. Learning and cognitive abilities remain intact in the absence of disease. Although the prevalence of chronic illness increases with age, many older people lead satisfying and active lives.

- Mental health disorders are a major problem that threaten the quality of life for older persons. Depression is the most common affective disorder of later life and is often responsive to treatment. Organic mental disorders or syndromes are associated with cognitive, physical, and behavioral dysfunctions that reflect pathologic changes of the brain. Alzheimer's disease is the most common organic mental disorder; it is chronic, progressive, and irreversible. Delirium, an acute, reversible confusion, requires immediate treatment of the underlying cause.

- Treatment of illnesses and relief of discomfort can be achieved with the prudent use of medications. Because of normal age changes that affect the absorption, distribution, metabolism, and elimination of drugs, the numbers and dosages must be carefully monitored. Drug interactions and drug toxicities occur commonly.

- Chronic illness is often accompanied by symptoms that cause discomfort. Commonly occurring health problems include urinary incontinence, fatigue, headaches, back pain, sleep disturbances, indigestion, dyspnea, and foot problems. Medical evaluation, necessary treatment, and life-style changes may be necessary to increase comfort.

- The family is the main source of social support for the older adult. Most elderly live near at least one of their children. There is mutual support between the generations, and adult children care very much about the welfare of their parents. In combination with community supports and services, the family can often enable the older person to stay in the community despite some dependency needs. Modification of the environment can enhance function and foster independence. Falls, the major cause of accidents in older adults, can sometimes be prevented with reduction of environmental hazards. To preserve future autonomy the older person should be encouraged to give advance directives regarding financial and personal decisions to be made in the event of incapacitation.

- Older people have increased susceptibility to serious infectious diseases, including pneumonia, urinary tract infections, tuberculosis, gastrointestinal infections, and skin infections. The manner in which older adults manifest signs of acute illness differs physically, emotionally, and systemically from that of younger persons. Reserve capacity, the body's ability to continue efficiently in the presence of stress, is diminished.

- If at some point the older adult needs an alternative living arrangement, the family must allow him or her to share in the decisions if at all possible. Retirement communities, continuing care communities, and nursing homes are among the choices available. Finances, state of health, individual needs, and availability are all factors to be considered in the decision-making process. Prevention and planning ahead can ease the many transitions that are evident in the life of the older adult.

Chapter 13   Pain Management

- Pain is an unpleasant sensory or emotional experience that occurs with many disease processes or during some diagnostic tests or treatments.

- Pain may be acute (lasting from a few seconds to 6 months) or chronic (lasting more than 6 months).

- The nociceptive system controls the transmission and perception of pain.

- Chemicals such as histamine, bradykinin, and acetylcholine increase the transmission or perception of pain. Endorphins and enkephalins are morphine-like substances produced by the body to inhibit the transmission and perception of pain.

- The gate control theory proposes that the stimulation of nerve fibers that transmit non-painful sensations blocks or decreases the transmission of pain impulses.

- Assessing pain is based on the person's verbal description of the pain, his or her behavioral reactions, and how he or she rates the pain on a pain scale.

- Pain is influenced by past experience with pain, anxiety, culture, age, and one's expectation about how pain relief measures will work.

- The preventive approach in pharmacologic interventions for pain relief advocates maintaining a therapeutic level of medication by administering pain medication at set intervals.

- Patient-controlled analgesia allows the patient to self-administer continuous infusions of medication within limits of safety.

- Analgesics are administered through the following routes: parenteral, oral, rectal, transdermal, and intraspinal.

- Common side effects of narcotics include respiratory depression, nausea, vomiting, constipation, and tolerance to the drug.

- Non-pharmacologic measures for managing pain include cutaneous stimulation, massage, ice and heat therapies, transcutaneous electrical nerve stimulation (TENS), distraction, relaxation techniques, guided imagery, and hypnosis.

- Body fluids, consisting of water and electrolytes, make up 60% of the weight of an average adult. The fluid is divided between the intracellular and extracellular fluid compartments, with the balance being regulated by a series of complex mechanisms, including the action of osmosis and diffusion, the concentration or osmolality of the dissolved electrolytes, the sodium–potassium pump, and the function of the kidneys, lungs, skin, and gastrointestinal tract.

- The main electrolytes in body fluid are cations, which are negatively charged ions, and anions, which are positively charged ions. The major cations are sodium, potassium, calcium, and magnesium. The major anions are chloride, bicarbonate, phosphate, and sulfate. Sodium is the major cation found in extracellular fluid; potassium is the major cation in intracellular fluid. The balance of sodium and potassium is a key factor in maintaining fluid and electrolyte balance.

- Key laboratory tests to evaluate fluid status include osmolality, urine specific gravity, blood urea nitrogen (BUN), creatinine, hematocrit, and urine sodium values.

- In addition to the role of the kidneys and lungs in maintaining fluid balance, the release of antidiuretic hormone (ADH) from the pituitary and aldosterone and cortisol from the adrenal glands, along with parathyroid hormone from the parathyroids, controls the levels of water, sodium, potassium, calcium and phosphate, respectively. Renin, an enzyme, also affects fluid balance.

- Fluid volume disturbances are categorized as fluid volume deficit (hypovolemia) or fluid volume excess (hypervolemia).

- Fluid volume deficit (FVD) occurs most frequently with the loss of water and electrolytes through vomiting, diarrhea, fever, blood loss, burns, and gastrointestinal suctioning, or with decreased fluid intake. Some of the signs of FVD include decreased urine output, decreased blood pressure, rapid pulse, weakness, dizziness, increased pulse, and decreased skin turgor. Increasing fluid intake, either orally or by IV, is the usual treatment, depending on the cause and the patient's condition.

- Nursing management of FVD includes carefully monitoring fluid intake and output; watching for excessive urination, diarrhea, or vomiting; taking daily weights; and checking vital signs, skin turgor, and mental function.

- Fluid volume excess (FVE) can result from renal failure, congestive heart failure, cirrhosis, administration of too much IV fluid containing sodium, severe stress, and hyperaldosteronism. Major manifestations include acute weight gain, edema, elevated blood pressure, bounding pulse, crackles, and distended neck veins. Diuretics and sodium restrictions are key management approaches.

- Nursing interventions for FVE include assessing for fluid retention by monitoring intake and output, weight, breath sounds, and edema; implementing sodium and fluid restriction; and administering diuretics as prescribed.

- Electrolyte imbalances include sodium deficits or excesses (hyponatremia or hypernatremia), potassium deficits or excesses (hypokalemia or hyperkalemia), calcium deficits or excesses (hypocalcemia or hypercalcemia), magnesium deficits or excesses (hypomagnesemia or hypermagnesemia), and phosphorus deficits or excesses (hypophosphatemia or hyperphosphatemia).

- Because these imbalances can be severe and life threatening, nursing care must involve monitoring those patients at risk and carrying out astute assessments to detect their occurrences and prevention. Vital signs; urine output; fluid intake; mentation; respiratory function; breath sounds; weight; skin turgor; the presence of diarrhea, vomiting, or nausea; and gastric suctioning are part of the daily assessment parameters for detecting possible problems.

- The four types of acid–base imbalances are metabolic acidosis, metabolic alkalosis, respiratory acidosis, and respiratory alkalosis.

- Maintaining plasma pH (hydrogen ion concentration) in the normal range of 7.35 to 7.45 is essential for acid–base balance and is carried out by hemostatic mechanisms related to chemical buffering (bicarbonate–carbonic acid ratios) and the functions of the kidneys and lungs.

- In the bicarbonate–carbonic acid buffering system, the normal ratio is 20 parts of bicarbonate to 1 part of carbonic acid. Carbon dioxide dissolved in water becomes carbonic acid.

- In respiratory acidosis and metabolic acidosis, the kidneys excrete hydrogen ions and conserve bicarbonate. In respiratory and metabolic alkalosis, the kidneys retain hydrogen ions and excrete bicarbonate.

- Metabolic acidosis is a base bicarbonate deficit with a low pH. Loss of bicarbonate from diarrhea and excess chloride intake are possible causes.

- Metabolic alkalosis is a base bicarbonate excess with a high pH and is frequently caused by vomiting and gastric suctioning with loss of hydrogen and chloride ions or by conditions that cause potassium loss.

- Respiratory acidosis is an excess of carbonic acid with a low pH and elevated $PaCO_2$, usually due to inadequate ventilation, which leads to elevated carbon dioxide and carbonic acid levels. Causes include pulmonary edema, atelectasis, pneumothorax, pneumonia, and adult respiratory distress syndrome, among others. Treatment is aimed at improving ventilation.

- Respiratory alkalosis is a carbonic acid deficit with elevated pH and decreased $PaCO_2$, due to hyperventilation possibly from anxiety, hypoxemia, or excessive ventilation by mechanical ventilation.

- IV solutions may be isotonic, with osmolality close to extracellular fluid and electrolyte content of 310 mEq/L; hypotonic, with electrolyte content less than 250 mEq/L; or hypertonic, with electrolyte content exceeding 375 mEq/L.

- Nursing responsibilities in IV therapy include selecting the appropriate site and cannula for the venipuncture, preparing the site, making a clean entry into the vein, setting and monitoring the flow or drip rate, and assessing for complications.

- Systemic complications include fluid overload, air embolism, septicemia, and infection. Local complications include infiltration, phlebitis, thrombophlebitis, hematoma, and clotting.

Chapter 15   Shock and Multisystem Failure

- Shock is a complex condition that results in an inadequate blood flow to body tissues.

- Shock occurs along a continuum across which the patient struggles to survive using all of the body's mechanisms of homeostasis.

- Shock can be classified according to its etiology as hypovolemic, cardiogenic, or distributive. All organ systems are affected by the shock syndrome, requiring ongoing systematic assessment.

- Management of shock involves fluid administration, careful titration of medications, and use of a variety of supportive modalities and technologies to preserve function and prevent complications.

- Nursing care of the shock patient requires a thorough understanding of physiologic processes, the ability to anticipate necessary treatments, and astute assessment skills. In addition to addressing the patient's physiologic needs, the nurse also must address the emotional and psychologic needs of the patient and family.

Chapter 16   Oncology: Nursing the Patient With Cancer

- Cancer is considered a systemic disease with multiple factors implicated in its etiology, including environmental, infectious, dietary, and hereditary influences.

- Carcinogenesis can be caused by a variety of factors. Certain viruses, genetic characteristics, and hormonal status are thought to play a role. In addition, environmental factors such as chemical exposure, diet, and physical phenomena are associated with cancer development. It is likely that a combination of several of these agents may be necessary to initiate and propagate malignant tumors.

- A major role of the nurse is in the area of prevention and screening. Teaching patients and others about risk factors, early detection strategies (*e.g.*, breast self-examination and testicular examination), warning signs, and health promotion measures is an important factor in cancer prevention and detection.

- Both the patient diagnosed with cancer and his or her family confront a major crisis. Although they may equate cancer with inevitable pain and death, successful cure or long-term control of cancer is increasing with advances in therapeutic modalities.

- The patient may undergo surgery for diagnosis and staging, for excision of the tumor, or for relief of symptoms.

- Additional cancer treatments include chemotherapy and radiation therapy. The patient who receives such treatments and the family require expert nursing care to deal effectively with the physiologic and psychologic consequences of cancer and its treatments.

- Effective rehabilitation of the patient with cancer requires that the nurse consider the long- and short-term needs of the patient and his family. Support persons and groups can be consulted before surgery or treatment is initiated as well as after treatment begins.

- Psychosocial and sexual needs of the patient and his family are as important as physiologic needs and require attention and skill from the nurse and other members of the health care team.

- For the patient with progressive disease, oncologic emergencies pose a significant threat to well-being and survival. The nurse must be aware of the risks for these complications and knowledgeable and skilled in assessing their occurrence; early detection increases the likelihood of early and successful treatment.

Chapter 17   Chronic Illness

- Chronic illness is a pervasive problem in modern society, affecting all ages and all groups.

- Chronic illness is a health problem that requires long-term management and affects many facets of a person's life.

- Adhering to the treatment regimen for a chronic illness is often difficult for the person with the illness.

- Chronic illness affects the whole family, causing adjustment in family relationships, roles, and daily living.

- Persons with chronic illness must assume major responsibility for the day-to-day management of the illness.

Chapter 18   Principles and Practices of Rehabilitation

- Rehabilitation is an integral part of nursing. It is a dynamic process that assists an individual, ill or disabled, in achieving his or her highest level of functioning and an acceptable quality of life with dignity, self-respect, and independence. Rehabilitation begins with the initial contact with the patient. Abilities, not disabilities, are emphasized. An interdisciplinary team approach is required. The individual with a disability is the key member of the rehabilitation team and an active participant in the rehabilitation process.

- The rehabilitation nurse develops a therapeutic relationship with the patient. Within the nursing process, the nurse helps the individual with a disability identify strengths and abilities, actively listens to and encourages him or her, and shares in the rehabilitation process. The nursing assessment may include a functional abilities index (*e.g.*, PULSES, Barthel Index, FIM, PECS). On the basis of the assessment and subsequent plan, the nurse helps the patient cope and adjust to the disability. The nurse focuses on facilitating self-care, improving mobility, promoting skin integrity, and managing bladder and bowel problems. In rehabilitation, the nurse assumes many roles, including caregiver, teacher, counselor, client advocate, consultant, and case manager.

- In facilitating self-care the nurse teaches, guides, and supports the patient and encourages his or her participation. Adaptive/assistive devices may be used to attain self-care goals. The patient is assisted in recognizing situations in which he or she needs assistance and in learning how to secure such assistance without overdependency.

- A goal of rehabilitation is reentry into the community. Transitions between levels of health care and resumption of independent self-care (or with necessary and appropriate assistance) in the community are planned. The community health nurse works with the rehabilitation team, the patient, the patient's support system, and available community services to optimize the transition.

- The Americans With Disabilities Act is civil rights legislation aimed at providing equal rights in employment, access, accommodation, and communication for persons with disabilities. The nurse can advocate for compliance with this law to eliminate discriminatory practices.

Chapter 19   Preoperative Nursing Management

- Perioperative nursing involves the use of the nursing process during the patient's surgical experience and encompasses three phases: preoperative (before surgery), intraoperative (during surgery), and postoperative (after surgery).

- The goals of preoperative nursing are to reduce patient anxiety and provide patient education.

- Common fears that contribute to preoperative patient anxiety are fear of the unknown and of possible death, fear of anesthesia, and fear of change in body image.

- Listening to and answering questions reduce the patient's anxiety.

- The content and teaching approach in patient education are individualized. Generally, preoperative patient education includes a description of the surgical procedure, the patient's role, a review of postoperative exercises, a discussion of preoperative procedures and pain medication, and expectations of postoperative care.

- The history and physical assessment performed in the preoperative phase provide the baseline for evaluating the intraoperative and postoperative courses. The nutritional status, degree of obesity, age, and data obtained from the review of systems and medication history are collectively considered when assessing surgical risk factors and planning specific interventions.

- Routine interventions include altering nutrition and fluid intake, skin preparation of surgical site, administration of preoperative medication, and completion of the preoperative checklist.

- Careful attention to psychologic and physical interventions prepares the patient optimally for the intraoperative phase.

Chapter 20   Intraoperative Nursing and Anesthesia

- The intraoperative phase, the second phase of perioperative nursing, focuses on the patient receiving anesthesia and undergoing surgery.

- The intraoperative nurse, anesthesiologist or nurse anesthetist, and surgeon work collaboratively to provide a safe outcome for the patient.

- Before surgery, the intraoperative nurse may visit the patient to establish rapport, discuss the experience, and answer questions.

- In the operating room, the nurse may assume a managing role as the circulating nurse or an assistant role as the scrub nurse. In either role, the intraoperative nurse maintains surgical asepsis by adhering to the operating room dress code and scrubbing procedure, identifying breaks in sterile technique, and using good health practices.

- The patient's safety needs are the primary concern. For the elderly patient this involves considerations of higher risk, including decreased response to stress, reduced gas exchange, and longer anesthetic effect.

- During surgery, the anesthesiologist or nurse anesthetist administers anesthesia and monitors vital signs, cardiac status, anesthesia levels, and adequacy of respiratory function and gas exchange.

- Anesthesia is classified as general or specific to a portion of the body. General anesthesia is usually administered by inhalation or intravenously; local anesthesia is injected directly into the tissues.

- General anesthesia is described in four stages of physiologic change: stages I, II, and III are normal, whereas stage IV is life threatening.

- Intravenous anesthetic agents have a rapid onset of action and are used for short procedures or as adjuncts to inhalation anesthesia in surgery of longer duration.

- Local anesthetic agents are used in spinal, regional, and local anesthesia. Other agents include neuromuscular blockers that promote relaxation during surgery.

- The nurse's observations, prompt reporting, and appropriate intervention in the intraoperative phase reduce the chance of complications and positively affect the postoperative course.

Chapter 21   Postoperative Nursing Management

- The postoperative phase, the third and last phase of perioperative nursing, centers on the recovery of the patient following surgery. Critical nursing assessment and prompt intervention promote the patient's return to optimal function and decrease the occurrence of postoperative complications that delay recovery. Nursing management in the postoperative phase includes the following: (1) patient care in the PACU and in the surgical nursing unit, (2) wound care and wound complications, and (3) other postoperative complications.

- Nursing management of the patient in the PACU focuses on adequate respiratory exchange, stabilization of vital signs, observation of the incision site, and comfort. In the PACU and after the patient's transfer from the PACU, nursing efforts focus on promotion of comfort, relief of pain, nausea and vomiting, and prevention or relief of abdominal and bladder distention.

- Wound healing is promoted in the postoperative phase by meticulous wound care, aseptic dressing change, and attention to factors that influence wound healing and skin integrity. Nursing assessment and intervention focus on postoperative complications that can prolong recovery and adversely affect the surgical outcome: shock; hemorrhage; deep vein thrombosis; pulmonary embolism; respiratory, urinary, and intestinal dysfunction; and psychologic disturbances.

- The increasing emphasis on ambulatory surgery and short hospital stays has reduced the preoperative and postoperative time available for preparation of the patient for surgery, postoperative teaching, and preparation for hospital discharge. Nurses are developing new strategies to prepare patients for surgery and to assist them in planning for postoperative care at home.

Chapter 22   Assessment of Respiratory Function

- Diagnosis of respiratory diseases is determined after a complete history, physical exam, and diagnostic studies. A variety of diagnostic tests may be performed to assist in the determination of respiratory conditions, including chest x-ray, CT scan, PET scan, pulmonary angiography, bronchoscopy, thoracentesis, sputum studies, arterial blood gas studies, pulse oximetry, lung scan, and lymph node biopsy. After identifying critical portions of the history, alterations in the physical examination, and abnormal findings in diagnostic studies, the physician will make a determination of the underlying respiratory disease.

- The patient undergoing extensive diagnostic evaluation for respiratory disorders is often short of breath, fatigued, and anxious about the results of the diagnostic tests. Support and psychologic preparation for the tests often reduce the patient's fears and anxieties. Repeated tests may add to the patient's fatigue and discomfort; therefore, the patient may require assistance in performing activities of daily living.

Chapter 23   Management of Patients With Conditions of the Upper Respiratory Tract

- A variety of disorders can affect the upper airway. These include upper airway infections, upper airway obstruction and trauma, and cancer of the larynx.

- Some of these disorders, such as upper airway infections, are more bothersome than threatening to life and well-being. Their high incidence and the time lost from usual activities make them clinically important.

- Although less common than infection, upper airway obstruction, trauma, and cancer of the larynx have serious implications for the health and well-being of the individual. The patient with cancer of the larynx faces potential major alterations in the ability to speak, alterations in life style, and often a prolonged rehabilitative phase.

- Nursing assessment and management are important in the preoperative, postoperative, and rehabilitative phases of care and focus on providing required treatment, comfort measures, support, and patient education.

Chapter 24   Management of Patients With Conditions of the Chest and Lower Respiratory Tract

- Atelectasis occurs when the alveoli in the lungs collapse, usually as a result of bronchial obstruction. A major cause is accumulation of secretions in the tracheobronchial tree. Pressure from accumulated fluid, air, an enlarged heart, or tumor growth may also restrict lung expansion and contribute to alveolar collapse.

- Treatment of atelectasis is directed at removing the obstruction or relieving the pressure to allow the patient to breathe more easily.

- Preventive nursing measures include frequent coughing and turning, postural drainage, chest physiotherapy, nasopharyngeal suctioning, early ambulation, and incentive spirometry.

- Pneumonia is an inflammatory pulmonary disease, generally caused by an infectious agent. It may be classified as bacterial or atypical, depending on the cause. Mortality and morbidity from pneumonia are high.

- Preventive measures include promoting coughing and expectoration in patients at risk, initiating precautions against infection, changing position frequently, employing tracheobraonchial suctioning and chest physical therapy, administering sedatives judiciously, promoting oral hygiene, and encouraging people to stop smoking.

- Signs of pneumonia depend on the causative agent but generally include sudden chills; high fever; rapid, bounding pulse; chest pains; cough and purulent sputum; and difficulty breathing. Abnormal breath sounds can be detected upon auscultation. Chest x-rays reveal consolidated areas in the lung, and sputum cultures identify the causative organism.

- Treatment includes antibiotics, rest, and oxygen if necessary.

- Nursing measures include maintaining a patent airway through suctioning, hydration, chest physical therapy, oxygen therapy, and positioning; promoting rest and conservation of energy; promoting fluid intake; and monitoring for signs of atelectasis, pleural effusion, and respiratory failure.

- The incidence of tuberculosis (TB) is increasing as a result of the development of strains that are multi-drug resistant. TB is an airborne disease transmitted by droplets emitted from an infected person. People at risk are those in close contact with the carrier, the elderly, immunosuppressed persons, IV drug users, alcoholics, the undernourished, the poor who live in crowded, substandard housing, and those with pre-existing diseases.

- TB is diagnosed primarily by a significant reaction to the Mantoux test and is treated with specific chemotherapeutic agents. Nonadherence to the drug regimen is a major problem in combating the spread of TB.

- Chronic obstructive pulmonary disease (COPD) is a broad classification for a group of disorders including chronic bronchitis, bronchiectasis, emphysema, and asthma. Reduced or obstructed airflow is common in each of these conditions. COPD is a slowly progressive disease that is associated with exacerbation and remissions.

- Environmental factors, including cigarette smoking, air pollution, and occupational exposure, are associated with the development of COPD. Genetic factors have also been implicated in some cases

- Chronic bronchitis is characterized by accumulation of thick secretions in the bronchioles and a long-lasting cough. Smoking is a key contributing factor in its development.

- Bronchiectasis results from a chronic dilation of the bronchioles with excessive secretions that block the bronchioles and cause atelectasis in sections of the lung.

- Emphysema occurs from abnormal distention of the air spaces in the lungs, leading to destruction of the alveolar walls and collapse of the alveoli. Impaired oxygen diffusion results along with impaired carbon dioxide elimination. The patient develops classic signs of extended expiration—labored breathing and a barrel chest.

- Asthma is reversible (unlike other COPD diseases) and is caused by a narrowing of the bronchioles resulting from hyperreaction to certain stimuli. The bronchial restriction results in cough, dyspnea, and wheezing. More severe attacks can result in status asthmaticus, which can prove fatal.

- Nursing actions for COPD include improving gas exchange with bronchodilators, humidification, and oxygen; removing bronchial secretions by promoting high fluid intake, postural drainage, and suctioning; preventing respiratory infections; teaching breathing exercises; encouraging self-care activities; supporting coping measures; and advocating smoking cessation.

- Adult respiratory distress syndrome is a type of noncardiogenic pulmonary edema associated with a variety of clinical disorders, resulting in alveolar capillary membrane injury, causing leakage of fluid into the alveolar interstitial spaces and capillary bed. As a result, gas exchange is disrupted and alveolar collapse occurs, leading to hypoxia, hypocapnia, and respiratory failure.

- Ventilation is supported with oxygen and then mechanical ventilation.

- Nursing care encompasses providing support through oxygen therapy, chest physiotherapy, endotracheal intubation, suctioning, and ventilator management. If neuromuscular blocking agents are used while the patient is on the ventilator, relieving anxiety and fear related to the resulting paralysis is essential.

- Pulmonary embolism is the obstruction of one or more pulmonary arteries by a thrombus or thrombi, resulting in a ventilation–perfusion imbalance and disruption in gas exchange. Unless ventilation is reinstated, the episode can be fatal.

- Prevention measures in people at risk for pulmonary embolism include frequent turning, active leg exercises, early ambulation, elastic stockings, anticoagulant therapy in some cases, use of intermittent pneumatic leg compression devices, elevation of the leg, and avoidance of leg dangling and leg crossing.

- Anticoagulation and thrombolytic therapy and possible surgery to remove the clot or prevent further emboli from entering the pulmonary system represent the main treatment strategies.

- Lung cancer is the most common cause of cancer deaths among men and is increasing in frequency among women. Smoking has been identified as a major cause of this disease. A cough that changes in character should be investigated as a symptom of lung cancer.

- Treatment may include surgical resection, radiation therapy, and chemotherapy.

- Attention is given preoperatively and postoperatively to pain management, nutritional support, relief of dyspnea, and maintenance of a patent airway. Psychologic support provides an opportunity for the patient and family to express their fears and concerns about the future.

- Chest trauma may be blunt or penetrating, as in knife and gunshot wounds, and may result in rib fractures, flail chest, hemothorax and pneumothorax, tension pneumothorax, open pneumothorax, pulmonary contusion, and cardiac tamponade.

- Since respiratory function is disrupted in each of these types of trauma, the goal of therapy is to return the system to as normal a state as possible. If fluid or air has collected in the chest, it must be removed; any opening into the chest wall must be closed; and any instability in the supporting structures of the chest must be stabilized.

- People experiencing chest trauma are in need of effective emergency treatment and expert nursing care to overcome the respiratory difficulty and deal with the emotionally traumatic reactions.

Chapter 25   Respiratory Care Modalities

- Hypoxia is the major reason for administering oxygen and is defined as hypoxemic, circulatory, anemic, and histotoxic.

- Oxygen therapy is given to raise the arterial oxygen pressure back to the patient's normal baseline.

- Oxygen toxicity can occur when too high a concentration of oxygen is given and can result in destruction of surfactant and in the development of pulmonary edema.

- Incentive spirometry is a means of promoting respiratory function and avoiding accumulation of secretions in the bronchioles and is especially effective for postoperative patients and those on forced bed rest.

- Chest physiotherapy includes postural drainage, chest percussion and vibration, breathing exercises, and effective coughing.

- Postural drainage uses specific positions that allow gravity to assist in removing bronchial secretions. The patient's chest may be percussed and vibrated to help dislodge mucus.

- Pursed-lip breathing and diaphragmatic breathing are two breathing techniques that can be taught to the patient to improve ventilation and gas exchange.

- Endotracheal intubation and tracheostomy are two measures to provide a patent airway for patients experiencing respiratory distress.

- The major objectives of nursing care for a patient with a tracheostomy are to alleviate the patient's apprehension, maintain a clear airway by suctioning secretions, and provide a means of communication for the patient.

- Mechanical ventilation is indicated for patients who are unable to maintain adequate ventilation and who have low arterial oxygen levels, high carbon dioxide levels, and a persistent acidosis.

- Nursing care is directed at assuring that the ventilator is operating properly to optimize gas exchange, that the settings are appropriate for the patient's needs, and that measures have been taken to help relieve pain and discomfort, prevent infection, and promote optimal communication.

- Frequent problems encountered with mechanical ventilation include cardiovascular compromise, pneumothorax, and pulmonary infection. Monitoring the patient for the development of these problems is an important nursing function.

- It is important for the nurse to work closely with other members of the health care team to assess the patient closely and monitor the functioning of the ventilator and oxygen delivery system. It is equally important to focus on the patient's physiologic and psychologic reactions and responses to treatment.

Chapter 26   Assessment of Cardiovascular Function

- The extent of the assessment of cardiovascular function varies depending on the setting, the acuity of the patient, and the situation. For the patient complaining of chest pain, the focus of the initial nursing assessment is primarily to identify the cause of the pain and to determine the severity of the problem.

- A basic cardiac examination always includes an assessment of heart rate and rhythm, blood pressure, general appearance, and level of comfort and alertness.

- Blood pressure measurement is important for all patients, because hypertension is silent but exceedingly common.

- The hands are also assessed for signs of peripheral cyanosis, pallor, temperature and moistness, capillary refill time, edema, turgor, and clubbing of the fingers.

- Jugular vein distention is an important indication of cardiac dysfunction and indicates increased filling volume and pressure on the right side of the heart.

- The health history of patients with cardiac problems centers on questions related to breathing difficulties; circulation-related problems, such as pain, weight gain, swelling, and dizziness; an increase or decrease in urination; and possible changes in mentation.

- Prevention of cardiac problems through patient teaching includes exploring methods to modify risk factors such as elevated cholesterol levels, blood pressure, smoking, obesity, inactivity, and stress.

- The heart is examined by inspection, palpation, percussion, and auscultation.

- The six areas of the chest wall examined in evaluating cardiac function include the aortic area, the pulmonary area, Erb's point, the right ventricular or tricuspid area, the left ventricular or apical area, and the epigastric area.

- The point of maximal impulse (PMI)—also called the apical impulse—is normally detected over the apex of the heart. An abnormal PMI can indicate an enlarged left ventricle due to heart failure or a ventricular aneurysm.

- Normal heart sounds include the first heart sound (S1) and second heart sound (S2). A gallop or third heart sound (S3) may be normal in children or young adults but is abnormal in patients with myocardial infarction or congestive heart failure.

- Other heart sounds include snaps, clicks, murmurs, and friction rubs.

- Pulmonary assessment in patients with cardiac disorders includes evaluating for breathing difficulties, Cheyne-Stokes respiration, hemoptysis, cough, crackles, and wheezes.

- The abdomen is evaluated for an enlarged liver indicating hepatojugular reflux and for bladder distention.

- A wide range of tests are used to evaluate cardiac function, including cardiac enzyme levels, such as creatine kinase and its isoenzymes, which assist in diagnosing myocardial infarction.

- Blood chemistry studies reflect lipid and cholesterol levels.

- Serum electrolyte tests help detect abnormal levels of sodium (hyponatremia or hypernatria), calcium (hypocalcemia or hypercalcemia), and potassium (hypokalemia or hyperkalemia).

- Other tests include evaluation of BUN and glucose levels, electrocardiography, cardiac catheterization, echocardiography, and radionuclide imaging.

- Nursing responsibilities in all these tests include offering explanations for the purpose of the test and the procedure involved and helping to alleviate the patient's anxiety and fears.

Chapter 27   Management of Patients With Dysrhythmias and Conduction Problems

- A dysrhythmia is a disorder of the heartbeat that includes a disturbance of rate of rhythm or both. Dysrhythmias are named according to the site of origin of the impulse and the mechanism of conduction involved.

- Cardiac muscle possesses the physiologic properties of excitability, automaticity, conductivity, and contractility.

- An electrocardiogram (ECG) views the electrical activity of the heart when electrodes or leads are placed at specific points on the body. The electrical activity is captured and recorded on a strip of ECG paper.

- The ECG is composed of several waveforms, including the P wave, the QRS complex, the T wave, the ST segment, the PR interval, and possibly a U wave.

- The following are types of dysrhythmias: sinus node dysrhythmias (which consist of sinus bradycardia and sinus tachycardia), atrial dysrhythmias (which consist of premature atrial contractions, paroxysmal atrial tachycardia, atrial flutter, and atrial fibrillation), ventricular dysrhythmias (which consist of premature ventricular contractions, ventricular bigeminy, ventricular tachycardia, and ventricular fibrillation), and conduction abnormalities (which consist of first-degree AV block, second-degree AV block, and third-degree AV block).

- Although dysrhythmias are most commonly treated with medication therapy, several types of adjunctive mechanical therapies are available. The three most common are elective cardioversion, defibrillation, and pacemakers. Other treatments include the use of implantable devices, electrophysiologic studies, and cardiac conduction surgery.

Chapter 28   Management of Patients With Cardiac Disorders and Related Complications

- Coronary heart disease caused by atherosclerosis is the most commonly occurring heart disease. In atherosclerosis, atheromas or fatty plaques form on the interior of the arteries, reducing blood flow.

- Coronary arteries, because of their anatomic structure, are particularly vulnerable to the formation of atheromas.

- Angina pectoris and myocardial infarction are the two clinical problems caused by coronary atherosclerosis.

- Risk factors for coronary heart disease may be nonmodifiable (family history, age, sex, race) or modifiable (cholesterol levels, high blood pressure, smoking, obesity, physical inactivity, stress, and overly competitive and aggressive behavior). Prevention is directed at changing the modifiable risk factors.

- Anginal pain results from an imbalance between the demand for and the supply of oxygen to the myocardium.

- Pharmacotherapy for angina includes nitroglycerin (or other nitrates), beta blockers, and calcium ion antagonists or blockers.

- When medication fails to relieve anginal pain, the patient may be a candidate for revascularization of blood flow to the myocardium either through percutaneous transluminal coronary angioplasty (PTCA) or coronary bypass surgery (CABG). Other possible measures include intracoronary stents, shunt catheters, and lasers.

- Patient teaching is an essential part of nursing management of the patient with angina and provides an opportunity for promoting preventive measures through life-style changes.

- Myocardial infarction (MI) involves the destruction of myocardial tissue as a result of reduced coronary blood flow.

- The primary symptom of MI is the sudden, unprovoked onset of severe vise-like chest pain, accompanied by pallor, shortness of breath, and diaphoresis.

- Diagnosis of MI is based on signs and symptoms, ECG findings, and serial serum enzymes.

- The goals of medical management of MI are to minimize damage to the affected cardiac tissue, preserve the unaffected tissue (by relieving pain, promoting rest to reduce the workload on the heart and the demand for oxygen, and administering medication to enhance blood flow), and prevent lethal complications.

- Continual nursing assessment of the MI patient focuses on monitoring physical signs to assure adequate heart rate and rhythm, urinary output, and level of consciousness.

- Nursing interventions for the MI patient are directed at relieving chest pain and reducing anxiety.

- Pharmacotherapy for pulmonary edema includes morphine (to reduce anxiety and dyspnea and to decrease peripheral resistance so blood can be distributed from the pulmonary circulation to the rest of the body); diuretics (to increase urine output and thus decrease fluid retention and to promote vasodilation); digitalis (to improve heart contractility); and bronchodilators (to relieve bronchospasm).

- Placing the patient in an upright position can also help reduce venous return to the heart.

- Congestive heart failure results from fluid volume overload caused by cardiac decompensation and is a leading cause of death in heart disorders.

- Damaged cardiac muscle impairs cardiac output by disrupting stroke volume—a function of preload, afterload, and contractility.

- Management of congestive heart failure is directed at improving cardiac contractility and reducing fluid volume overload.

- Acute episodes of cardiac failure may be minimized through patient education. An important nursing role is to provide education in regard to medications, diet, and weight control.

- Decreased mobility and impaired circulation in cardiac patients contribute to thromboembolic episodes, especially pulmonary embolism.

- The major signs of pulmonary embolism are chest pain, cyanosis, shortness of breath, rapid respiration, and hemoptysis.

- A systemic embolism may result in stroke or renal infarction.

- Pericardial effusion may accompany pericarditis, advanced congestive heart failure, or cardiac surgery. The signs are pressure in the chest, shortness of breath, and a drop or fluctuation in blood pressure.

- Pericardiocentesis or pericardial aspiration, in which the pericardial sac is punctured to remove the fluid, may be done to prevent tamponade.

- Cardiac arrest is an emergency situation requiring immediate cardiopulmonary resuscitation.

Chapter 29 **Management of Patients With Structural, Infectious, or Inflammatory Cardiac Disorders**

- The function of the heart valves is to maintain the forward flow of blood from the atria to the ventricles and from the ventricles to the great vessels.

- Valvular damage may interfere with valvular function by stenosis (narrowing) of the valve or by impaired closure that allows backward leakage of blood (valvular insufficiency, regurgitation, or incompetence).

- Acquired valvular disease often is the result of previous rheumatic endocarditis that has damaged one or more heart valves. The mitral valve is involved most frequently, followed by the aortic, tricuspid, and pulmonic valves.

- Although a valve may be badly damaged, the heart muscle may remain strong enough to allow it to adjust and maintain efficient function. Such compensatory changes include modification of the heartbeat, hypertrophy, and redistribution of blood.

- Valves may be repaired through commissurotomies (to relieve stenosis caused by the valve commissures adhering to one another). Commissurotomies may be closed or opened.

- Other forms of valve repair include balloon valvuloplasty, leaflet repair, and chordoplasties.

- Valve replacement is performed for stenosis or regurgitation when valve repair is not an alternative and when symptoms become severe.

- Nursing care involves assisting the patient to recover from anesthesia, maintain hemodynamic stability, and learn about the disorder and how to comply with treatment.

- Nursing assessment includes monitoring for such postoperative complications as bleeding, thromboembolism, infection, congestive heart failure, hypertension, dysrhythmias, hemolysis, and mechanical obstruction.

- Cardiomyopathies affect the structure and function of the myocardium and are classified as dilated or congestive and hypertrophic or restrictive.

- The pumping action of the left ventricle is affected, leading to similar failure of the right ventricle and general heart failure.

- Management of cardiomyopathies is directed at preventing heart failure. Heart transplantation or a ventricular assistive device may be necessary.

- The heart is vulnerable to the toxic effects of microorganisms that can invade the bloodstream. Resulting problems include infective endocarditis, rheumatic endocarditis, myocarditis, and pericarditis.

- The responsible organism migrates to an area of the heart tissue and attaches itself there, serving as a site for fiber, bacteria, and platelets to aggregate. Eventually scar tissue forms and the tissue becomes thick, stiff, and deformed.

- Symptoms depend on the side of the heart affected.

- Infective diseases of the heart are preventable; therefore, patient teaching becomes a major nursing function in promoting healthy behavior to avoid such problems.

Chapter 30   **Management of the Cardiac Surgery Patient**

- Cardiopulmonary bypass maintains blood circulation and tissue perfusion while the patient undergoes heart surgery. It oxygenates the blood and regulates temperature while allowing for a "bloodless" heart during surgery.

- Complications of cardiopulmonary bypass may result from coagulation changes, high blood viscosity, fluid overload, and increased capillary permeability leading to edema.

- Heart transplantation is a treatment option for some patients with end-stage cardiac disease.

- Medications to suppress rejection of the transplanted heart must be carefully balanced to avoid increasing the patient's susceptibility to infection.

- Patients who undergo heart transplantation must maintain lifelong compliance with a variety of regimens for diet, activity, medication, and follow-up.

- Postoperative nursing care of the cardiac surgery patient focuses on maintaining cardiac output, promoting adequate oxygenation, maintaining fluid and electrolyte balance, preventing infection, reducing pain, and relieving sensory perception problems.

- A major facet of nursing care of the patient who has undergone cardiac surgery is to monitor for potential complications such as hypovolemia, bleeding, cardiac tamponade, fluid overload, hypothermia, hypertension, dysrhythmias, cardiac failure, myocardial infarction, renal failure, electrolyte imbalances, hepatic failure, and infection.

- Home care may include nursing visits to change dressings, monitor for vital signs, provide diet counseling, and carry out ongoing teaching for the patient and family.

Chapter 31   **Assessment and Management of Patients With Vascular Disorders and Problems of Peripheral Circulation**

- The delivery of adequate amounts of oxygen and nutrients to the cells and tissues of the body depends on the structural and functional integrity of the cardiovascular system. The peripheral vascular system provides the avenue for the delivery of oxygen and other nutrients to the cells and tissues, and the metabolic demands of the cells dictate the utilization of these nutrients.

- Patent and intact arteries, capillaries, veins, and lymphatic vessels constitute the structural elements of the vascular system. Cellular requirements, neuronal and hormonal control of the vessels, and the availability of oxygen and other nutrients make up the functional components. When any of these elements is disrupted, the potential for tissue ischemia exists.

- Atherosclerosis is a generalized disorder of the intimal layer of the arteries. Plaque, a lesion that consists of collagen fibers, lipids, and other blood components, accumulates on the intimal layer and obstructs the flow of oxygenated blood to distal tissues. These lesions may form in the coronary arteries, cerebrovascular system, aorta, or the arteries of the extremities.

- The clinical manifestations of atherosclerosis depend on the organ or tissues affected. At present the cause of atherosclerosis is unknown; however, several theories have been proposed. Both genetic and controllable risk factors have been determined.

- Hypertension is defined as an elevation in blood pressure that exceeds 140/90 mmHg when taken two or more times on two or more occasions.

- Although the exact cause of hypertension is unclear, it is known that there is an increase in vascular resistance at the arteriolar level. As resistance is sustained, vessels in the eyes, heart, kidneys, and other organs are damaged. Eventually the left heart will thicken and hypertrophy in an attempt to supply the blood to the tissues.

- Initially a hypersensitive patient may not exhibit any overt manifestations of this disease; however, physical findings may reveal vascular or end-organ damage.

- Prevention of associated morbidity and mortality is the goal of all treatment programs. Reduction in blood pressure values can be accomplished by a combination of pharmacologic and nonpharmacologic approaches.

- Venous disorders are characterized by stasis, hypercoagulability of the blood, and vessel wall injury. An inflammation of the vein wall can occur with the subsequent formation of a clot. Clots may occur anywhere but are most commonly found in the veins of the lower extremities. Clinical findings are variable and may include edema, pain, and warmth. The goal of management is to resolve the thrombus and prevent recurrence. Resolution can be accomplished by anticoagulation or thrombolytic medications or by surgery.

- Leg ulcers, necrotic skin tissue of the leg, are frequently caused by arterial or venous insufficiency. Vascular insufficiency does not allow for an adequate supply of oxygen and nutrients to the tissues. When cellular metabolic needs can no longer be satisfied, cellular death (necrosis) ensues.

- Manifestations of leg ulcers are dependent on the type, duration, and extent of the insufficiency. Typical signs include an open wound, swelling of the extremity, and pain. Prevention of wound infection and promotion of the healing process are the goals of treatment.

- Disorders of the lymph system are generally considered to be treatable but not curable. The guiding principle for all therapy is the reduction of edema through increased muscular activity and enhanced venous return. This can be accomplished by a variety of therapies, including limb elevation, elastic stockings, and external pneumatic compression devices.

Chapter 32   Assessment and Management of Patients With Hematologic Disorders

- The hematologic system comprises the blood and the sites where blood is produced. Blood is composed of a straw-colored fluid, the plasma, in which are suspended the red and white blood cells and platelets.

- Through the vascular system, nutritive substances and oxygen needed for repair, growth, and metabolic actions are circulated to the body, and metabolic waste products, including carbon dioxide, are eliminated from the body.

- Blood has an intricate protective clotting mechanism that controls the excessive loss of blood from the body. Maintenance of the normal fluidity of the blood in the body is achieved through the fibrinolytic system.

- Anemia is a reduction in the number of red cells or the amount of hemoglobin. It can be a result of blood loss, accelerated destruction by hemolysis, problems with production due to either a deficiency in the necessary building blocks (*e.g.*, iron, vitamin B_{12}, folic acid) or a structural problem in the marrow resulting from a tumor or lack of erythropoietin.

- Iron deficiency anemia is the most common anemia. The total body iron content is decreased below normal. In most adults it is associated with a history of bleeding or poor diet. The red cells appear microcytic and hypochromic. The patient presents with fatigue, irritability, numbness and tingling of the extremities, and soreness of the tongue.

- Megaloblastic anemias are caused by a lack of vitamin B_{12} or of folic acid, both of which are required for normal DNA synthesis. Vitamin B_{12} deficiency can be caused by any of the following: dietary factors, gastric injury, lack of intrinsic factor, sprue, certain drugs (*e.g.,* neomycin, trimethoprim, phenytoin, KCl), transport and utilization problems, and increased demand (pregnancy, hyperthyroidism, certain neoplasms). Folic acid deficiency also occurs from decreased dietary intake, in malabsorption syndromes similar to those producing vitamin B_{12} deficiency, and through interference by drugs.

- Hereditary hemolytic anemias are caused by membrane, metabolic, or hemoglobin defects of the red blood cell. Although knowledge of the pathophysiology of these disorders is extensive, equivalent progress in therapy has not been achieved.

- The lymphomas are neoplasms that involve the cells of the immune system. They include Hodgkin's disease, which originates in lymphoid tissue, and non-Hodgkin's disease, which refers to all other malignant lymphomas not diagnosed as Hodgkin's disease.

- Prognosis for all lymphomas varies, and primary complications resulting from both the disease and treatment include increased risk for infection, anemia, pain, and the possibility of developing a second malignancy.

- Careful assessment for disease progression and complications and the provision of education and emotional support are essential components of nursing care.

- Thrombocytopenia can be a result of decreased production, increased destruction, or increased utilization of platelets. Treatment is aimed at the underlying disease. Idiopathic thrombocytopenic purpura is thought to be mediated by autoantibodies that shorten the life span of platelets. Corticosteroids, splenectomy, and immunosuppressive drugs are possible treatment modalities.

- Hemophilia is a sex-linked recessive disorder that affects blood clotting. Factor VIII deficiency results in hemophilia A, whereas a low level of absence of factor IX results in the less frequent hemophilia B. Both disorders are manifested by bleeding into muscles, joints, and soft tissues. Treatment consists of replacement therapy.

- Nursing management includes education of the patient and family about the disease process, prevention and management of bleeding episodes, and strategies for coping with chronic illness.

- Von Willebrand's disease is usually inherited as an autosomal dominant trait caused by a deficiency of factor VIII, part of which is necessary for normal platelet function. Severity may vary, and treatment consists of replacement therapy or desmopressin.

- The most common acquired coagulation disorders are vitamin K deficiency, liver disease, and disseminated intravascular coagulation (DIC). Vitamin K deficiency results in hypoprothrombinemia. Malabsorption, liver dysfunction, biliary obstruction, medications such as coumarin, and surgery can cause a decrease in vitamin K. Bleeding is dependent on the severity of the deficiency.

- Treatment in the form of replacement therapy or changes in medications depends on the underlying causative factor. DIC occurs secondary to another disease process.

- Overstimulation of the normal coagulation system leads to bleeding and thrombosis. Severity can be mild to acute, depending on the depletion of coagulation factors. Treatment is directed at the underlying disease process.

- Blood transfusions of whole blood or blood components are given to restore blood volume in instances of hemorrhage or certain injuries, to combat shock, and to treat certain disorders such as anemia or infection.

- Before a transfusion is started, the nurse must double check to assure that the labeling on the blood container matches the patient's blood type; that the correct patient is receiving the transfusion; and that the blood does not contain gas bubbles, is not cloudy, and is the appropriate color.

- During a transfusion the nurse observes the patient frequently for any signs of adverse reactions, such as circulatory overload, sepsis, febrile non-hemolytic reaction, allergic reaction, or acute hemolytic reaction.

- Should any transfusion reactions occur, the transfusion is stopped and the event is reported immediately; the IV line is kept open with normal saline; the blood container and tube are saved; the blood bank is notified; and treatment protocols are implemented as prescribed.

Chapter 33   Assessment of Digestive and Gastrointestinal Function

- During normal gastrointestinal functioning, food passes through the component structures of the gastrointestinal tract, where it is digested, absorbed, and eliminated. Each component structure of the tract is specialized to assist in these functions. The overall goal of this process is to provide nutrients to the body's cells so that they can perform their functions effectively.

- Many diagnostic tools and procedures are available to assist in assessing the structure and function of the gastrointestinal tract. This chapter provides specific information about some of the more commonly seen procedures, including the method, preparation, special instructions, and follow-up care. It also identifies some of the newer techniques and procedures that will become more commonplace.

Chapter 34   Management of Patients With Ingestive Problems and Upper Gastrointestinal Disorders

- Alterations in the oral cavity may be the result of a localized disease or a systemic disease that has oral manifestations. Several specific causes for these changes may include (1) neoplasms, (2) immunosuppression from drug therapy or human immunodeficiency virus (HIV) infection, (3) trauma, (4) diabetes, and (5) infectious lesions of bacterial, viral, or fungal origin. Treatment is dependent on the type, location, and extent of the oral condition.

- Persons at risk for developing esophageal cancer include those who smoke cigarettes and drink alcohol and the elderly. If the malignancy is detected early, its removal is simplified and the continuity of the digestive system is easily maintained. The mortality rate among patients with esophageal cancer is high because the patient is often an older person with increased risk for pulmonary and cardiovascular disorders; the tumor has already invaded surrounding structures, making its removal impossible; and the unique relationship of the esophagus to the heart and lungs makes these organs the site of extension of the tumor.

- Neck dissection is a surgical procedure that may be used in patients with head and neck cancer. The patient is instructed in the potential preoperative and postoperative complications. Often these patients require home care after hospitalization.

Chapter 35   Gastrointestinal Intubation and Special Nutritional Management

- Short nasogastric tubes are used for decompression of the stomach, removal of gastric contents, and feedings. Size, diameter, and length vary depending on the indications for use and length of time needed. The Sengstaken-Blakemore tube is used to control bleeding from esophageal varices.

- Long nasoenteric decompression tubes have single or double lumina and are used for decompression and gas and fluid removal. The tubes are used prophylactically before bowel surgery or to treat small bowel obstruction.

- Feeding tubes can be used for total diet administration, for supplemental feedings, and for postoperative feedings given to promote positive nitrogen balance. They are useful for long-term therapy because they are pliable and comfortable for the patient.

- A gastrostomy tube is for long-term use and total feeding supplementation. The risk of regurgitation is less frequent with this procedure than with nasogastric or nasoenteric feedings.

- Total parenteral nutrition (TPN) is used to provide short- and long-term nutritional supplementation when the gastrointestinal tract cannot be used. Nutritional solutions provide the essential nutrients needed to improve nutritional status and promote weight gain and healing ability.

- Various methods are used to administer TPN solution in clinical practice: peripheral venous, central venous, and right atrial routes. The avenue chosen depends on the patient's condition and length of therapy. Subclavian central catheters are inserted by the physician at the bedside and require nurses to assist in patient preparation, initiation, and monitoring of the TPN solution and maintenance of patent catheter lines.

- Goals for patients receiving TPN include attainment of optimal nutrition, absence of infection, maintenance of adequate fluid volume, achievement of optimal activity, knowledge of and skill in self-care, and absence of complications. Ongoing assessment is directed toward monitoring the patient's response to the therapy: weight, intake and output, laboratory values, signs of infection at the site of the catheter, and level of mobility and activity. The physician's order for the TPN solution is changed as appropriate to meet the patient's individual needs.

- Some patients receive parenteral nutrition at home. These patients and their families and significant others must be motivated and able to learn the skills necessary for successful management of the therapy in the home setting. Follow-up supervision by health care personnel is essential to assure that the patient's care is satisfactory and that all physical and psychosocial needs are being met.

Chapter 36   Management of Patients With Gastric and Duodenal Disorders

- Gastritis is an irritation of the stomach mucosa that occurs in an acute and chronic form. Acute gastritis generally results from ingesting irritable substances and usually subsides in a few days. Chronic gastritis is divided into two types: A and B.

- Type A gastritis is associated with pernicious anemia and is usually treated with vitamin B_{12}.

- Type B gastritis is associated with gram-negative bacilli *H. pylori* and is treated with antibiotics and bismuth salts.

- Patient teaching for patients with gastritis includes advising against drinking alcohol and eating irritating foods.

- Gastric ulcers may be caused by bacterial infection. However, ulcers are frequently associated with stress, smoking, or alcohol.

- Clinical manifestations of ulcers include pain, heartburn, vomiting, and possible constipation and bleeding.

- Ulcers are treated with H_2-receptor antagonists, antacids, cytoprotective drugs, antibiotics, bismuth salts, and diet modification.

- Nursing interventions for patients with ulcers include relieving pain, reducing anxiety, and providing patient education to encourage life-style changes and diet modification.

- Complications of ulcers include possible hemorrhage, shock, perforation, and obstruction.

- Gastric cancer may be linked to diet, hereditary factors, chronic inflammation of the stomach, and pernicious anemia. Prognosis is usually poor since metastasis has usually occurred by the time the cancer is diagnosed.

- Nursing care is directed at reducing anxiety, implementing nutritional measures, relieving pain, providing information, and supporting coping efforts.

- Gastric surgery may be an emergency treatment for gastric hemorrhage, perforation, obstruction, or trauma. It is also a designated treatment for patients with gastric cancer and those with gastric ulcers who do not respond to medications.

- Patients who undergo gastric surgery are usually anxious and in pain. Nursing interventions attempt to relieve the anxiety and pain and provide supportive teaching measures in the pre- and postoperative periods.

- Nursing assessment in the postoperative period is directed at detecting possible signs of hemorrhage, dysphagia, dumping syndrome and possible regurgitation, and other dietary problems.

Chapter 37   **Management of Patients With Intestinal and Rectal Disorders**

- Two problems that occur frequently with intestinal and rectal disorders are constipation and diarrhea. Patients with constipation (abnormal infrequency of defecation) or diarrhea (increased frequency of defecation) require nursing interventions directed toward maintenance of fluid and electrolyte balance, relief of discomfort and anxiety, and restoration of normal bowel pattern.

- Appendicitis, diverticulitis, and peritonitis are acute inflammatory disorders manifested by many of the same signs and symptoms. Each, however, involves a different infectious pathophysiology. Nursing goals for patients with these disorders are similar: relief of pain, maintenance of fluid and electrolyte balance, reduction of anxiety, and prevention of complications.

- Regional enteritis and ulcerative colitis are chronic inflammatory disorders with resultant changes in the physiologic function of the area of the intestine involved. Initially both conditions are generally treated medically, but they may eventually require surgical intervention.

- Nursing goals for patients with regional enteritis and ulcerative colitis are similar: relief of anxiety and pain; attainment and maintenance of fluid, electrolyte, and nutritional balance; and ability to cope with the effects of the illness and any required surgical procedure (*e.g.,* ileostomy).

- Bowel obstruction may result from pathology in the small or large intestine. Symptoms of pain and abdominal distention are similar in both situations. Diagnosis must be based on x-ray findings. Treatment varies from decompression of the bowel to surgical resection.

- Colorectal cancer causes an abnormality in the physiologic functioning of the lower gastrointestinal tract and therefore changes in bowel habits. Surgery is the primary treatment and may result in a colostomy. Preoperative and postoperative nursing care is directed toward psychosocial support and patient and family education related to the management of the colostomy.

- Diseases of the anorectum cause similar signs and symptoms even though the pathophysiologic basis differs with each disease entity. Nursing interventions in each case are directed toward assisting the patient to obtain normal elimination patterns, experience less pain and anxiety, and avoid complications.

Chapter 38   **Assessment and Management of Patients With Hepatic and Biliary Disorders**

- Disease of the liver may be acute or chronic in nature; however, chronic liver disease is common and is often associated with alcohol abuse.

- Liver disease causes systemic problems that range from mild flulike symptoms to gastrointestinal hemorrhage and hepatic coma.

- Management of liver disease ranges from symptomatic treatment of symptoms such as ascites, jaundice, and gastrointestinal bleeding to replacement of a severely damaged liver through liver transplantation.

- Nursing care of the patient with chronic liver dysfunction is focused on assisting the patient with cirrhosis to cope with chronic symptoms and promoting healthy life-styles.

- Nursing management of the patient with acute liver disease and liver failure may focus on relieving the systemic effects of the dysfunction; assessment and early intervention for life-threatening symptoms such as gastrointestinal hemorrhage; and assisting with recovery from liver transplantation.

- Education regarding avoidance of alcohol, drugs, and other agents that may harm the liver and other health-promotion strategies is an important aspect of the nurse's role in health promotion and prevention of liver disease.

- Surgery for the treatment of gallstones is the most common surgical procedure performed in the United States.

- A variety of surgical and nonsurgical approaches to treatment of gallstones are available.

- Same-day surgery and early discharge programs have enabled some patients undergoing elective cholecystectomy to return home within 24 hours of surgery and make it essential that patients and their families receive instructions about signs and symptoms of complications as well as measures to prevent them.

Chapter 39   **Assessment and Management of Patients With Diabetes Mellitus**

- Diabetes mellitus is a group of disorders characterized by abnormalities in the metabolism of carbohydrate, protein, and fat. These abnormalities are related to a lack of insulin or a decrease in the amount of insulin produced by the pancreas.

- In addition to the metabolic disorders, many vascular and neurologic complications are associated with diabetes mellitus that may contribute to such problems as blindness, renal failure, amputation, and an increased rate of strokes and heart attacks.

- Treatment of diabetes involves diet management, monitoring glucose levels in blood and sometimes urine, monitoring urinary ketones in patients with type I diabetes, exercise, and medications such as oral hypoglycemic agents and insulin.

- Major advances in treatment modalities over the last decade have allowed diabetic patients to achieve near-normal blood glucose levels and to have more flexibility in life-style.

- The most important aspect of diabetes treatment is education. Nurses play a vital role in providing patients and their families with the tools and knowledge necessary for successful management of diabetes. Patients must learn skills for the daily management of diabetes, the avoidance and treatment of acute complications such as hypoglycemia and hyperglycemia, and the avoidance of long-term complications.

- Nurses play an important role in promoting psychosocial well-being in patients and families who are dealing with this chronic illness.

Chapter 40 **Assessment and Management of Patients With Endocrine Disorders**

- The endocrine glands secrete substances known as hormones directly into the circulation where they work with the nervous system to regulate organ function.

- The concentration of the hormones in the bloodstream is normally maintained at a relatively constant level through feedback mechanisms. When the concentration of a hormone is reduced, production or secretion is increased until a normal concentration is restored. When the hormone level rises in the bloodstream, production or secretion is reduced until a normal concentration is achieved.

- Disorders of the endocrine glands generally result from overproduction (hyper-) or underproduction (hypo-) of hormones. Dysfunction of any of the endocrine glands results in major disturbances throughout the body.

- Hypofunction of the endocrine glands is generally treated with replacement of the specific hormone that is affected.

- Hyperfunction is usually treated by removal of part or all of the gland that is overproducing the hormone(s).

- Pancreatitis and cancer of the pancreas are the most common disorders of the pancreas, other than diabetes mellitus, and are accompanied by nutritional disorders and abdominal pain.

- Treatment of pancreatic disease may be surgical or nonsurgical, depending on the etiology.

- Nursing management of the patient with pancreatic disease focuses on assisting him or her to cope with the diagnostic and treatment regimens, promoting a healthy life-style and supportive environment, and monitoring for and managing potential complications.

Chapter 41 **Assessment of Urinary and Renal Function**

- Normal function of the urinary and renal system is essential for life.

- Dysfunction of the kidneys and urinary tract has the potential to cause systemic manifestations, including fluid and electrolyte disturbances, acid–base imbalance, and elevated blood pressure.

- Diagnostic tests of urinary and renal function may focus on the specific structures of the lower urinary tract or may be directed toward the effects of the disorder on electrolyte concentrations in the blood.

- Disorders of renal or urinary function and required diagnostic studies may cause the patient to be uncomfortable or embarrassed because voiding is usually a private function.

Chapter 42 Management of Patients With Urinary and Renal Dysfunction

- Disorders of the renal and urinary tract may occur across the life span; they range in severity from being inconvenient and embarrassing to life threatening.

- Treatment of renal and urinary tract disorders may be limited to medication and temporary use of urinary catheters to treat infection or relieve obstruction or retention, or it may involve long-term dialysis therapy to sustain life.

- Asepsis and meticulous care are necessary to prevent infection and possible sepsis when a patient has an indwelling urinary catheter or another urinary drainage system in place.

- Urinary incontinence is often transient and is not an inevitable consequence of aging.

- All patients with urinary incontinence should undergo assessment and treatment as most cases can be successfully controlled.

- Treatments used with renal and urinary tract disorders relieve symptoms, often improve the patient's well-being, and prolong life; however, they do not duplicate kidney function, may not cure the disorder, and are often accompanied by side effects and complications.

- The nurse caring for the patient with urinary or kidney disorders must understand the physical, social, psychologic, and economic impact of the disorders and their treatment on the patient and family.

- Renal surgery is performed to remove an obstruction, to reestablish drainage of the urinary tract, or to remove the kidney itself.

Chapter 43 Management of Patients With Urinary and Renal Disorders

- Disorders of the urinary tract and kidneys have the potential to alter the function of many body systems as well as fluid and electrolyte and acid–base balance.

- The nurse caring for the patient with disorders of the urinary tract and kidneys must understand the complex functions of the kidneys and lower urinary tract.

- An understanding of fluid and electrolyte imbalances that may occur secondary to urinary tract and renal dysfunction is essential.

- Although disorders may be limited to uncomplicated urinary tract infections that are usually easily treated, the nurse has an important role in patient education to assure compliance with therapy and follow-up if indicated.

- When renal dysfunction or urinary tract disorders necessitate complex treatments such as dialysis, transplantation, lithotripsy, or urinary diversion, the nurse is responsible not only for major aspects of patient teaching but also for many high-technology aspects of care.

- As patients who undergo such treatments are hospitalized for shorter periods of time, home care considerations take on increasing importance to assure continuity of quality care, preservation of remaining renal function, and patient recovery.

Chapter 44   Assessment and Management of Patients With Problems Related to Female Physiologic Processes

- An important role of the nurse is promotion of positive practices and behaviors related to women's health.

- The nurse strives to provide women with information about the importance of regular gynecologic examinations to promote health, detect health problems at an early stage, assess problems related to gynecologic and reproductive function, and discuss questions or concerns related to gynecologic function, reproductive function, sexual function, and sexuality.

- The nurse also provides an open, nonjudgmental environment, which is crucial if the woman is to feel comfortable discussing these personal issues.

- The woman who experiences a tubal ectopic pregnancy may have a mild, nonsurgical experience treated medically as an out-patient or may experience manifestations of pain and physiologic shock due to hemorrhage and grief simultaneously.

- In addition to providing expert physical care to the patient, the nurse also must be sensitive to the crisis of loss and grief that often occurs with ectopic pregnancy. The patient may express feelings of self-blame and concern for her future childbearing capacity. The patient's partner may also experience these concerns and reactions as well and should be included in the care plan.

- The nurse also is alert to signs and symptoms of abuse and screens all patients in a private and safe environment. The nurse is ever mindful that the patient who experiences a disorder related to the reproductive system is usually distressed, anxious, and embarrassed because of the personal or private nature of reproduction and sexuality. The woman who experiences such disorders requires knowledgeable nursing care, which always includes understanding and sensitivity.

Chapter 45   Management of Patients With Disorders of the Female Reproductive System

- Although most female reproductive tract infections are not life threatening, they do cause discomfort and embarrassment. Moreover, symptoms of these infections raise anxiety about their occurrence and fear about possible life threatening disorders such as AIDS. Whereas some pelvic infections (for example, toxic shock syndrome) may cause pain, disability, and other serious problems, vaginal infections may leave the patient mistrustful of her sexual partner, posing a threat to her intimate relationships.

- The patient with a pelvic infection may require interventions to relieve symptoms and instructions to perform self-care measures, particularly safer sexual practices and hygiene. Both kinds of patients may need help in dealing with infection-related emotional reactions (*e.g.*, distrust, anger, depression) and adequate information about the possible effects of the infection on future childbearing.

- The emotional trauma imposed by a diagnosed genital infection (*e.g.*, herpes simplex virus) requires such nursing interventions as reassurance, support, and education about the meaning of this virus for the patient's future.

- The current epidemic of human papilloma virus (or genital warts) with its potential for causing premalignant cervical changes challenges nurses to implement patient education programs and to encourage patients to use condoms and practice safer sex.

- Structural disorders of the female reproductive tract may affect the vagina, uterus, rectum, or bladder. These disorders are commonly attributed to aging or trauma, especially from childbirth. Long-standing consequences may include vaginal discharge, infection, and excoriation.

- Smyptoms of urinary or gastrointestinal tract involvement may occur with structural disorders and range from occasional or mild to severe. Surgical intervention may be required if structural disorders disrupt normal activities. Otherwise, Kegel's exercises may be practiced to strengthen the pelvic floor muscles and decrease the incidence of disorders related to childbirth and aging.

- Because malignant cells may develop in any female reproductive organ, awareness of those at risk for cervical, uterine, and ovarian cancer provides a starting point for patient education. Individual patient counseling includes information about warning signs and symptoms and prevention.

- Although early detection has increased as a result of adhering to American Cancer Society recommendations (for regular gynecologic examinations, breast self-examination, and mammograms), many women still do not follow these recommendations or they ignore or deny unusual symptoms. The nurse who provides care for women during hospitalization— or in a clinic, long-term care facility, or at home—has an opportunity to teach and counsel women about practices that may protect them from an undetected cancer.

- The patient with female reproductive cancer feels anxious and fearful about the diagnosis and its implications for the future. She often has realistic fears about her treatment options and their potential effects on her survival as well as her ability to care for her family and pursue her usual activities.

- Nurses who are sensitive to the impact of the cancer diagnosis and knowledgeable about standard and investigational treatment options (including potential benefits, risks, and side effects) are better able to provide quality patient care.

- The gynecologic health of older women is receiving much attention at present. Nurses are important sources of preventive and supportive education as they provide care to women throughout the life span.

- Sensitivity to fears of death and mutilation are always considered in care planning and in response to patient behavior. Women who have helped friends or relatives through radiation or chemotherapy may have preconceived notions about outcomes that need to be explored.

- Provision of adequate care and access to care for women of all ages and life-styles, including the homeless, financially restricted, HIV infected, young, old, abused, or any other woman, is a challenge for today's nurse. This challenge requires skill, compassion, and constant continued education and review of the nursing literature.

Chapter 46   Assessment and Management of Patients With Breast Disorders

- Although breast examinations and diagnostic studies are recommended to detect problems early, many patients feel anxious and uncomfortable during these procedures. The nurse who understands this and discusses the issues and procedures with the patient in a sensitive, routine manner can help relieve the patient's anxiety.

- Teaching patients to perform breast self-examination and informing them of current treatment and research programs are hallmarks of cancer prevention, health promotion, and sensitive nursing care.

- When a problem is detected and the patient requires more extensive diagnostic testing or surgery to correct or treat a breast disorder, the nurse must consider the physical and psychologic impact on the patient. Providing accurate information about the tests and procedures and giving emotional support can help to alleviate some of the patient's distress.

- Clinical breast examinations, mammography, and diagnostic studies are recommended to evaluate any abnormal breast lesion. Nurses can best prepare patients by providing accurate written and verbal instruction, delineating differences between benign and malignant breast conditions, explaining sensations that the patient may experience during diagnostic procedures, and following up on patient concerns promptly.

- Although certain breast conditions, such as fibrocystic breast changes, fibroadenomas, and fat necroses, are rarely life threatening, they produce discomfort and distress, especially if the patient detects them and interprets the mass as a serious disorder. Providing understanding about the impact of such a discovery, helping the patient grasp the significance of the disorder, and exploring coping strategies can help the patient adjust effectively.

- The patient with breast cancer requires nursing care for emotional as well as physiologic needs related to diagnosis and treatment. In the early postoperative period, the patient requires the nurse's assistance with positioning, self-care activities, and pain management. Additionally, she requires understanding and assistance in dealing with the cancer diagnosis and its implications for treatment, prognosis, and well-being. The nurse can help the patient manage more effectively by helping to coordinate care and by identifying appropriate support services.

- By preparing the patient for discharge and subsequent therapies (*e.g.,* chemotherapy or radiation therapy), the nurse can help her deal with treatment and increase the likelihood of compliance with follow-up treatment regimens. Sensitivity to the patient's feelings and responses to her threatened self-esteem, sexuality, and life are important throughout this period.

- Rapid changes in treatments and results of research demand constant study and review of nursing and medical literature. Optimism and hope for more and better treatment modes are realistic and should be conveyed to patients.

Chapter 47

Assessment and Management of Patients With Disorders of the Male Reproductive System

- Male sexual dysfunction results from various factors requiring specific treatment strategies. Regardless of its cause, sexual dysfunction has vast psychologic and social implications for most men, making it imperative to listen and offer empathy and support to the patient and his partner.

- Male genitourinary tract infections are usually related to sexually transmitted diseases (STDs). Anti-infection measures include identifying and screening men at risk for such diseases, especially human papilloma virus (HPV), and teaching them how to avoid acquiring or spreading these diseases or how to minimize their effects.

- Prostate disorders, especially those requiring surgery, call for a thorough understanding of both the procedure and the genitourinary system. Appropriate perioperative interventions focus on ensuring patient comfort, relieving anxiety, preventing complications, promoting bladder control with perineal exercises, providing sensitive support for potential erectile dysfunction and issues of sexuality and self-esteem, and preparing the patient and family for possible rehabilitation.

- Patients with prostate cancer, their families, and partners need assistance coping not only with the diagnosis but also with alterations in their usual activities and an uncertain future.

- Management measures for the patient with a testicular disorder are similar to those for prostate cancer. The patient needs careful verbal and written instructions, especially about early detection and regular follow-up evaluations.

- Disorders affecting the penis are usually not life threatening, but they do threaten the patient's body image and sexuality. Management includes assessing for anxiety and providing the necessary support and education to help the patient cope effectively.

- Although testicular cancer accounts for about 1% of all cancers, it is the major cause of cancer death in men 25 to 35 years of age. Teaching patients how to perform testicular self-examinations is one way to promote early detection of this problem.

Chapter 48   Assessment of Immune Function

- The immune system protects the body against foreign substances and the proliferation of malignant cells.

- The normal immune response is activated by invasion by bacteria or viruses, by ingestion or injection of foreign substances, and by other modes of contact with antigens.

- Disorders of the immune system occur when the immune response is directed at the body's own tissues (*e.g.,* in autoimmune disorders), when the immune response is excessive (*e.g.,* in anaphylaxis), or when the immune response is depressed (by cancer or radiation or in AIDS).

- Immune disorders may be genetically determined or acquired through bacterial, viral, fungal, or protozoan infections.

- An alteration in the immune system may occur from medications used to treat other disorders (*e.g.,* antibiotics, corticosteroids, or nonsteroidal anti-inflammatory drugs).

- Alteration of the immune system also occurs as a result of the aging process.

- In planning comprehensive nursing care, a detailed history and physical assessment of the patient must be obtained by the nurse to identify threats to immune system function.

Chapter 49   Management of Patients With Immunodeficiency Disorders

- Immunodeficiencies are characterized by severe depression of one or more components of the immune system and can be primary or secondary disorders.

- Primary immunodeficiencies are rare, usually fatal diseases that are primarily genetic in origin and often occur in infancy and early childhood.

- Treatment of primary immunodeficiencies may include bone marrow transplantation, intravenous immunoglobulin, thymus-derived factor, and thymus gland transplantation.

- Prevention and management of infection are important in all immunodeficiency states.

- Secondary immunodeficiency diseases are more common than primary disorders and occur as a result of underlying disease processes (malnutrition, chronic stress, burns, and certain viral infections) or from treatment for these diseases.

- Management of secondary immunodeficiency disorders includes treatment of the underlying cause and prevention and treatment of infection; it may include antibiotic and intravenous gamma globulin therapy.

- The nursing care of secondary immunodeficiency disorders includes assessment for infection and interventions to prevent and manage infection.

Chapter 50   Acquired Immunodeficiency Syndrome

- Acquired immunodeficiency syndrome (AIDS) is a disorder characterized by severe suppression of the immune system; it is the symptomatic stage along the continuum of HIV infection.

- The virus responsible for HIV infection is a retrovirus transmitted by sexual contact, contaminated blood, and perinatal transmission from mother to fetus.

- The virus enters the helper T lymphocytes, a type of T4 lymphocyte, where it replicates.

- As T lymphocytes are destroyed by the HIV virus, the infected person is unable to mount an immune response against common or ordinarily harmless pathogens or abnormal cells. The result is the appearance of opportunistic infections and malignancies.

- The severity of physical symptoms, the poor prognosis, and the emotional, psychologic, and social consequences of AIDS exact a toll on the patient, the family, and often the health care provider.

- The nurse caring for the patient with HIV infection and AIDS requires expert assessment, communication, and interpersonal skills; the ability to deal with a wide range of physical problems and psychologic reactions; and commitment to and respect for the dignity of patients from all walks of life who have contracted AIDS.

Chapter 51   Management of Patients With Allergic Disorders

- The human body has a vital defense mechanism equipped with weapons (antibodies) to protect itself against invaders (antigens). Allergy disorders occur when the body produces an inappropriate or exaggerated response to antigens that are not necessarily harmful. Allergic reactions can range from mild to life threatening.

- Chemical mediators are released when cells are stimulated by antigens. Primary chemical mediators include histamine, eosinophil chemotactic factor of anaphylaxis (ECF-A), platelet-activating factor (PAF), and prostaglandins. Secondary chemical mediators include leukotrienes, bradykinin, and serotonin.

- Hypersensitivity reactions can be classified as one of four types: anaphylactic (type I) hypersensitivity, cytotoxic (type II) hypersensitivity, immune complex (type III) hypersensitivity, and delayed-type (type IV) hypersensitivity.

- Atopic allergic disorders can be characterized as type I hypersensitivity reactions. There is a strong genetic factor in susceptibility to these diseases. Anaphylaxis, allergic rhinovitis, atopic dermatitis, urticaria, angioedema, gastrointestinal allergy, and asthma are all atopic allergic disorders.

- Allergies affect approximately 40 million children and adults in the United States. A thorough history and physical examination are important elements in diagnosing allergic disorders. Educating patients about the various types of allergic disorders is an important detection and prevention strategy. Patients with life-threatening allergies and their families require explicit instruction on avoiding allergic responses, recognizing their onset, and initiating emergency measures.

Chapter 52   Management of Patients With Rheumatic Disorders

- The rheumatic diseases that are systemic in nature are disorders of the autoimmune system with inflammation as the pathologic process. Those rheumatic diseases that are more localized in nature reflect degeneration of a specific portion of the musculoskeletal system but may have an autoimmune component. Other than the crystal arthropathies (such as gout) and infectious arthritis, the etiology of most rheumatic diseases is unknown but is thought to be some combination of genetic, environmental, and possibly viral factors.

- The rheumatic diseases include a wide group of conditions that vary in manifestations and severity. The conditions representative of the rheumatic diseases include not only those readily thought of as "arthritis" (*e.g.,* rheumatoid arthritis or osteoarthritis) or closely associated with arthritis (*e.g.,* gout) but also those conditions that have a significant articular impact (*e.g.,* neoplasms, hemophilia, hyperthyroidism, regional enteritis, or chronic active hepatitis).

- Rheumatic diseases are manifested in a wide variety of ways, including not only the expected joint involvement but also major organ system involvement (central nervous system, kidney, heart, vascular system, lungs, and skin). The severity of these diseases ranges from mild but annoying symptoms relating to joint involvement to life-threatening organ involvement.

- Complications of treatment can also have a sudden and significant impact on health status, such as happens with bone marrow suppression. The impact on quality of life cannot be overlooked. Many people can adapt and cope to a significantly changed lifestyle; others find even minor side effects from medications or limitations in activities intolerable.

- This diversity challenges the nurse in identification of the patient problems (rather than the disease), in the determination of the nursing diagnoses, in the application of appropriate nursing interventions and collaboration with other members of the care team, and in realistic expected outcomes.

Chapter 53   Assessment of Integumentary Function

- The integument is the largest organ of the body. Because it is the body system that is most visible, it is said to be the reflection of a person's overall state of health.

- The skin is involved in many complex functions necessary to maintain homeostasis: protection from environmental agents and conditions, normal sensation, water balance, temperature regulation, and the immune response.

- Skin function can be affected by many environmental factors and by the normal aging process to a degree.

- Systemic disease and one's emotional state are typically manifested by changes in the appearance and condition of the skin, hair, and nails. These visible consequences affect body image and self-esteem, and their effects can lead to social isolation and stigma, as well as the loss of significant relationships and occupational opportunities.

- Because eliciting a comprehensive health history requires probing and intimate inquiry and because diagnostic procedures and tests may cause embarrassment and discomfort, the nurse needs to convey support and acceptance during the interview.

- Evaluating the integumentary system requires the nurse to have a basic understanding not only of anatomy and physiology but also of common skin conditions and their diagnosis. Additional skills needed in conducting the physical examination include sensitivity and a thoughtful approach to the individual and the dermatologic problem.

- Acne vulgaris can affect anyone, but it occurs mostly in teenagers. It usually subsides spontaneously a few years after onset. Severe, disfiguring acne and acne that continues into adulthood are associated with considerable psychologic and social distress.

- Herpes zoster (shingles), a virus that affects the nerves and that is caused by varicella zoster, the chicken pox virus, is becoming more prevalent, especially in persons who are immunocompromised (*e.g.*, transplant recipients, patients with AIDS) and susceptible to opportunistic infections. The disease is self-limiting.

- Tinea (ringworm) is a fungus infection that grows in body areas prone to excessive perspiration (skin folds, feet). Ringworm is contagious and can be spread by direct contact or by contact with objects (comb, towel). Scratching spreads tinea on the body. Treatment includes meticulous cleanliness and antifungal medications.

- Scabies results from infestations by the female *Sarcoptes scabiei (var hominis)* mite, which burrows under the skin and lays eggs that hatch and reach adulthood in 10 days. Clinical symptoms include intense itching in affected areas, especially at night. Common treatment is application of 1% gamma benzene hexachloride (lindane) lotion.

- Contact dermatitis, a nonallergic, inflammatory response by the skin to a chemical or physical irritant, is more common than allergic contact dermatitis. Signs range from mild erythema to inflammation, vesicle formation, and pain. Most contact dermatitis affects the hands, face, and eyelids and does not spread. Removing or avoiding the irritant usually results in resolution of symptoms. Allergy patch testing should be performed if the rash does not clear within a short time.

- Psoriasis is a chronic, noninfectious dermatosis characterized by unrestricted proliferation of the basal cells of the epidermis. Signs include reddened, thick scales or plaques of epidermal tissue. The cause is unknown, although heredity may play a role, and no cure is available. Current therapy can control lesions. The disease has devastating psychologic effects on self-esteem and body image and calls for sympathetic concern and support.

- Pemphigus vulgaris is a serious autoimmune disorder characterized by blisters that rupture easily, heal poorly, and involve the mucous membranes and the skin. Diagnosis is confirmed by histologic and immunofluorescent studies. Primary treatment is systemic oral corticosteroid therapy. Additional treatments include topical steroids and immunosuppressants. Although incurable, the disease can be controlled. Psychologic and emotional support are vital.

- Toxic epidermal necrosis (TEN) causes widespread erythema, blisters, serious eye inflammation, and possibly death. The disease is thought to result from an infection or an allergic reaction to drugs or chemicals. Treatment includes systemic corticosteroids, debridement of necrotic skin, correction of fluid and electrolyte imbalances, symptomatic relief, and prevention of complications.

- Skin cancers, such as basal cell carcinoma and squamous cell carcinoma, tend to be related to sun exposure. They affect light-skinned people who do not tan. When detected early, the disease is easily cured by surgical excision or similar therapies.

- Malignant melanoma, a potentially deadly skin cancer, can be cured or controlled if detected and treated early. Treatment includes surgery, isolation limb perfusion techniques (isolating the involved limb and infusing chemotherapeutic agents locally), chemotherapy, and immunotherapy.

- Facial reconstructive and plastic surgery includes such complex techniques as skin grafting. The patient undergoing this surgery requires skillful nursing care for the graft site and the donor graft site if the skin comes from another part of the patient's body. The aim is to avoid complications and to promote the patient's positive outlook and recovery. Patient education is important as well.

- Other facial treatments include planing, such as chemical peeling and dermabrasion; face lifts; and removal of skin lesions by laser surgery. Important nursing care measures for patients having planing or face lifts include patient education in preparation for the procedures and meticulous care later to avoid infection or other complications. For procedures involving laser beams, the patient and health care staff need to wear protective eye gear.

- Androgenetic alopecia is hair loss in men and women and is related to androgen (hormone) levels. Of special importance is educating the patient about over-the-counter and prescribed (minoxidil) hair-restoring products and about restorative surgical hair transplantation techniques.

Chapter 55   **Management of Patients With Burn Injury**

- The severity and extent of a burn injury may vary from a superficial burn on a fingertip to a full-thickness burn covering most of the body surface, destroying the skin layers, and triggering a massive systemic response.

- The patient with extensive burns has a multisystem injury that may require multiple surgeries and procedures for wound closure, debridement, skin grafting, and joint mobility.

- Of the three phases of wound care, the emergent/resuscitative phase focuses on patient survival through replacing fluid losses (fluid resuscitation); correcting acute life-threatening problems, such as compromised pulmonary, cardiovascular, and renal function; and taking initial steps to prevent such complications as sepsis, contractures, and other serious problems.

- Nursing assessment and communication expertise are essential skills for identifying physical and psychologic changes in the patient in the emergent/resuscitative phase.

- The acute, or intermediate, phase of burn care begins 48 to 72 hours after the burn injury and extends until the burn wounds close satisfactorily.

- Nursing priorities in the acute phase are recognizing and preventing infection, sepsis, and other complications as well as pain management and informing the patient and family about care and planning for the future.

- Advanced assessment and wound care skills, psychologic assistance and support, and collaborative management of any pulmonary, cardiovascular, and renal complications are essential elements of nursing care during the acute phase.

- The rehabilitation phase of burn care begins with the patient's admission and may extend for years, depending on the extent of injury. Throughout this phase, nursing attention focuses on the patient's fluid and electrolyte status, nutrition, activity, and psychosocial adjustment.

- Additional nursing responsibilities in the rehabilitative phase include the coordination of health care services in preparation for the patient's discharge to home or to another health care center. Knowledge of community resources and supportive services as well as collaboration with other health care professionals are key to nursing care in this phase.

Chapter 56   **Assessment and Management of Patients With Vision Problems and Eye Disorders**

- The eye is the organ of vision. It provides one of the five senses, sight. The various parts of the eye work in harmony to allow light rays to enter, converge, and register as nerve impulses, thus producing an image. Disease, trauma, and the aging process account for changes in vision.

- Examination of the eye involves inspection and specialized instruments to visualize its structure and assess the function of vision. Visual acuity is the most important initial assessment of the eyes, since vision is the primary function of the eyes. Knowing the level of visual acuity and how a person maneuvers within his environment is helpful in identifying potential problems associated with activities of daily living and safety issues. Other tests include those that evaluate ocular tension (pressure), extraocular muscle movement, the field of vision, and the internal eye.

- Refractive errors, problems in focusing light rays (*e.g.*, presbyopia, myopia, hyperopia, and astigmatism), are corrected by lenses. Corrective lenses include eyeglasses, contact lenses, and intraocular lenses (IOL).

- The eyelids can develop inflammation, infectious lesions, and tumors. Blepharitis, chalazion, and hordeolum are the most common eyelid conditions for which treatment is sought. Entropion, ectropion, blepharoptosis, and exophthalmus are common disorders of the lid position and can affect the external eye.

- Conditions of the lacrimal system usually involve disorders of tear production and drainage. Inadequate tear film may result in dryness of the eyes and structural and inflammatory consequences. Dacryocystitis is an infection of the lacrimal sac secondary to nasolacrimal duct obstruction.

- Conjunctivitis is the inflammation of the conjunctiva. Trachoma, a chlamydial conjunctivitis, is seen most often in third-world countries. Pterygium is an outgrowth of tissue extending to the cornea, thought to be caused by ultraviolet light. Conjunctival hemorrhages are usually benign and heal over a period of weeks.

- Conditions of the cornea include microbial keratitis, exposure keratitis, corneal dystrophies, and keratoconus. Various corneal transplantation procedures are used to restore vision in patients suffering from corneal conditions. Corneal transplantation surgery has restored sight for many people; many others could also be helped if more donor tissue were available.

- A cataract is a progressive condition of the lens of the eye generally occurring with aging. As the lens opacifies, vision is blurred or dimmed with distortions of images and poor night vision. Severe visual loss and eventual blindness occur unless surgery is performed. Two surgical techniques used to remove cataracts are intracapsular and extracapsular extraction. Because the focusing power of the eye is altered after cataract extraction, correction is made by aphakic spectacles, contact lenses, or an IOL implant.

- Uveitis is inflammation of one or all three structures of the uveal tract. Sympathetic ophthalmia is an inflammation of the uveal tract of the fellow eye occurring after injury to the uveal tract of one eye. Enucleation, the complete surgical removal of the eyeball, is a surgical alternative following penetrating injuries to the eye to prevent sympathetic ophthalmia.

- Glaucoma is the leading cause of blindness in the United States. Although there is no cure for glaucoma, it can often be controlled with medication. Laser or incisional surgery may be required; the goal of these procedures is to arrest the progression of the condition. It is imperative that the nurse stress to the patient and family the importance of regular eye examinations and the consistent and proper use of medications prescribed for glaucoma.

- Conditions of the adult retina and vitreous body include retinal detachment, infectious endophthalmitis, diabetic retinopathy, age-related macular degeneration, retinitis pigmentosa, and defective color vision.

- Safety precautions are the best prevention for ocular trauma, since trauma is often the result of accidents. Once injury is suspected, it is imperative that no pressure be applied to the eye globe. Inspection of the outer structures of the eye may indicate a minor injury; however, this should be treated as a serious injury until severe ocular injury can be excluded. It is estimated that 90% of all eye injuries are preventable.

- Legally blind refers to visual acuity (with glasses) that is 20/200 or worse in the better eye, or when the visual field is restricted to a 20-degree diameter.

- Low vision or partially sighted refers to visual impairment that cannot be corrected with lenses. Low-vision treatment should be initiated when the patient experiences problems in daily life. It is vital that the patient be referred to appropriate health care providers and agencies that will help with the adjustment needed for the patient to live as normal a life as possible.

Chapter 57   Assessment and Management of Patients With Hearing Problems and Ear Disorders

- Hearing impairment affects more than 20 million people in the United States. The sense of hearing plays a significant role in a person's ability to participate in activities of daily living and to communicate with others through speech. Therefore, hearing deficits must be identified so that measures can be taken to promote hearing and communication.

- Assessment of the ear involves inspection and palpation of the external ear and use of an otoscope to examine the middle ear. Estimation of auditory acuity can be accomplished by assessing the patient's ability to hear a whispered phrase or a ticking watch. A variety of procedures are available for measuring the auditory and vestibular systems and diagnosing hearing loss. These tests are usually performed by the audiologist. The most important diagnostic instrument for measuring hearing loss is the audiometer.

- The ear, although encompassing a relatively small portion of the human body, is a very complex organ. It is responsible for the senses of hearing and balance.

- Problems of the external ear, middle ear, and inner ear can occur, and the symptoms that frequently accompany them include hearing loss, tinnitus, and balance disturbance. Infection, masses, and the aging process are frequent otologic disorders that affect quality of life.

- A variety of medical and surgical therapies are available for treating these disorders. Fortunately, it is extremely rare for an otologic condition to be life threatening.

- Conductive hearing loss results from an impairment of sound transmission through the outer ear, middle ear, or both. The inner ear is not involved in this type of loss because it can clearly analyze sounds.

- Sensorineural hearing loss is produced from a disorder of the inner ear or nerve pathways that impairs sensitivity to and discrimination of sounds.

- Sounds may be conducted properly through the external and middle ear but are not efficiently converted to electrical energy and transmitted to the central nervous system by the inner ear and/or cochlear nerve.

- When hearing loss occurs, aural rehabilitation is important and can include auditory training, speech reading, speech training, and the use of hearing aids. In addition, implanted hearing devices (cochlear implant, bone conduction device, semi-implantable hearing device) are available and are appropriate for some persons with hearing loss, as are specially trained hearing guide dogs.

Chapter 58

Assessment of Neurologic Function

- The nervous system consists of the brain, spinal cord, and peripheral nerves and controls the major functions throughout the body. Many disorders have their origins in neurologic dysfunctions. An understanding of the anatomy and physiology of the neurologic system is an important knowledge base for nurses working with patients with these problems.

- The neurologic examination evaluates five areas: cerebral functions, motor functions, sensory functions, reflexes, and cranial nerve functions.

- Cerebral function is assessed by evaluating mental status, intellectual function, thinking ability, emotional status, perception of physical objects, motor ability, and language ability.

- The Glasgow Coma Scale provides a method for assessing level of responsiveness and consciousness in three aspects of behavior: eye opening, verbal response, and motor responses. Numerical values are assigned to the type of responses elicited in each area and can serve as a guide to changes in the patient's status.

- Cranial nerve function is assessed in relation to sense of smell, visual acuity, eye movement, facial sensation, corneal reflex, chewing ability, facial movement and expression, taste, hearing and equilibrium, pharyngeal contraction and soft palate movement, vocal cord movement, movement of the sternocleidomastoid and trapezius muscles, and tongue movement.

- The motor system is primarily assessed by evaluating muscle strength, balance, and coordination. Techniques include testing alternating movements and point-to-point coordination. The Romberg test is used to evaluate balance.

- Reflexes are evaluated by testing reflexes in the following major areas: biceps, brachioradialis, triceps, patellar, and ankle or Achilles. Hyperactive reflexes may be reflected in a clonus type response.

- The Babinski response is a key reflex reaction used to determine central nervous system disease. When the sole of the foot is stroked, the toes should contract and draw together. In an abnormal response, the toes fan out and draw back.

- Sensory function is assessed in terms of tactile sensation, pain and temperature sensations, vibration and proprioception, and position sense.

- Neurologic functions undergo change with age and can result in a variation in responses in elderly people, especially in relation to hearing, vision, taste, smell, temperature sensitivity, tactile sensation, and mental acuity.

- Major diagnostic tests conducted to detect neurologic disorders include computed tomography scanning (CT), position emission tomography (PET), magnetic resonance imaging (MRI), cerebral angiography, myelography, radionuclide imaging studies (brain scans), echoencephalography, electroencephalography, evoked potential studies, electromyography, nerve conduction studies, and lumbar puncture.

- The nurse's role in diagnostic studies is to explain to the patient the purpose and function of the studies, to answer questions, and to reduce patient anxiety by providing reassurance and understanding.

Chapter 59

Management of Patients With Neurologic Dysfunction

- The altered function in patients with neurologic disorders affects a wide range of physiologic and psychologic functions, including breathing patterns, swallowing ability, skin integrity, physical mobility, self-care activities, vision and oral abilities, thought processes, urinary and bowel elimination, and coping abilities for the individual and the family.

- Nursing care of these patients involves providing care and support measures to deal with these dysfunctions and to avoid more severe complications, such as respiratory failure, pneumonia, aspiration, pain, contractures, and pressure sores.

- Intracranial pressure (ICP) is the result of the amount of brain tissue, intracranial blood volume, and cerebrospinal fluid (CSF) within the skull. Normally, ICP is less than or equal to 15 mmHg.

- Pathologic conditions such as head injury, stroke, tumors and inflammatory lesions, and intracranial surgery can alter the relationship between the volume of the brain, blood volume, and CSF, leading to ICP. Herniation, in which increasing pressure forces brain tissue to shift, can occur and adversely affects cerebral blood flow. Other complications, aside from herniation, include diabetes insipidus and syndrome of inappropriate antidiuretic hormone (SIADH).

- Signs of increased ICP include changes in mental status or level of consciousness and in vital signs with bradycardia, widening pulse pressure, and respiratory changes. Posture changes may also occur with decortication, decerebration, and flaccidity.

- Management of increased ICP includes decreasing cerebral edema with osmotic diuretics, reducing the amount of CSF by draining it, controlling temperature, and reducing metabolic demands by administering barbiturates and possibly muscle relaxants.

- Nursing assessment to detect increasing ICP includes evaluating the three criteria of the Glasgow Coma Scale: eye opening, verbal response, and motor response. Other subtle changes include headache, forced breathing or respiratory irregularities, purposeless movements, mental cloudiness, changes in vital signs, widening pulse pressure, pupillary changes, and vomiting.

- Unconsciousness may be caused by neurologic problems (head injury, stroke, increased intracranial pressure), toxic substances (drug overdose, alcohol intoxication), or metabolic imbalances (hepatic or renal failure, diabetic ketoacidosis).

- Management is directed at securing a patent airway, perhaps with intubation or tracheostomy. Mechanical ventilation may be necessary for patients who cannot breathe on their own. An IV line may be instituted to maintain fluid balance and nutritional support provided with a feeding tube or gastrostomy tube when unconsciousness is of long duration.

- Complications of prolonged unconsciousness include respiratory failure, pneumonia, aspiration, and pressure ulcers.

- Nursing assessment of the unconscious patient includes evaluating level of consciousness, respiration patterns, pupil size, eye movement, corneal reflexes, facial symmetry, swallowing reflex, response to noxious stimuli, possible Babinski sign, and abnormal positioning.

- Nursing measures are to maintain the airway with proper positioning, periodic suctioning, chest physical therapy, auscultation of breath sounds, and appropriate care if the patient is intubated or on a mechanical ventilator. IV therapy and tube feedings are carried out as prescribed. Mouth care is given to maintain the oral membranes; skin integrity is protected through frequent turning and skin care. Eye care is directed at removing encrustations and avoiding corneal injury. Temperature regulation is assured, along with bowel and bladder function. Family concerns are addressed by answering questions and providing an opportunity for expression of feelings.

- Stroke results from thrombosis or embolism, ischemia, or cerebral hemorrhage. The interruption in blood supply to the brain causes temporary or permanent loss of movement, thought, memory, speech, or sensation.

- Major risk factors for stroke include hypertension, cardiac problems, smoking, high cholesterol, excess weight, diabetes, and oral contraceptives.

- Clinical manifestations of stroke include motor dysfunction in the form of hemiplegia or hemiparesis; communication loss as evidenced by aphasia, dysarthria, or apraxia; perception disturbances in vision, vision–spatial relationships, and sensory loss; mental impairment; bladder dysfunction; and emotional fragility.

- Nursing measures are directed at monitoring to assure cerebral blood flow and oxygenation; evaluating level of consciousness and orientation to time, place, and person; and assessing for signs of increased ICP. Proper positioning is important to prevent contractures, possible shoulder adduction, and hip rotation. Range-of-motion exercises are carried out to avoid contracture and to begin retraining. Frequent turning helps maintain skin integrity and avoid pressure sores. The patient is assisted in preparing for ambulation, in developing self-care abilities, and in dealing with the frustrations of neurologic impairment.

- The goals of postoperative management following a craniotomy are to reduce cerebral edema with osmotic diuretics, relieve pain and prevent convulsions, prevent infection, and detect any signs of increasing ICP.

- Major complications following craniotomy include increased ICP and hypovolemic shock; fluid and electrolyte disturbances, including diabetes insipidus and SIADH; infection; CSF leakage; and seizures.

- Nursing measures include assessing respiratory function and arterial blood gases to detect any evidence of hypoxia, monitoring vital signs and levels of consciousness for signs of increasing ICP, and tracking rectal temperature to determine any dysfunction of the hypothalamus. Assessment of neurologic status focuses on level of responsiveness, eye signs, motor responses, and vital signs.

Chapter 60   Management of Patients With Neurologic Disorders

- The complexity of the central nervous system and its important role in mediating cognitive, motor, and sensory function make neurologic disorders particularly devastating to patients and their families.

- Neurologic disorders range from occasional headaches that may cause no disruption in activities to acute and chronic disorders that may be debilitating and life threatening.

- The nurse caring for the patient with a neurologic disorder must have an appreciation of the complex functions of the nervous system, highly developed assessment skills, and an understanding of and sensitivity to the anxiety and fear experienced by the patient and his or her family.

- Although many patients with neurologic disorders are initially treated in acute care facilities, including neurologic/neurosurgical intensive care units, they also require consideration of their rehabilitation needs from the moment of entry into the health system.

- Management of the patient with neurologic disorders requires the collaboration and cooperation of all members of the health care team; the health care team is frequently involved in the care of an individual for many years, and that care often extends into the home and community.

- An important role for the nurse is coordination of the services required by the patient and his or her family, as it is easy to lose sight of the complex regimens that are often required in coping with neurologic disorders.

Chapter 61   Assessment of Musculoskeletal Function

- The 206 bones in the human body, which constitute the bony skeleton, protect vital organs, support body structures, and store minerals. Bone is composed of cells, protein matrix, and mineral deposits. Blood cells are produced in the bone marrow.

- Bone is highly vascular, living tissue that is maintained and repaired by bone cells (*i.e.*, osteocytes, osteoblasts, osteoclasts).

- Healing of fractured bone generally occurs in stages: inflammation, cellular proliferation, callus formation, callus ossification, and remodeling.

- The skeletal muscles contract to move the body, maintain posture, and maintain body temperature. Tendons attach the muscles to the bones. Joints allow for and control the extent of movement. Ligaments provide stability to the musculoskeletal system. Movement and muscle tone are coordinated through the nervous system.

- Exercise maintains muscle strength and function. Atrophy and contracture occur with immobility and disuse.

- Aging is reflected in the musculoskeletal system by the development of osteoporosis, decreased range of motion, thinned intervertebral discs, and weakened muscles.

- Physical assessment and multiple diagnostic studies are used to evaluate the musculoskeletal system. The nurse prepares and supports the person undergoing various diagnostic procedures and reviews the diagnostic findings for nursing care implications.

- Altered function of the musculoskeletal system affects the person's ability to carry out activities of daily living. The nurse and the patient develop strategies to meet the patient's basic human needs that have been compromised by alterations in the musculoskeletal system.

Chapter 62   Management Modalities for Patients With Musculoskeletal Dysfunction

- Individuals with musculoskeletal dysfunction are assessed to determine the impact of the condition on their ability to maintain health, accomplish activities of daily living, and manage the treatment modality. Using knowledge of various treatment modalities, the nurse applies the nursing process to assist the patient in meeting identified health needs. Treatment modalities frequently used for patients with musculoskeletal dysfunction include casts, external fixation devices, traction, and surgery.

- Casts are rigid, external immobilizing devices that encase a body part to maintain a specific position. They are most frequently used to treat fractures and to support weakened joints and muscles. They may be used for immobilization after orthopedic surgery (*e.g.*, bone grafting, bone fusion, internal fixation). Complications that can result from a cast include compartment syndrome, pressure ulcers, and disuse atrophy.

- Compartment syndrome results from an increase of tissue pressure within the cast and resulting compromise of circulation. Loss of motor and sensory function results from tissue anoxia if compartment syndrome is undetected and untreated.

- Pressure ulcers result from pressure of the cast on soft tissues. If not detected early, excessive loss of tissue may occur.

- Disuse syndrome results from inadequate exercise of muscles and muscle atrophy. The use of isometric muscle contraction exercises is important in maintaining muscle tone and strength and reducing muscle atrophy.

- External fixation devices are special frames attached to the bone by pins or wires. They are used primarily for treatment of open fractures. Special fixators (*e.g.,* Ilizarov device) may be used for correction of deformity and nonunion and for limb lengthening. Care of the tissues in the area of the pin or wire is essential for preventing infection.

- Traction is the application of a pulling force to the skin or bony skeleton to minimize muscle spasm; to reduce, align, and immobilize fractures; to lessen deformity; and to increase space between opposing joint surfaces. Traction must be applied in the desired direction and appropriate magnitude to achieve the therapeutic effect. Skin traction, such as pelvic and cervical traction, used to reduce muscle spasm is usually prescribed as intermittent traction. Conversely, skeletal traction is not to be interrupted and must be continuous.

- Surgical procedures (*e.g.,* open reduction, internal fixation, bone grafting, amputation, arthroplasty, meniscectomy, joint replacement, tendon transfer, fasciotomy) are used to treat a variety of musculoskeletal disorders. In the early postoperative period the nurse focuses on pain management, promotion of tissue perfusion, and prevention of complications: shock, atelectasis, pneumonia, urinary retention, infection, and deep vein thrombosis.

- Patient education and preparation to care for himself or herself in the home setting are essential. The patient is encouraged to actively participate in the progressive rehabilitation program.

Chapter 63   Management of Patients With Musculoskeletal Disorders

- Low back pain is experienced by many individuals during their lives. The most frequent of the multiple causes of low back pain is musculoskeletal in origin. Frequently, the pain is due to strain of weak back muscles as a result of using improper body mechanics. Conservative therapy includes bed rest to promote healing of weakened structures, progressive strengthening exercises, instruction in the use of proper body mechanics, and weight reduction if appropriate. Analgesics, anti-inflammatory agents, and muscle relaxants are useful in reducing the discomfort. At times a multidisciplinary approach is needed to help the patient to modify pain perception and to cope with changes in role performance and prolonged disability.

- Musculoskeletal conditions of the upper extremities are in many cases a result of acute or long-standing stress on the involved structure or trauma. Pain and difficulty in performing activities of daily living are the most common concerns expressed by patients with these conditions. Painful shoulder syndrome and "tennis elbow" respond to rest, thermal therapies, and gradual resumption of activity after healing has occurred. Other conditions (*e.g.,* ganglion, carpal tunnel syndrome, Dupuytren's contracture) may require surgery for symptom relief.

- Common foot conditions (*e.g.,* corns, calluses, ingrown toenails) and common deformities of the foot (*e.g.,* flatfoot, hammer toes, bunion, pes cavus, Morton's neuroma) affect the individual's comfort and mobility. Therapy is designed to correct the underlying problem. Frequently, appropriate supportive footwear is needed to relieve the discomfort. If surgery is required, the patient is assisted in controlling pain, improving mobility through safe use of assistive devices, and preventing infection.

- Metabolic bone disorders (osteoporosis, osteomalacia, and Paget's disease) affect the amount and quality of bone. Osteoporosis can result in vertebral compression fractures, fractures of the hip, and fractures of the wrist, particularly in small-framed, non-obese, postmenopausal Caucasian women. Preventive education includes increasing the intake of calcium; avoiding smoking, caffeine, and alcohol; performing weight-bearing exercise; and preventing falls. At menopause, hormone replacement therapy may retard bone loss and prevent occurrence of fractures in women at risk. When a fracture occurs, efforts are directed toward pain relief, stabilization and healing of the fracture, and prevention of further fractures.

- Osteomalacia is characterized by softening of bone, pain, bowing of bones, and pathologic fractures. Nursing management focuses on pain management and improvement of the patient's body image and self-concept.

- Paget's disease is characterized by deformity, weakness, and risk of pathologic fracture. Symptoms are varied; treatment approaches are individualized and may include nonsteroidal anti-inflammatory agents or suppressive therapy to inhibit bone resorption.

- Musculoskeletal infections include osteomyelitis and septic arthritis. Prevention of infection is the goal since the infection may affect the quality of life or result in the loss of an extremity. Osteomyelitis may be associated with open fracture, bone surgery, and soft-tissue or blood-borne infection. It may be evident soon after orthopedic injury or surgery or not until months or years afterwards. The patient is assisted to understand and comply with the therapeutic regimen, including long courses of antibiotic therapy and surgical debridement, pain management, and mobility limitations. Septic arthritis requires prompt treatment to preserve joint function.

Chapter 64 Management of Patients With Musculoskeletal Trauma

- Injury to the musculoskeletal system includes trauma to the bones and muscles and to associated soft tissues (*i.e.*, cartilage, tendons, ligaments, blood vessels, nerves). Contusions from blunt blows result in bleeding into the soft tissues. Strains are muscle pulls; sprains are injuries to the ligament structures surrounding a joint.

- All soft-tissue injuries require immobilization of the injured part and elevation to control edema. Gradual resumption of activities is essential for successful rehabilitation.

- Joint dislocations are medical emergencies because of possible injury to associated blood vessels and nerves. Prompt reduction and gradual resumption of activities are necessary for restoring joint function.

- Sports injuries are most common in individuals participating in recreational sports without adequate training. Proper equipment (*e.g.*, running shoes) and conditioning can help prevent sports injuries. Individuals who experience sports-related injuries are highly motivated to return to the pre-injury level of activity; they may have difficulty complying with gradual resumption of prescribed activities, which is essential for healing.

- Fractures in the continuity of the bone occur when the stress on the bone is greater than it can absorb. Clinical manifestations of fracture include pain, loss of function, false motion, deformity, shortening, crepitus, local swelling, and discoloration. Treatment includes reduction (reestablishment of length and alignment) and immobilization (*e.g.*, cast, traction, splint, brace, bandage, external fixation, internal fixation). The patient is monitored for the development of fracture complications, response to treatment, and resumption of activities. Resumption of activities depends on the location of the fracture and the specific rehabilitation prescribed.

- Amputation may be necessary because of progressive trauma, peripheral vascular disease, congenital deformity, or malignancy. Amputation is performed to improve the patient's quality of life. The patient may encounter difficulties, including pain, phantom limb sensations, altered skin integrity, disturbed body image, grieving, self-care deficit, and impaired mobility as well as hemorrhage, infections, and skin breakdown. Rehabilitation after amputation is a multidisciplinary effort. The nurse focuses on the patient's physical and psychologic responses, adjustment to the amputation, and promotion of health.

Chapter 65　Management of Patients With Infectious Diseases

- Knowledge of infectious diseases is important in all aspects of health care, particularly because of the increased incidence of infectious diseases such as HIV and AIDS, TB, and sexually transmitted diseases and the growing problem of antibiotic-resistant infectious organisms.

- An understanding of the complexity of many serious, contagious, or common infections is vital. In addition, it is important to effectively rely on the resources of infectious disease specialists, epidemiologists, and guidelines from the Centers for Disease Control (CDC) for assistance in less common diseases.

- The outcome of infectious diseases can range from absence of symptoms to fatality. Prevention of the spread of infection requires breaking the chain of transmission.

- Controlling and preventing infection requires the practices of handwashing and glove use, adhering to standards and guidelines of the CDC and the Occupational Safety and Health Administration (OSHA), and practicing Universal Precautions and Body Substance Isolation.

- Infectious diseases can be grouped into several categories and subcategories: nosocomial infections, sexually transmitted diseases, community infections, diarrheal diseases, hepatitis viruses, herpes viruses, meningitis, rickettsial infections, and vaccine-preventable diseases.

- Understanding the natural history of the human immunodeficiency virus is important for all health care workers. HIV has a very long incubation period and can influence the health status of an individual for a decade or longer. The dismal outcome associated with HIV infection demands intense educational and supportive efforts to decrease the risk of transmission from the patient to others.

- Nurses and other health care workers can protect themselves from occupational acquisition of infectious diseases by practicing Universal Precautions, by obtaining hepatitis B and influenza vaccination, and by strictly adhering to CDC and OSHA standards and prevention guidelines.

- Research for more and better antibiotics and other pharmacologic advances continues. Microorganisms have proved their adaptability by developing resistance to antibiotics. It would be a potentially catastrophic scenario if common infectious diseases became untreatable, as they were throughout history.

Chapter 66　Emergency Nursing

- Management of patients who present to emergency departments with acute drug abuse, psychiatric emergencies, or after sexual assault is complex and requires a multidisciplinary team approach.

- The patient's physiologic, psychologic, and emotional status is continuously assessed and managed. Precautions are taken to assure the safety of both the patient and the hospital personnel involved in his or her care.

- Specific protocols are followed for victims of sexual assault; these provide for crisis intervention and for measures that ensure that the requirements for subsequent legal proceedings are met.

- Once the patient's acute needs have been met, provisions are made for ongoing treatment as appropriate.

Answer Key

Chapter 1

I. Knowledge-Based Questions

Multiple-Choice

1. d (p. 8)
2. a (p. 8)
3. d (p. 11)
4. d (p. 11)

5. b (pp. 4–5)
6. a (pp. 4–5)
7. b (pp. 4–5)
8. a (p. 15)

9. c (pp. 4–5)
10. d (pp. 11–13)
11. d (pp. 9–11)
12. d (pp. 9–11)

Fill-In

1. Legislative and sociologic changes that are impinging on nursing care are chronic illnesses, the increase in those older than 65, the shift from disease cure to health promotion, and cost control and resource management. (pp. 4–5)

2. Human responses requiring nursing intervention are (b) self-image changes, (c) impaired ventilation, and (d) anxiety and fear. Answers may also include pain and discomfort, grief, and impaired functioning in areas such as rest and sleep. (pp. 8–9)

3. Answer may include any of the following: (a) stop/don't smoke, (b) exercise at least three times weekly for 30 to 45 minutes, (c) decrease salt, sugar, and fat intake, (d) find some time to relax each day, and (e) find ways to manage and cope with stress. (pp. 8–9)

4. Declining in-patient hospital days, shorter lengths of hospital stay, increased acuity of patients, expansion of ambulatory care, and an explosion of community-based care. (pp. 7–8)

5. The role of the independent nurse practitioner is to provide nursing services in her office or in the patient's home for the purpose of health assessment, counseling, teaching, and making referrals to other health professionals and agencies. The boundaries of the independent practitioner role are determined by state nurse practice acts. (pp. 12–14)

6. The major purpose of the nurse practice acts is to set rules and regulations for nursing practice within each state. (pp. 8–9)

7. In Maslow's hierarchy of needs, needs are ranked as follows: (pp. 11–12, Figure 1–1)

Need	*Example*
Physiologic	Food
Safety and security	Financial security
Belongingness and affection	Companionship
Esteem and self-respect	Recognition by society
Self-actualization	Achieved potential in an area
Self-fulfillment	Creativity (painting)
Knowledge and understanding	Information and explanation
Aesthetics	Attractive environment

8. Case management focuses on managing the care of an entire caseload of patients and the personnel who care for the patients. The goals include quality care, appropriate and timely care delivery, and cost reduction. (pp. 7–8)

9. Clinical pathways list the sequencing of tests, treatments, activities, medications, and such, that a patient must progress through per diagnosis, within a set time period from admission to discharge. (pp. 9–10)

II. Critical Analysis Questions

Supporting Arguments

1. Values are personalized and influenced by your society's ideals and customs. Therefore, your answers will be individualized. However, for your reference, some common values found in the nursing profession are: compassion, equality, honesty, integrity, respect for human dignity, and selflessness. (pp. 8–9)

2. Share your data and discuss your response with your instructor and classmates. There are no specific right or wrong answers. The validity of your response is determined by your ability to consciously support your argument. (pp. 4–12)

Recognizing Contradictions

1. A person with chronic illness can attain a high level of wellness if he or she is successful in meeting his or her health potential within the limits of the chronic illness. (p. 4)

2. The majority of health problems today are chronic in nature. (pp. 4–5)

3. The elderly in the United States will constitute 20% of the total population by the year 2000. (pp. 4–5)

4. A patient may refuse medical and nursing care according to the AHA's Patient Bill of Rights. (p. 6, Chart 1–1)

5. Health care costs will be 15% to 22% of the GNP by 2000. (pp. 7–8)

Generating Solutions: Clinical Problem Solving

1. Flow Chart: Smoking (pp. 6–7 plus reference your current knowledge about anatomy and physiology)

Smoking   *Illnesses*

Respiratory changes
- ↓ciliary action
- ↑mucous production =
- ↑airway resistance

- Coronary artery disease
- Emphysema
- Lung cancer

Cardiovascular change
- ↑CO levels
- ↑arterial vasoconstriction
- ↑blood pressure

2. Flow Chart: Radial pulse assessment (pp. 6–7 plus reference your knowledge of fundamental skills)

Radial Pulse Assessment

1.0	2.0	3.0	4.0	5.0
Patient ID	Explain Procedure	Identify Site	Palpate Pulse	Document Results

1.0	2.0	3.0	4.0	5.0
1.1 ID Patient 1.2 Ask patient his name 1.3 Check patient's name on bed.	2.1 Give instruction at level of patient's learning.	3.1 Extend forearm 3.2 Locate pulse on inner thumb-side of wrist	4.1 Place pads of index and middle finger over radial artery. 4.2 Palpate for rate, rhythm, amplitude, and symmetry. 4.3 Count rate for 60 seconds if irregular, 30 seconds × 2 if regular. 4.4 Reassess for any abnormalities.	5.1 Note rate and character. 5.2 Record on graphic sheet on patient chart. 5.3 Report appropriate information.

Chapter 2

I. Knowledge-Based Questions

Multiple-Choice

1. d (pp. 18–20)
2. d (pp. 18–20)
3. c (pp. 18–20)

4. c (pp. 18–20)
5. b (p. 19)
6. d (pp. 19–20)

Fill-In

1. Nurses will need to be expert, independent decision-makers who are self-directed, flexible, adaptable, and competent in independent decision making. (pp. 19–22)

2. Call the patient to obtain permission for a visit, schedule the visit and verify the address. (p. 20)

3. During the initial home visit, the patient is evaluated and a plan of care established. (p. 20)

4. Ambulatory health care can be provided in medical clinics, ambulatory care units, urgent care centers, cardiac rehabilitation programs, and nurse-managed centers. (p. 22)

5. Nurse practitioners can specialize in gerontology, midwifery, pediatrics, and family planning. (pp. 22–24)

Chapter 3

I. Knowledge-Based Questions

Multiple-Choice

1. d (pp. 27–29)
2. d (pp. 28–30)
3. c (p. 29 [Table 3–1])
4. a (p. 30 [Chart 3–2])
5. a (pp. 31–33)

6. d (pp. 31–33)
7. b (pp. 33–35)
8. c (pp. 33–34)
9. b (pp. 33–34)
10. a (pp. 34–36)

Fill-In

1. The nurse has many roles during the interview process. Your answer may include any four of the following. The nurse should:
   a. maintain privacy and promote comfort.
   b. establish rapport based on trust and respect.
   c. listen and question.
   d. observe and interpret.
   e. synthesize and plan.
   f. assume a dominant role throughout, guide the interaction, and set time limits. (pp. 27–29)

2. Suggested statements include: "Please tell me what brought you to the hospital," "Please tell me what you think your needs are," and "Please tell me about your past history." (pp. 27–29 [Chart 3–1])

3. A complete health assessment identifies physical, psychological, and emotional parameters of functioning, to determine whether a nursing need exists. (pp. 27–29)

4. A nursing diagnosis identifies actual or potential health problems that are amenable to resolution by nursing actions. Collaborative problems are physiologic complications that nurses monitor, in collaboration with a physician, to detect onset or changes in a patient's status. The nursing diagnosis and collaborative problems are the patient's nursing problems. A medical diagnosis identifies diseases conditions or pathology that can be medically managed. (pp. 30–31)

5. A nursing diagnosis is a clinical judgment about individual, family, or community responses to actual or potential health problems or life processes. Nursing diagnoses provide the basis for selecting nursing interventions to achieve outcomes for which the nurse is accountable. (pp. 30–31)

6. Expected outcomes of nursing intervention should be stated in behavioral terms and should be realistic as well as measurable. Expected behavioral outcomes serve as the basis for evaluating the effectiveness of nursing intervention. (pp. 33–35)

II. Critical Analysis Questions

Generating Solutions: Clinical Problem Solving

Outcomes per Nursing Diagnosis

1. Patient will be able to walk from his room to the nursing station every morning with respiratory rate within normal limits.

2. Patient will move from bed to chair on second postoperative day with legs abducted.

3. Patient will achieve a balance between fluid intake and output without a weight gain > 1 lb per week.

4. Patient will eat 1800 cal/day to maintain a desired weight of 135 lb.

5. Patient will sleep 6 to 8 hours, without interruption, every evening.
   (Reference pages 33–35)

Nursing Diagnoses and Collaborative Problems

1. N	**6.** N
2. N	**7.** C
3. C	**8.** C
4. C	**9.** N
5. N	**10.** C (pages 30–31)

Chapter 4

I. Knowledge-Based Questions

Multiple-Choice

1. d (p. 40)	**6.** a (pp. 41–43)
2. d (pp. 40–45)	**7.** a (pp. 41–43)
3. b (pp. 40–45)	**8.** a (p. 43)
4. d (pp. 41–42)	**9.** b (pp. 43–45)
5. a (pp. 41–43)	**10.** a (pp. 44–45)

Fill-In

1. People with chronic illness need as much health care information as possible to actively participate in and assume responsibility for the management of their own care. Health education can help the patient adapt to illness and cooperate with a treatment regimen. The goal of health education is to teach people to maximize their health potential. (p. 40)

2. *Adherence* implies that a patient assumes a more active role in determining and altering his or her health behaviors. (pp. 40–41)

3. Factors influencing adherence include demographic variables, such as age, sex, and education, illness variables, such as the severity of illness and the effects of therapy, and psychosocial variables, such as intelligence and attitudes toward illness. (pp. 40–41)

4. The teaching–learning process requires the active involvement of teacher and learner, both striving to achieve the goal of changing patient behavior. The teacher serves as a facilitator of learning. (pp. 41–42)

5. The effects of a learning situation are influenced by a person's physical, emotional, and experiential readiness to learn. *Physical readiness* implies the physical ability of a person to attend to a learning situation. Basic physiologic needs are met so that higher-level needs can be addressed. *Emotional readiness* involves the patient's motivation to learn and can be encouraged by providing realistic goals that can be easily achieved so that self-esteem needs can be met. A person needs to be ready to accept the emotional changes (anxiety, stress) that accompany behavior modification resulting from the learning process. *Experiential readiness* refers to a person's past experiences that influence his or her approach to the learning process. Previous positive feedback and improved self-image reinforce experiential readiness. (pp. 41–42)

6. Both processes are cyclic and recurrent with each step related to the others. Continuous evaluation supports the processes and helps maintain accountability. (pp. 43–45)

II. Critical Analysis Questions

Recognizing Contradictions

1. Health education is an independent function of nursing practice that is a primary responsibility of the nursing profession. (p. 40)

2. Although diseases in children and those of an infectious nature are of utmost concern, the largest group of people today that need health education are those with chronic illness. (p. 40)

3. Patients are encouraged to adhere to their therapeutic regimen. Adherence connotes active, voluntary, collaborative patient efforts whereas compliance is a more passive role. (pp. 40–41)

4. Evaluation should be continuous throughout the teaching process so that the information gathered can be used to improve teaching activities. (p. 45)

Chapter 5

I. Knowledge-Based Questions

Multiple-Choice

1. b (p. 52)
2. c (p. 53)
3. b (pp. 53–54)
4. d (p. 54)

5. a (p. 54)
6. d (p. 54)
7. d (p. 56)
8. c (pp. 56–58)

Fill-In

1. A moral decision exists when there is a clear conflict of two or more principles or competing moral claims. One must choose "the lesser of two evils." (p. 53)

2. *Ethical pluralism* refers to ethical reasoning and decision making tht combines utilitarianism and formalism. (pp. 54–55)

3. Ethical behavior based on "virtues" means that moral conduct is directly related to an individual's character traits. (pp. 55–56)

4. Two types of "advanced directive" are a living will and a durable power of attorney. (p. 61)

5. An "advanced directive" provided health care practitioners with information about the person's wishes for health care before their illness. (p. 61)

Matching

1. d
2. e
3. b
4. f
5. a
6. c

(p. 55, Chart 5–1)

II. Critical Analysis Questions

Analyzing Comparisons

1. a personal commitment to values (p. 52)

2. understanding concepts (pp. 52–53)

3. normative ethics (p. 53)

4. behaviors based on individual character traits (pp. 54–56)

Recognizing Contradictions

1. Nursing ethics is a distinct form of applied ethics because nursing is its own separate profession. (p. 53)

2. A moral problem infers no conflict of moral principle. (p. 53)

3. Moral distress exists when a nurse is prevented from doing what she believes is correct. (p. 53)

4. A request for withdrawal of food and hydration necessitates an evaluation of harm and may not be routinely supported even for competent patients. (pp. 58–59)

5. Living wills are not always honored because they refer to terminal illnesses and patients frequently change their perspectives as they become sicker. (p. 61)

Supporting Arguments

1–3. Answers are individualized, there are no right or wrong responses. (reference pp. 52–56)

Generating Solutions: Clinical Problem Solving

CASE STUDY: Ethical Analysis

Assessment: Your answer should include the conflict between the nurse's professional obligation to provide treatment to all and the unpleasant outcome of choosing "the lesser of two outcomes." (pp. 52–53)

Planning: You should be able to analyze the medical and political data that influences the treatment options. Because of the vast numbers of refugees relative to medical personnel, everyone cannot be cared for. Refer to pages 54–55 for a discussion of utilitarian versus deontological theories of decision making.

Implementation: You need to carefully analyze the outcomes of both theories for your decision making. There is no right or wrong answer. You just need to support your decision with an ethical theory. (pp. 54–55)

Evaluation: Your evaluation needs to show logical sequencing of problem solving based on an ethical theory. There is no right or wrong response. (reference p. 59, Chart 5–3)

Chapter 6

I. Knowledge-Based Questions

Multiple-Choice

1. d (p. 68)
2. d (pp. 68–70)
3. d (pp. 68–70)
4. c (pp. 68–70)
5. b (pp. 68–69)

6. a (pp. 72–73; Chart 6–1)
7. b (pp. 72–73; Chart 6–1)
8. b (p. 74; Chart 6–2)
9. b (pp. 74–75)
10. d (pp. 73–76)

Fill-In

1. The nursing database is a combination of the traditional medical history and the nursing assessment. The systems review and patient profile are expanded to include individual and family relations, lifestyle patterns, health practices, and coping strategies. (p. 68)

2. Health professionals work together so that each member of the health care team can maximize his or her skills in contributing to the resolution of the patient's problems. Health professionals include physicians, nurses, nutritionists, social workers, pharmacists, respiratory therapists, and others. (p. 68)

3. When an atmosphere of mutual trust and confidence exists between an interviewer and a patient, the patient becomes more open and honest and is more likely to share personal concerns and problems. (pp. 68–69)

4. During an interview, a nurse is inquiring when she allows the patient to communicate freely. The interview becomes therapeutic when the nurse directs the conversation toward specific goals. The interview becomes more nurse-directed and nurse-controlled with a therapeutic approach. (pp. 68–70)

5. The term *chief complaint* refers to that issue that brings the patient to seek help. When documenting a patient's chief complaint, exact words should be recorded in quotation marks. (p. 71)

6. The focus of information obtained for a patient profile is personal and subjective. Content areas that should be covered include past development, education and occupation, environmental influences (physical, spiritual, and interpersonal), lifestyle, self-concept, and stress responses. (p. 71)

II. Critical Analysis Questions

Recognizing Contradictions

1. A major role for nurses is the <u>diagnosis and planning of appropriate interventions</u> that can be met through nursing care. (p. 68)

2. <u>Nonverbal communication</u> is always more effective than verbal communication. (p. 70)

3. The <u>interviewer</u> needs to <u>assume</u> a <u>dominant leadership role</u>. (pp. 68–70)

4. <u>Continual documentation</u> is <u>distracting</u> to the patient. It also interferes with eye contact and may imply an attitude of disinterest. (pp. 7–10)

5. The most personal area of assessment on the patient profile is the section on <u>sexuality</u>. (p. 75)

6. A person's ability to handle stressful situations is influenced by his <u>past coping patterns</u> and the <u>type and duration of a stressor</u>. (pp. 75–76)

Chapter 7

I. Knowledge-Based Questions

Multiple-Choice

1. b (pp. 80–81)
2. a (p. 81)
3. d (p. 82)
4. a (p. 82)
5. a (pp. 82–83)

6. d (pp. 83–84, Figure 7–7)
7. b (p. 89, Figure 7–7)
8. c (p. 85, Figures 7–5 and 7–6)
9. a (pp. 85–86)
10. a (pp. 88–90)

Matching

1. h
2. c
3. d
4. e
5. g
6. b

(p. 87, Table 7–3)

Fill-In

1. inspection and palpation (pp. 80–82)

2. Your answer may include any of the five diseases related to dietary excess: obesity, coronary artery disease, osteoporosis, cirrhosis, diverticulitis, and eating disorders. (pp. 87–91)

3. upperarm and arm muscle (pp. 84–85)

4. Negative nitrogen balance occurs when nitrogen output (urine, feces, perspiration) exceeds nitrogen intake (food) (pp. 85–86)

5. maintain nutrition and replace any nutrient loss within the framework of the patient's condition and environment (pp. 88–90)

Correlation

1. inspection ⎫
2. inspection ⎬ (pp. 80–81)
3. palpation ⎫
4. palpation ⎬ (pp. 81–82)

5. percussion (p. 82)
6. auscultation ⎫
7. auscultation ⎬ (pp. 82–83)
8. palpation (pp. 81–82)

II. Critical Analysis Questions

Generating Solutions: Clinical Problem Solving

CASE STUDY

Part I: Estimate Ideal Body Weight

Mrs. Alred's Situation

1. b, medium frame, height to wrist (p. 84, Chart 7–2) circumference is 10.4

2. IBW = 130 lb; lose 50 lb (p. 84, Chart 7–1)

Part II: Calculate a Balanced Diet Using the Food Guide Pyramid as a Reference

1. 50 kg
2. 1418 cal
3. 1985 cal (1418 + 567)
4. 993 cal from carbohydrates
   595 cal from fat
   397 cal from protein
5. 248 g of carbohydrates
   66 g of fat
   99 g of protein

(pp. 88–90, Figure 7–7)

Chapter 8

I. Knowledge-Based Questions

Multiple-Choice

1. b (pp. 96–100)
2. a (pp. 96–100)
3. d (pp. 96–100)
4. d (pp. 96–97)
5. d (p. 98)
6. a (pp. 99–100)

7. d (pp. 98–100)
8. d (pp. 99–100)
9. d (p. 100)
10. c (p. 100)
11. d (pp. 100–101)
12. d (p. 101)

13. d (p. 101)
14. b (p. 101)
15. a (pp. 101–102)
16. a (pp. 102–103)
17. d (pp. 102–103)
18. d (pp. 102–103)

II. Critical Analysis Questions

Analyzing Comparisons

1. adaptation (pp. 98–99)

2. perpetuation of activity and noncompensation (p. 98)

3. decreased cellular size (*e.g.*, secondary sex organs) (pp. 98–99)

4. cellular infiltration, necrosis, and fibrosis (pp. 101–103)

Generating Solutions: Clinical Problem Solving

CASE STUDY

Use the "Representative Pathophysiologic Process: Hypertensive Heart disease (pp. 103–104) as a guide.

Selected Compensatory Mechanisms	*Nursing Implications*	*Rationale*
A. Renal blood flow is decreased as a result of hypertensive heart disease.	*Assessment*	
	A. Blood pressure	A. Changes in the cardiovascular system are reflected in the blood pressure.
	B. Urinary output	
	1. Amount	1. Output decreased with decreased blood flow.
	2. Characteristics	2. Color changes occur with increased density.
	3. Urine chemistry values	
	a. Osmolality	a. Osmolality increases with heart failure.
	b. Electrolytes	b. Potassium increases with renal failure.
	C. Ability to cope with stress	C. Stress results in increased resistance to cardiac output.
	Nursing Diagnosis/ Collaborative Problem	
	A. Fluid volume excess related to renin–angiotensin stimulation	A. Renin–angiotensin has a direct vasoconstriction effect on arterioles which leads to water retention.
	Planning	
	A. Plan time for assessment around patient's need for rest.	A. Rest lowers metabolic rate and facilitates the healing process.
	B. Plan an individual program of stress reduction.	B. Compliance with a stress-management program will be higher if the program is individualized.

Selected Compensatory Mechanisms	Nursing Implications	Rationale
	Implementation	
	A. Teach various relaxation techniques.	A. Stress tends to increase epinephrine secretion, which causes vasoconstriction. This, in turn, increases the heart rate and resistance to cardiac output.
	B. Develop specific ways to help the patient cope with and reduce stress.	B. Stress reduction tends to reduce epinephrine secretion.
	C. Modify diet to reduce sodium intake.	C. Lowered sodium levels tend to decrease fluid retention, which decreases the work load of the heart.
	Evaluation	
	A. Stress-reduction measures	A. Blood pressure reduction may be indicative of successful stress-reduction measures.
	B. Dietary compliance relative to lowered sodium intake	B. Weight estimates, serum sodium levels, and the presence of edema are indicators of fluid retention and possible excess intake of sodium.

(Refer to pp. 103–104 for help in completing this case plan.)

Chapter 9

I. Knowledge-Based Questions

Multiple-Choice

1. d (p. 106)
2. c (pp. 106–109)
3. a (pp. 106–109)
4. d (pp. 107–109)
5. d (pp. 107–108)
6. b (p. 108)

7. a (p. 108)
8. b (pp. 109–111 [Table 9–1])
9. b (pp. 109–111 [Table 9–1])
10. d (pp. 110–111)
11. c (pp. 110–111)
12. b (p. 110)

13. d (p. 110)
14. d (pp. 107–109)
15. d (pp. 108–109)
16. d (pp. 108–109)

Matching

1. b
2. a
3. a
4. a
5. b   (pp. 106–111)
6. a
7. b
8. a

Fill-In

1. Hans Selye (p. 106)

2. Hans Selye stated that "stress is essentially the rate of wear and tear on the body." He also defined stress as being a "nonspecific response" of the body regardless of the stimulus producing the response. (p. 3)

3. Answer may include any of the following: traffic jam, sick child, missed appointment, car won't start, train is late (day-to-day stressors), earthquakes, wars, terrorism, events of history (major events that affect large groups of people); and marriage, birth, death, retirement (infrequently occurring major stressors). (pp. 106–107)

4. Adolph Meyer, in the 1930s, first showed a correlation between illness and critical life events. A Recent Life Changes Questionnaire (RLCQ) was developed by Holmes and Rahe that assigned numerical values to life events that required a change in an individual's life pattern. A correlation was seen between illness and the number of stressful events; the higher the numerical value, the greater the chance for becoming ill. (p. 107)

5. *Cognitive appraisal* refers to the evaluation of an event relative to what is at stake and what coping resources are available. *External resources* consist of money to purchase services and materials and social support systems that provide emotional and esteem support. (pp. 106–109)

II. Critical Analysis Questions

Generating Solutions: Clinical Problem Solving

General body arousal

		Rationale
$\uparrow$norepinephrine =	$\uparrow$ blood coagulability	vasoconstriction
	$\uparrow$ heart rate	$\uparrow$ myocardial contractility
	$\uparrow$ blood pressure	peripheral vasoconstriction
	$\uparrow$ blood glucose levels	$\uparrow$ glycogen breakdown

$\downarrow$

Skeletal muscles	increased tension	$\uparrow$ muscle excitation
Pupils	dilated	$\uparrow$ awareness
Ventilation	rapid and shallow	oxygen preservation

(pp. 109–111, Table 9–1)

373

Chapter 10

I. Knowledge-Based Questions

Multiple-Choice

1. b (p. 120)
2. c (p. 121)
3. d (p. 122)
4. a (pp. 122–123)
5. b (pp. 122–123)
6. d (pp. 124–125; NCP 10–1)
7. b (p. 123)

8. a (pp. 123–125)
9. a (pp. 125–127)
10. a (pp. 128–129)
11. a (p. 130)
12. d (p. 130)
13. b (pp. 128–130)
14. d (pp. 128–130)

15. b (pp. 123–127)
16. b (pp. 120–121)
17. d (pp. 120–127)
18. d (pp. 120–123)
19. c (pp. 120–121)

II. Critical Analysis Questions

Generating Solutions: Clinical Problem Solving

CASE STUDY: Hodgkin's Disease

Joan's Situation

1. a
2. b
3. d
⎬ (pp. 120–121)

CASE STUDY: Radical Mastectomy

Kathy's Situation

1. a
2. b
3. b
4. d
⎬ (pp.120–121)

Chapter 11

I. Knowledge-Based Questions

Multiple-Choice

1. d (p. 134)
2. b (pp. 134–135)
3. d (p. 135)
4. d (pp. 136–137)

5. a (pp. 136–137)
6. d (p. 137)
7. a (p. 137)
8. a (p. 137)

9. c (pp. 137–138 [Table 11–1])
10. b (pp. 138–139)

Fill-In

1. The four basic characteristics of culture reflect the fact that it is learned from birth through langauge and socialization, it is shared by all members of the group, it is influenced by specific environmental factors, and it is ever-changing. (p. 134)

2. Subcultures can be grouped accordingly by religion, occupation, age, sexual orientation, geographic location, and race. (p. 134)

3. Four strategies include changing the subject, nonquestioning, inappropriate laughter, and nonverbal cues. (pp. 135–136)

4. The Catholics, Mormons, Buddhists, Jews, and Muslims routinely abstain from eating as part of their religious practice. (pp. 137–138)

5. The yin and yang theory of illness proposes that the seat of energy in the body is within the autonomic nervous system where balance is maintained between the key opposing forces. *Yin* represents the female and negative energy, while *yang* represents warmth and the male. (pp. 138–139)

Chapter 12

I. Knowledge-Based Questions

Multiple-Choice

1. d (p. 142)
2. b (pp. 143–145)
3. d (pp. 143–144)
4. b (p. 144)
5. b (pp. 144–145)
6. d (pp. 145–146)

7. b (p. 146)
8. a (p. 148)
9. c (p. 149)
10. a (p. 150)
11. b (pp. 151–152)
12. d (pp. 151–152)

13. d (pp. 165–167 [Table 12–7])
14. b (pp. 165–167 [Table 12–7])
15. a (pp. 168–169)
16. a (p. 169)

II. Critical Analysis Questions

Recognizing Contradictions

1. The muscles, composed of postmitotic cells, diminish in size and lose strength, flexibility, and endurance with decreased activity and advanced age. (pp. 150–151)

2. Osteoporosis can be arrested or prevented, but not reversed. (pp. 150–151)

3. If the symptoms of delirium go untreated and the underlying cause is not treated, permanent, irreversible brain damage or death can occur. (p. 24)

4. It is a myth that older people should avoid vigorous activity. Activity is a desired state in older adults. (pp. 158–159)

5. Back pain can accompany a number of chronic problems and may be an early sign of osteoporosis. (p. 167)

Generating Solutions: Clinical Problem Solving

CASE STUDY: Loneliness

Suzanne's Situation

1. d (pp. 145–146)
2. d (pp. 148–149)
3. a (pp. 149–150)
4. d (pp. 149–150)
5. d (pp. 168–169)

CASE STUDY: Dehydration

Vera's Situation

1. d (pp. 147–149 [Table 12–3])
2. c (pp. 147–149 [Table 12–3])
3. d (pp. 149–150)
4. d (p. 148)

CASE STUDY: Alzheimer's Disease

Thomas' Situation

1. a
2. c
3. d   (pp. 157–165 [NCP 12–1])
4. d

Chapter 13

I. Knowledge-Based Questions

Multiple-Choice

1. d (pp. 182–183)
2. d (pp. 182–183)
3. a (p. 184)
4. c (p. 187)
5. c (p. 187)

6. d (pp. 188–189)
7. b (pp. 182–183)
8. b (p. 180)
9. b (pp. 180–181)
10. c (pp. 180–181)

11. a (pp. 184–185)
12. a (pp. 185–186)
13. d (pp. 188–190)
14. d (pp. 192–193)
15. d (pp. 192–193)

16. c (pp. 192–193)
17. b (p. 195)
18. d (p. 196)
19. d (pp. 190–191)

II. Critical Analysis Questions

Generating Solutions: Clinical Problem Solving

CASE STUDY: Pain Experience

Courtney's Situation

1. a (p. 180)
2. c (pp. 185–187)
3. d (pp. 196–197)
4. d (p. 198)

Chapter 14

I. Knowledge-Based Questions

Multiple-Choice

1. d (p. 208; [Table 14–2])
2. b (pp. 208, 212; [Table 14–4])
3. a (p. 213 [Table 14–5])
4. a (p. 214)
5. b (pp. 217–218)
6. a (p. 218)
7. b (p. 218)
8. b (pp. 218–219)

9. c (pp. 218–220)
10. c (p. 219)
11. a (p. 221)
12. b (p. 222–223)
13. c (pp. 220–222)
14. c (pp. 224–225)
15. b (pp. 225–227)
16. b (p. 228)

17. c (pp. 228–229)
18. d (pp. 233–235)
19. c (p. 232)
20. a (pp. 232–233)
21. c (p. 233)
22. b (pp. 233–234)
23. a (pp. 234–235)

Fill-In

1. potassium; sodium. (pp. 206–207 [Table 14–1])

2. *Colloidal osmotic pressure* refers to the pressure exerted by plasma proteins to hold fluid within vessels. The osmotic pressure is a pulling force. (pp. 207–208)

3. kidney. (pp. 223–224)

4. Calcium levels are primarily regulated by the combined actions of parathyroid hormone and vitamin D. (pp. 61–62)

5. 7.35 to 7.45. (p. 232)

6. Blood pH levels incompatible with life are about 6.8 on the lower range and 7.8 on the upper range. (p. 232)

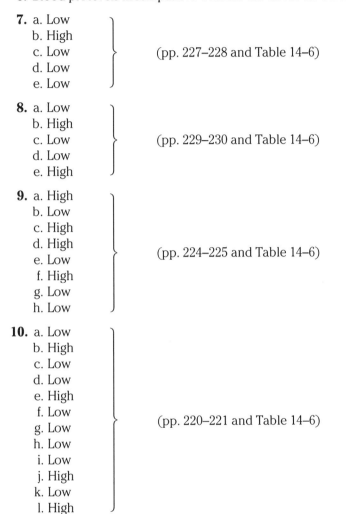

7. a. Low
   b. High
   c. Low
   d. Low
   e. Low   (pp. 227–228 and Table 14–6)

8. a. Low
   b. High
   c. Low
   d. Low
   e. High   (pp. 229–230 and Table 14–6)

9. a. High
   b. Low
   c. High
   d. High
   e. Low   (pp. 224–225 and Table 14–6)
   f. High
   g. Low
   h. Low

10. a. Low
    b. High
    c. Low
    d. Low
    e. High
    f. Low
    g. Low   (pp. 220–221 and Table 14–6)
    h. Low
    i. Low
    j. High
    k. Low
    l. High

11. a. Low
  b. Low
  c. High
  d. High
  e. High
  f. Low
  g. High
  h. Low
  i. Low
  j. High
  k. High
  l. Low

(pp. 217–218 and Table 14–6)

12. a. R-acid
  b. M-acid
  c. M-acid
  d. R-acid
  e. R-alka
  f. R-acid
  g. M-acid
  h. M-alka
  i. M-alka
  j. R-alka

(pp. 233–235 and Table 14–7)

13. Intense supervision is required because only small volumes are needed to elevate the serum sodium from dangerously low levels (pp. 236–238)

14. dyspnea, cyanosis, a weak pulse, hypotension, and unresponsiveness. (p. 243)

15. infection. (pp. 243–244)

II. Critical Analysis Questions

Generating Solutions: Clinical Problem Solving

CASE STUDY: Congestive Heart Failure

George's Situation

1. b
2. d
3. d
4. b

(pp. 214–216)

CASE STUDY: Extracellular Fluid Deficit

Harriet's Situation

1. b
2. b
3. a
4. b

(pp. 211–214)

CASE STUDY: Diabetes Mellitus

Isaac's Situation

1. a
2. a
4. c

(pp. 233–234)

Chapter 15

I. Knowledge-Based Questions

Multiple-Choice

1. d (pp. 248–249)
2. c (pp. 248–249)
3. b (pp. 249–250)
4. d (pp. 249–250)
5. d (pp. 249–250)

6. b (pp. 250–252)
7. d (pp. 250–252)
8. d (pp. 252–253)
9. d (p. 258)
10. a (pp. 258–259)

11. d (pp. 258–259)
12. d (pp. 258–259)
13. a (p. 260)
14. a (p. 260)
15. d (pp. 255–256)

16. b (pp. 255–256)
17. c (pp. 258–259)
18. a (pp. 258–259)
19. d (p. 263)
20. d (p. 263)

Scramblegram

1. shock (p. 248)
2. ATP (p. 248)
3. renin (p. 249)
4. ADH (p. 249)
5. hypoxemia (p. 248)
6. preload (pp. 248–251)
7. oliguria (pp. 251–252, Table 15–1)
8. albumin (p. 253, Table 15–4)

9. dopamine (p. 258)
10. septic (p. 262)
11. CVP (p. 254)
12. pulmonary edema (pp. 259–260)
13. colloids (p. 255)
14. lungs (p. 263)
15. Nipride (p. 259)

D	A^8	O	L	E	R	^{12}P^6			R^3
	L				U			E	
	B				L		N^{15}		
	U				M	I			
	M				O	N			O^7
	I	S	P		N	S	G	N	U	L^{14}
A	N	D	T		A			I		I
I		I	^{4}A^2	D^9	H	R		P		G
M		O		O	Y		R		U
E		L		P	E		I		R
X		L		A	D		D		I
O		O		M	E	S^1	E		A
P	V	^{13}C^{11}		I	M		H		
Y				N	A		O		
H^5				E	S^{10}	E	P	T	I	C
									K

Matching

1. c

2. a

3. a

4. e

5. f

6. d

7. c

8. b

9. b

10. e

All answers can be found on pp. 255–263, Tables 15–2, 15–3, and 15–4.

II. Critical Analysis Questions

Generating Solutions: Clinical Problem Solving

CASE STUDY: Hypovolemic Shock

Mr. Mazda's Situation

1. c

2. 20

3. rise, decline

4. 90

5. 30

6. a. colloids, Ringer's lactate, and normal saline

b. elevating the lower extremities at a 20-degree angle

c. keeping the patient warm

d. providing supplemental oxygen therapy as ordered

e. maintaining strict intake and output measurements

All answers can be found on pp. 255–257.

Chapter 16

I. Knowledge-Based Questions

Multiple-Choice

1. b (p. 266)

2. d (p. 270)

3. d (pp. 270–272)

4. d (pp. 271–272)

5. c (p. 271)

6. a (pp. 275–276)

7. d (pp. 275–276)

8. c (pp. 276–277)

9. b (pp. 276–277)

10. c (pp. 277–278)

11. b (pp. 277–278)

12. a (pp. 278–279)

13. d (pp. 280–281)

14. b (pp. 281–282)

15. a (p. 281)

16. a (p. 284)

17. d (p. 284)

18. d (p. 287)

19. a (pp. 287–288)

20. a (pp. 290–291)

21. a (pp. 309–310)

22. b (pp. 312–313)

Matching

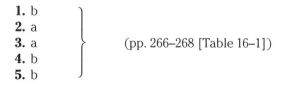

1. b

2. a

3. a   (pp. 266–268 [Table 16–1])

4. b

5. b

Fill-In

1. Men: lung, prostate, colorectal area
   Women: lung, breast, colorectal area (p. 266)

2. *Invasion:* The growth of the primary tumor into surrounding host tissues by mechanical pressure. *Metastasis:* direct spread of tumor cells to body cavities or through lymphatic and hematogenous circulation. (pp. 269–270)

3. carcinoembryonic antigen (CEA) and prostate specific antigen (PSA). (p. 268)

4. 85. (p. 270)

5. Answer may include cabbage, broccoli, cauliflower, brussel sprouts, and kohlrabi. (p. 271)

6. *Primary prevention* is concerned with reducing the risk or preventing the development of cancer in healthy people.

   Example:

   Teaching people the importance of stopping smoking to decrease the incidence of lung cancer.

   Secondary prevention involves detection and screening efforts to achieve early diagnosis and prompt intervention to halt the cancerous process.

   Example:

   Teaching principles of breast self-examination to facilitate the early detection of breast cancer. (p. 272)

7. *Cure* implies complete eradication of malignant disease.
   Control strives for prolonged survival with the presence of malignancy.
   Palliation implies relief of symptoms associated with the cancerous disease. (p. 274)

8. *Skin:* alopecia, erythema, desquamation; *Oral mucosal membrane:* xerostomia, stomatitis, decreased salivation, loss of taste; *Stomach or colon:* anorexia, nausea, vomiting, diarrhea; and *Bone marrow producing sites:* anemia, leukopenia, and thrombocytopenia. (pp. 277–280)

9. *Cell cycle–specific agents* destroy cells in specific phases of the cell cycle by interfering with DNA and RNA synthesis or by halting mitosis. *Cell cycle–nonspecific agents* exert prolonged effects on cells, independent of cell cycle phases, which lead to cell damage or death. (pp. 280–281)

10. An extravasation of an infusion of a cancer chemotherapeutic agent is believed to have occurred if redness, pain, swelling, a mottled appearance, phlebitis, loss of blood return, and resistance to flow are present. (p. 281)

11. *Hyperthermia,* the generation of temperatures greater than physiologic fever range, elicits tumoricidal effects by irreparably damaging the DNA and cell membranes, by increasing cellular metabolic demands to which the cancer cells are not able to respond, and by stimulating the body's immune system. (p. 287)

12. *Interferons* are biological response modifiers (BRMs), with antiviral and antitumor properties that stimulate an immune response. It is believed that the stimulated immune system will eradicate the malignant growth. (pp. 287–288)

Matching

1. e
2. c
3. a
4. f
5. a

6. b
7. d
8. a
9. c
10. e

(pp. 282–283 [Table 16–6])

II. Critical Analysis Questions

Analyzing Comparisons

1. care and rehabilitation after diagnosis and treatment (pp. 272–273)

2. tumor cell classification (pp. 273–274)

3. a donor from an identical twin (pp. 285–287)

4. the thinning or complete loss of hair (pp. 292–293)

5. appetite failure resulting in a wasting syndrome (p. 293)

Generating Solutions: Clinical Problem Solving

CASE STUDY: Cancer of the Breast

Kim's Situation

1. b (p. 271)
2. d (pp. 272–273)
3. a (pp. 291–292)
4. d (pp. 291–292)
5. d (pp. 277–280)

6. c (pp. 277–80)
7. a (pp. 280–283 [Table 16–7])
8. d (p. 285)
9. b (p. 285)

Chapter 17

I. Knowledge-Based Questions

Multiple-Choice

1. c (p. 318 [Table 17–1])
2. c (p. 319 [Table 17–2])
3. b (p. 319 [Table 17–2])
4. d (p. 319 [Table 17–2])

5. a (p. 319 [Table 17–2])
6. a (p. 319 [Table 17–2])
7. d (p. 321)
8. b (pp. 321–322 [Table 17–3])

Fill-In

1. Diets high in saturated fat and cholesterol, sedentary lifestyles, substance abuse, smoking, and high levels of stress. (pp. 318–319)

2. Answers may include preventing the occurrence of other chronic conditions, alleviating and managing symptoms, preventing and handling disabilities, preventing and managing crises and complications, adapting to re-

peated threats and progressive functional loss, living with isolation and loneliness, and any other conditions listed on pages 319–320.

3. The *Trajectory Framework* refers to the course of action taken by the ill person, his family, health professionals, and others to manage the course of the illness. (pp. 321–322)

4. *Trajectory phasing* represents the management of the different medical, biographical, and everyday living problems that arise with changes in the status of illness. *Trajectory scheme* denotes the plan of action chosen to handle the illness, identity, and everyday living problems. (p. 322)

5. Step 5. (pp. 322–323)

II. Critical Analysis Questions

Recognizing Contradictions

1. Chronic illnesses <u>increase</u> in frequency with age. (p. 318)

2. Individuals with a chronic illness <u>can lead</u> a fully <u>independent existence</u> and others may never know that they are sick. (pp. 318–319)

3. <u>Diabetes</u> is the least prevalent chronic illness in the United States (p. 318, Table 17–1)

4. Superimposing an "acute care framework" on a chronic condition <u>increases the risk</u> that medical problems will be ignored. (pp. 319–320)

5. In the Trajectory Framework, medical aspects of illness and management <u>are not separated</u> from the social and psychological components. (pp. 321–322)

Chapter 18

I. Knowledge-Based Questions

Multiple-Choice

1. d (p. 326)
2. d (p. 326)
3. b (p. 326)
4. d (p. 327)
5. b (p. 327)
6. a (pp. 327–328)

7. c (pp. 330–331 [Chart 18–2])
8. b (pp. 331–334 [Table 18–4])
9. d (p. 335)
10. a (p. 335)
11. d (pp. 341–343)
12. a (p. 342)

13. a (p. 342)
14. b (p. 345)
15. d (p. 348)
16. d (p. 348)

Matching

1. e
2. a
3. b
4. d
5. f

(pp. 332–334 [Chart 18–4])

Fill-In

1. The term *physiatrist* is used to describe a physician specialist in physical medicine and rehabilitation. (p. 327)

2. Weakened muscles, joint contractures, and deformity are common complications associated with prolonged immobility. (pp. 329–330)

3. Braces, splints, collars, corsets, supports, and calipers. (p. 330)

4. External rotation. (p. 330)

5. Prolonged bed rest, lack of exercise, incorrect positioning in bed, and the weight of the bedding. (p. 330)

6. 3. (pp. 330–331)

7. Right; right. (p. 340 [Chart 18–6])

8. A pressure sore is a localized area of infarcted soft tissue that occurs when pressure greater than normal capillary pressure is applied to the skin for a prolonged period. (pp. 342–344)

9. sepsis, osteomyelitis, pyarthrosis, and joint disarticulation. (pp. 344–346)

10. does not permit free drainage of the tissue. (pp. 344–346)

II. Critical Analysis Questions

Generating Solutions: Clinical Problem Solving

Clinical Situation: Impaired Skin Integrity

1. Pressure ulcers are localized areas of infarcted soft tissue that occur when pressure applied to the skin over time is greater than normal capillary closure pressure, approximately 32 mm Hg. (pp. 341–343)

2. erythema; reactive hyperemia (p. 342)

3. sacrum and heels (pp. 342–343 ([Fig. 18–5])

4. c. (pp. 344–346)

5. b. (pp. 344–346)

6. As the body sinks into the fluid, more surface area becomes available for weight-bearing, thus decreasing body weight per unit area. (Pascal's law). (pp. 344–345)

7. Increased elevation increases the downward-pulling force of body weight, which increases pressure on the skin, which results in localized blood flow reduction. (pp. 342–343)

CASE STUDY: Traumatic Amputation—Psychosocial Perspective

Oliver's Situation

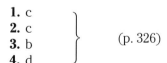

1. c
2. c
3. b
4. d

(p. 326)

CASE STUDY: Buck's Extension Traction

Patricia's Situation

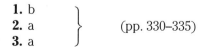

1. b
2. a
3. a

(pp. 330–335)

Chapter 19

I. Knowledge-Based Questions

Multiple-Choice

1. d (pp. 358–359)	**8.** d (p. 361)	**15.** a (p. 364)	**22.** c (pp. 369–370)
2. a (p. 359)	**9.** c (p. 363)	**16.** a (pp. 364–366)	**23.** b (p. 370)
3. a (p. 360)	**10.** d (p. 363)	**17.** d (p. 363)	**24.** b (p. 370)
4. a (pp. 360–361)	**11.** a (p. 363)	**18.** c (p. 368)	**25.** d (p. 370)
5. d (pp. 360–361)	**12.** a (p. 363)	**19.** a (p. 368)	
6. d (pp. 360–361)	**13.** c (p. 363)	**20.** a (p. 369)	
7. d (pp. 360–361)	**14.** d (p. 364)	**21.** c (p. 369)	

Fill-In

For assistance in completing this chart, see textbook page 364.

Matching

Sample

Column 1	*Column II*
Nursing Activity	*Nursing Goal*
Restriction of nutrition and fluids	Prevent aspiration

See textbook pages 368–371 for assistance in completing this chart.

II. Critical Analysis Questions

Recognizing Contradictions

1. About <u>60%</u> of surgeries are performed on an outpatient basis despite the use of advanced technology. (p. 358)

2. the intraoperative phase of perioperative nursing <u>ends</u> when the patient is admitted to the <u>recovery area</u>. (p. 358)

3. Cosmetic surgery is based on personal choice and is, therefore, classified as <u>optional</u> (p. 351)

4. <u>Vitamin C</u> is needed for collagen synthesis; vitamin K is used for <u>clotting</u> and <u>prothrombin production</u>. (p. 362)

5. Corticosteroids should <u>never be abruptly discontinued</u> before surgery because cardiovascular collapse may occur. (p. 370)

Chapter 20

I. Knowledge-Based Questions

Multiple-Choice

1. b (pp. 374)
2. d (p. 374)
3. d (pp. 376–377 [Table 20–1])
4. d (pp. 377–378)
5. d (pp. 378–379)

6. b (p. 380)
7. c (pp. 380–383 [Table 20–5])
8. a (pp. 22–23 [Table 20–5])
9. d (p. 25)
10. d (p. 27)

11. b (p. 28)
12. b (p. 30)
13. c (pp. 31–32)
14. d (pp. 33–35)

Fill-In

1. Answer should include four of these five: handling tissue, providing exposure at the operative field, using instruments, suturing and providing hemostasis. (p. 374)

2. cerebral ischema, thrombosis, embolism, infarction, and anoxemia, thermoregulatory problems; cerebral hypoxia; and an increased risk of pneumonia. (pp. 377–378)

3. thiopental sodium (Pentothal), respiratory depression. (p. 380)

4. the subarachnoid space at the lumbar level (usually at L-2) (p. 382)

5. Complete return of sensation in the patient's toes, in response to a pinprick, indicates recovery. (pp. 382–384)

II. Critical Analysis Questions

Recognizing Contradictions

1. The circulating nurse controls the environment, coordinates the activities of other personnel, and monitors aseptic techniques. (p. 374)

2. Whenever sterility is in question, an item is considered unsterile. (p. 376)

3. Only the top of a table that is draped is considered sterile. Drapes hanging over the edge are clean but not sterile. (p. 376)

4. The unsterile arm of the circulating nurse should never extend over a sterile area. (p. 376)

5. Older patients require less anesthesia and take longer to eliminate anesthetic drugs. (pp. 378–379)

Generating Solutions: Clinical Problem Solving

CASE STUDY: General Anesthesia	CASE STUDY: Intravenous Anesthesia
Anne's Situation	*Brian's Situation*

1. b
2. b } (pp. 378–380)
3. b

1. d
2. a } (pp. pp. 380–381 [Table 20–4])
3. b

Chapter 21

I. Knowledge-Based Questions

Multiple-Choice

1. d (p. 392)
2. c (pp. 392–394 [Figure 21–1])
3. a (pp. 392–394 [Figure 21–1])
4. c (p. 394)
5. d (p. 395)
6. d (p. 396)
7. a (p. 13)
8. d (pp. 398–399)
9. a (p. 399)

10. a (p. 400)
11. a (p. 400)
12. c (pp. 400–401)
13. b (p. 403)
14. d (p. 403)
15. b (p. 411)
16. c (p. 401)
17. c (p. 412)
18. c (p. 413)

19. c (pp. 413–414)
20. d (p. 414)
21. d (pp. 414–415 [Chart 21–1])
22. d (p. 420)
23. a (pp. 405–407)
24. d (pp. 406–408)
25. a (p. 408)
26. b (pp. 408–409)

Fill-In

1. Respiratory function and patency of the airway. (pp. 392–394)

2. The answer may include any of the following:
   - Medical diagnosis.
   - Type of surgery performed.
   - Patient's general condition: age, airway, patency, vital signs, blood pressure.
   - Anesthetic and other medications used.
   - Any untoward intraoperative problems that may influence postoperative care (shock, hemorrhage, cardiac arrest).
   - Any pathology encountered, whether patient or family informed.
   - Fluid administered, blood loss and replacement.
   - Tubing, drains, catheters, or other supportive aids.
   - Specific information about which surgeon or anesthesiologist wishes to be notified. (pp. 392–394)

3. Self-perception, personality, learning, ethnic and cultural factors, and environment. (p. 397)

4. Patient-controlled analgesia refers to self-administration of pain medication by way of intravenous or epidural routes within prescribed time/dosage limits. (p. 398)

5. Bowel sounds and the passage of flatus. (pp. 398–399)

6. Atelectasis and hypostatic pneumonia are reduced with early ambulation because ventilation is increased and the stasis of bronchial secretions in the lungs is reduced. (p. 401)

7. absence of nausea, absence of vomiting, and presence of bowel sounds. (pp. 402–403)

8. Your answer should include four of these eight organisms: *Staphylococcus aureus,* methicillin-resistant *Staphylococcus aureus, Escherichia coli, Pseudomonas, Klebsiella pneumoniae, Proteus,* and *Clostridium difficile.* (p. 403)

9. The correct way to apply adhesive tape is to place the tape at the center of the dressing and then press the tape down on both sides, applying tension evenly away from the midline. Adhesive should be removed by pulling it parallel with the skin surface and in the direction of the hair growth, not at right angles. (p. 417 [Figure 21–6])

10. *Primary hemorrhage* occurs at the time of the operation. Intermediary hemorrhage occurs within the first few hours after an operation and is due to the return of blood pressure to its normal level. *Secondary hemorrhage* occurs some time after the operation as a result of the slipping of a ligature, which may happen because of infection, insecure tying, or erosion of a vessel by a drainage tube. (p. 405)

II. Critical Analysis Questions

Supporting Arguments

Pain stimulates the stress response,   which increases muscle tension

and

local vasoconstricity

Noxious impulses stimulate
sympathetic activity   which increases myocardial demand

and

oxygen consumption

Hypothalmic stress responses increase   blood viscosity

which can lead to phlebothrombosis   and

and   platelet aggregation

pulmonary embolism

Benedetti (1992) found that cardiovascular insufficiency can be three times more frequent and infection five times greater with inadequate postoperative control. (pp. 397–399)

Recognizing Contradictions

1. Because of the negative impact of pain on recovery, nurses *need to think "pain prevention"* rather than control. Narcotic addiction rarely occurs for short-term pain control. (pp. 397–399)

2. Pain intensity is most severe for surgery on the *upper abdominal area* and the *back* and *lower extremities.* (pp. 397–399 [Table 21–1])

3. Signs of *hypovolemia* include hypotension, tachycardia, oliguria and CVP < 4 cm H_2O. (p. 405)

4. The presence of devitalized tissue in a wound causes a wound to be classified as *dirty* and *infected.* (p. 413)

5. Sutures are usually removed *before the seventh day,* after that they are of little value. (p. 417)

Generating Solutions: Clinical Problem Solving

CASE STUDY: Hypopharyngeal Obstruction   **CASE STUDY: Wound Healing**

Daena's Situation   *Elizabeth's Situation*

1. d   **1.** b
2. b)   **2.** c
3. d   pp. 392–394 [Figure 21–2])   **3.** d   (pp. 412–414 [Table 21–2])
4. c   **4.** b

Illustration Interpretation (Figure 21–4): Phlebothrombosis

(reference pp. 405–407)

1. The nurse is gently palpating the calf muscle for tenderness.

2. To assess for the presence of Homans' sign, the nurse would ask the patient to flex his knee and dorsiflex his foot. Calf pain is an early sign of phlebothrombosis.

3. Phlebothrombosis is blood clotting in a vein without marked inflammation.

4. The nurse assesses for calf swelling in the affected leg by measuring calf circumference in both legs and comparing the results.

Chapter 22

I. Knowledge-Based Questions

Multiple-Choice

1. b (pp. 432–433)	**8.** b (p. 434)	**15.** d (pp. 440–441)	**22.** d (p. 451)
2. b (pp. 432–433)	**9.** d (pp. 434–436)	**16.** a (p. 442)	**23.** b (pp. 452–453)
3. c (pp. 433–434)	**10.** b (pp. 436–437)	**17.** a (pp. 446–448)	**24.** c (pp. 453–454)
4. a (pp. 433–434)	**11.** d (pp. 436–438)	**18.** d (pp. 449–450)	**25.** d (pp. 454–455)
5. c (pp. 433–434)	**12.** c (pp. 437–438)	**19.** d (p. 450)	**26.** b (p. 456)
6. d (pp. 433–434)	**13.** b (pp. 439–440)	**20.** d (p. 450)	**27.** d (p. 457)
7. a (p. 434)	**14.** d (pp. 439–440)	**21.** a (pp. 450–451)	

II. Critical Analysis Questions

Generating Solutions: Clinical Problem Solving

CASE STUDY: Bronchoscopy

Mr. Kecklin's Situation

1. c
2. d
3. b   (p. 448)
4. d
5. a

CASE STUDY: Thoracentesis

Mrs. Lomar's Situation

1. d
2. b
3. b   (p. 456)
4. d
5. c

Chapter 23

I. Knowledge-Based Questions

Multiple-Choice

1. a (p. 462)
2. a (p. 462)
3. c (p. 462)
4. d (pp. 462–463)
5. a (p. 463)
6. d (pp. 463–464)
7. a (pp. 464–465)
8. d (pp. 464–465)

9. d (pp. 464–465)
10. a (pp. 466–467)
11. c (pp. 466–467)
12. d (pp. 467–468)
13. a (pp. 467–468)
14. a (pp. 469–470)
15. d (pp. 470–471)
16. b (pp. 470–471)

17. d (p. 471)
18. b (p. 471 [Figure 23–5])
19. a (p. 471)
20. b (p. 472)
21. d (pp. 473–474)
22. d (pp. 474–477)

II. Critical Analysis Questions

Generating Solutions: Clinical Problem Solving

CASE STUDY: Epistaxis

Gilberta's Situation

1. Gilberta should sit upright with her head tilted forward to prevent swallowing and aspiration of blood. She should also pinch the soft outer portion of the nose against the midline spectrum for 5 to 10 continuous minutes.
2. d
3. b   (pp. 469–470)
4. d

CASE STUDY: Tonsillectomy and Adenoidectomy

Isabel's Situation

1. d
2. c   (pp. 466–467)
3. a
4. c

CASE STUDY: Laryngectomy

Jerome's Situation

1. b
2. d
3. d   (pp. 472–477)
4. d
5. d

Chapter 24

I. Knowledge-Based Questions

Multiple-Choice

1. b (pp. 480–481)
2. d (pp. 480–481)
3. c (pp. 481–486)
4. d (pp. 495–496)
5. a (pp. 495–496)
6. d (p. 501)
7. d (p. 502)
8. d (pp. 502–503)

9. d (p. 504)
10. d (p. 504)
11. d (pp. 505–507)
12. b (pp. 507–508)
13. a (pp. 508–509)
14. c (pp. 509–511)
15. d (pp. 509–510)
16. b (pp. 509–510)

17. d (p. 511)
18. c (pp. 512, 518–520)
19. d (pp. 512, 518–520)
20. d (p. 520)
21. a (pp. 520–521)
22. d (pp. 521–523)
23. c (p. 523)
24. b (p. 525)

25. a (p. 526)
26. c (pp. 526–527)
27. b (pp. 526–527)
28. d (pp. 529–530)
29. a (pp. 531–534)
30. d (p. 532)
31. b (p. 539)

II. Critical Analysis Questions

Generating Solutions: Clinical Problem Solving

CASE STUDY: Bacterial Pneumonia

Theresa's Situation

1. d
2. b
3. d
4. d
5. b
6. d
} (pp. 481–487)

CASE STUDY: Adult Respiratory Distress Syndrome (ARDS)

Anne's Situation

1. d
2. d
3. c
4. d
5. d
} (pp. 521–523)

CASE STUDY: Bronchitis

Lois' Situation

1. c
2. b
3. a
4. d
5. b
6. d
} (pp. 507–508)

CASE STUDY: Pulmonary Embolism

Sandy's Situation

1. d
2. a
3. a
4. b
5. c
6. d
} (pp. 525–529 [Charts 25–7, and 24–8])

Chapter 25

I. Knowledge-Based Questions

Multiple-Choice

1. a (p. 544)
2. b (p. 544)
3. a (p. 544)
4. d (pp. 544–545)
5. d (p. 545)
6. d (pp. 545–546)
7. b (p. 545 [Table 25–1])
8. c (p. 545 [Table 25–1])
9. d (p. 545 [Table 25–1])
10. a (p. 547)
11. c (p. 547)
12. d (p. 547)
13. d (pp. 547–548 [Figure 25–3])
14. d (pp. 549–550)
15. a (pp. 549–550 [Figure 25–4])
16. c (pp. 549–550 [Figure 25–4])
17. a (pp. 550–551)
18. d (pp. 551–553)
19. a (p. 552 [Figures 25–5 and 25–6])
20. d (pp. 553–554)
21. c (p. 555 [G 25–3])
22. a (p. 555 [G 25–3])
23. c (pp. 555–557 [Chart 25–3])
24. d (pp. 555–557)
25. c (p. 557)
26. b (p. 567)
27. d (pp. 566–569)
28. d (pp. 569–571 [Figure 25–12])

Complete the Chart

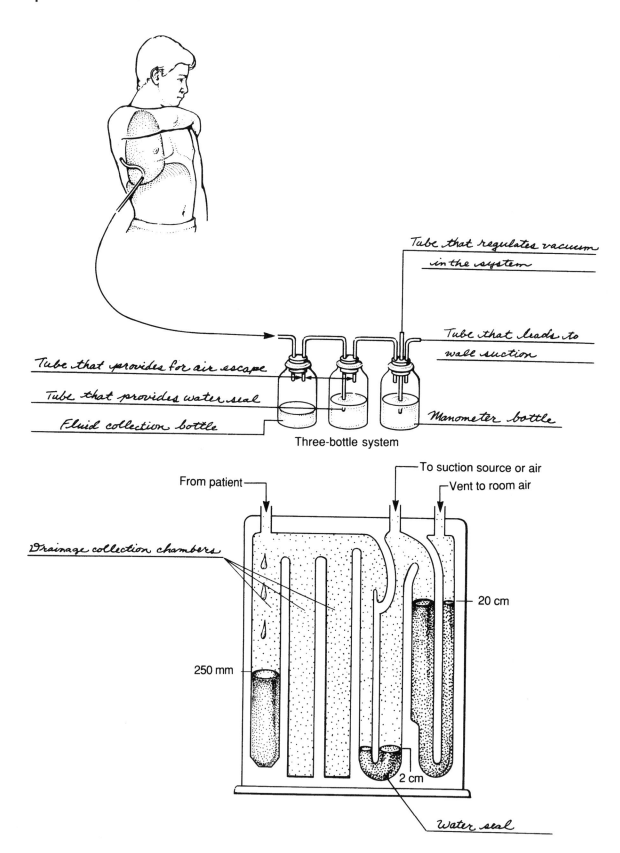

Tube that regulates vacuum in the system

Tube that leads to wall suction

Tube that provides for air escape

Tube that provides water seal

Fluid collection bottle

Manometer bottle

Three-bottle system

From patient

To suction source or air

Vent to room air

Drainage collection chambers

20 cm

250 mm

2 cm

Water seal

II. Critical Analysis Questions

Generating Solutions: Clinical Problem Solving

CASE STUDY: Pneumonectomy: Preoperative Concerns

Mrs. Miley's Preoperative Situation

1. d
2. a
3. d
4. a
} (pp. 566–569)

CASE STUDY: Pneumonectomy: Postoperative Concerns

Mrs. Miley's Postoperative Situation

1. a
2. b
3. d
4. a
} (pp. 569–572)

CASE STUDY: Ventilator Patient

Mr. Brown's Situation

1. d
2. a
3. d
4. d
} (pp. 555–562)

CASE STUDY: Weaning From Ventilator

Mr. O'Day's Situation

1. d
2. d
3. d
} (pp. 563–565)

Nursing Care Plan: Chest Tube Management

Nursing diagnosis: Ineffective breathing pattern, related to chest trauma.

Immediate goal: Maintain effective pulmonary ventilation with the aid of a chest drainage system.

Intermediate goal: Assist in restoring normal pulmonary dynamics.

Long-term goal: Return the patient to his maximum level of functioning.

Nursing interventions   *Expected outcomes*

References for completion of this nursing care plan are Chapter 2, and Chapter 25 pages 569–571, and Figures 25–12 and 25–13.

Chapter 26

I. Knowledge-Based Questions

Multiple-Choice

1. a (pp. 588–589 [Figure 26–2])
2. d (pp. 590–591 [Figure 26–3])
3. d (p. 593)
4. c (pp. 591–593)
5. d (p. 593)
6. d (p. 593)
7. c (p. 597)
8. a (pp. 597–598)
9. a (p. 598)
10. b (p. 602)
11. d (p. 606)
12. d (pp. 607–609)

Fill-In

1. The atrioventricular valves separate the atria from the ventricles. The tricuspid separates the right atrium and ventricle; the bicuspid separates the left atrium and ventricle. The AV valves permit blood to flow from the atria into the ventricles. The semilunar valves are situated between each ventricle and its corresponding artery. The pulmonic valve is between the right ventricle and the pulmonary artery; the aortic valve is between the left ventricle and the aorta. These valves permit blood to flow from the ventricles into the arteries. (pp. 588–589 [Figure 26–1])

2. Depolarization is said to have occurred when the electrical difference between the inside and the outside of the cell is reduced. The inside of the cell becomes less negative, membrane permeability to calcium is increased, and muscle contraction occurs. (pp. 590–591 [Figure 26–4])

3. Cardiac output would equal 5320 ml. (p. 593)

4. Starling's law of the heart refers to the relation between increased stroke volume and increased ventricular end-diastolic volume for a given intrinsic contractility. (p. 593)

5. Physiologic effects of the aging process may include reduction in the size of the left ventricle, decreased elasticity and widening of the aorta, thickening and rigidity of cardiac valves, and increased connective tissue in the sinoatrial and atrioventricular nodes and bundle branches. (pp. 593–594)

6. Cardiac catheterization is used most frequently to assess the patency of the patient's coronary arteries and to determine readiness for coronary bypass surgery. It is also used to measure pressures in the various heart chambers and to determine oxygen saturation of the blood by sampling specimens. (pp. 607–609)

7. Selective angiography refers to a technique of injecting a contrast medium into the vascular system to outline a particular heart chamber of blood vessel. (p. 608)

8. Echocardiography involves the use of high-frequency sound waves that are sent into the heart through the chest wall and recorded as they return. An ECG is recorded simultaneously to time events within the cardiac cycle. Motions of the echoes are traced on an oscilloscope and recorded on film. (p. 609)

9. A lowered central venous pressure reading indicates a patient is hypovolemic. Serial measurements are more reflective of a patient's condition and should be correlated with the patient's clinical status. (p. 611)

10. Complications of pulmonary artery monitoring may include infection, pulmonary artery rupture, pulmonary thromboembolism, pulmonary infarction, catheter kinking, dysrhythmias, and air embolism. (pp. 611–612)

Crossword Puzzle (reference pp. 594–597)

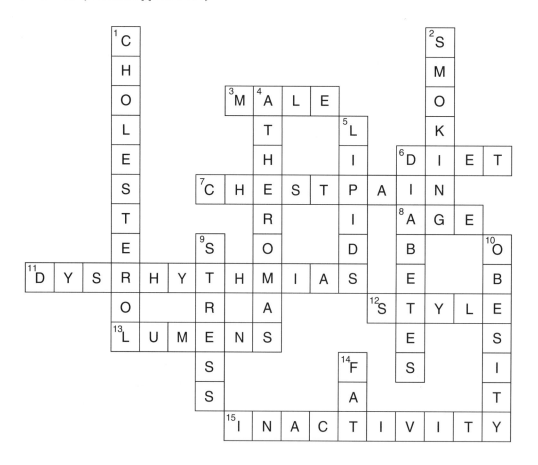

II. Critical Analysis Questions

Analyzing Comparisons

1. the remainder of the body. (pp. 588–589)
2. myocardium. (p. 589)
3. third intercostal space. (pp. 601–602)
4. the aortic and pulmonic valves. (p. 602)
5. abrasion of the pericardial surfaces. (pp. 603–604)

Generating Solutions: Clinical Problem Solving

	Myocardial Infarction	*Angina Pectoris*
Assessment	Substernal pain or pain over precordium. May spread widely throughout chest. Painful disability of shoulders and hands may be present.	Substernal or retrosternal pain spreading across chest. May radiate to inside of arm, neck, or jaws.
	Pain > 15 minutes.	Pain 5 to 10 minutes.
Precipitating events	Occurs spontaneously but may be sequelae of unstable angina.	Usually related to exertion, emotion, eating, cold.
Nursing intervention	Morphone sulfate, successful reperfusion of blocked coronary artery.	Rest, nitroglycerin, oxygen

Table 26–1, p. 595

Chapter 27

I. Knowledge-Based Questions

Multiple-Choice

1. d (p. 616)
2. d (pp. 618–619)
3. c (p. 621)
4. d (p. 622)
5. b (p. 623)
6. a (pp. 623–624)
7. d (p. 624)
8. c (pp. 624–625)
9. c (p. 628)
10. a (pp. 628–629)
11. d (p. 629)
12. d (p. 629 [Chart 27–2])
13. d (pp. 631–633)

Fill-In

1. *Excitability* is the ability of a myocardial cell to respond to a stimulus. *Automaticity* allows a cell to reach a threshold potential and generate an impulse without being stimulated by another source. *Conductivity* refers to the ability of the muscle to move an impulse to from cell to cell. *Contractility* allows the muscle to shorten when contracted. (p. 616)

2. Electrical conduction through the heart begins in the sinoatrial node (SA), travels across the atria to the atrioventricular node (AV), and then travels down the right and left bundle branches and Purkinje fibers to the ventricular muscle. (p. 616)

3. Sinus tachycardia can be caused by any of the following: fever, hypovolemia, anemia, exercise, pain, congestive heart failure, anxiety, and sympathomimetic or parasympatholytic drugs. (pp. 619–620)

4. The standard procedure is to place one paddle to the right of the upper sternum below the right clavicle and the other paddle just to the left of the cardiac apex. (pp. 628–629 [Figure 27–19])

5. A demand pacemaker is set for a specific rate and stimulates the heart when normal ventricular depolarization does not occur; the fixed rate pacemaker stimulates the ventricle at a preset constant rate, independently of the patient's rhythm. (pp. 629–632 [Figure 27–22])

II. Critical Analysis Questions

Generating Solutions: Clinical Problem Solving

Graph Analysis

1. a. T wave
   b. P-R interval
   c. P wave   (pp. 617–618)
   d. QRS complex
   e. ST segment

2. a. Q wave is larger
   b. ST segment is elevated   (pp. 617–618 [Figure 27–3])
   c. T wave is inverted

Graphic Recordings

1. Premature atrial contraction (PAC).

   P wave comes early in cycle and close to T wave of previous heartbeat. (pp. 620–621 [Figure 27–7])

2. Premature ventricular contraction (PVC).

   QRS complex is bizarre. P wave is hidden in QRS complex. (pp. 622–623 [Figure 27–11])

Chapter 28

I. Knowledge-Based Questions

Multiple-Choice

1. b (p. 636)	**12.** b (pp. 642–643)	**22.** d (p. 648)	**33.** a (pp. 670–671)
2. d (p. 636)	**13.** d (pp. 642–643)	**23.** c (pp. 648–649)	**34.** c (pp. 671–672)
3. a (pp. 637–638)	**14.** a (pp. 642–643)	**24.** c (pp. 650–651)	**35.** a (pp. 672–673)
4. c (p. 639)	**15.** d (pp. 644–645)	**25.** d (pp. 654–658)	**36.** b (p. 673)
5. d (p. 640)	**16.** b (p. 646)	**26.** d (p. 659)	**37.** c (p. 674 [Table 28–3])
6. c (p. 640)	**17.** b (p. 647)	**27.** d (p. 658)	
7. a (p. 640)	**18.** a (p. 647)	**28.** a (p. 663)	
8. b (p. 640)	**19.** b (pp. 647–648)	**29.** d (p. 665)	
9. d (p. 642)	**20.** d (pp. 647–648 [Table 28–1])	**30.** d (pp. 666–667)	
10. c (pp. 642–643)		**31.** a (p. 666)	
11. a (pp. 642–643)	**21.** c (p. 648)	**32.** b (p. 670)	

Matching

1. a
2. b
3. a
4. b
5. b
6. a   (pp. 662–663)
7. a
8. b
9. a
10. b

II. Critical Analysis Questions

Supporting Arguments

1. (a) Hemoglobin combines more readily with CO than with O_2, thereby limiting the oxygen being supplied to the heart. (b) Nicotine triggers the release of catecholamines, which cause arterial constriction and decreased oxygenation. (c) Smoking increases platelet adhesion, which increases thrombus formation. (p. 637)

2. Calcium ion blockers increase myocardial oxygen supply (a) by dilating the smooth muscle wall of the coronary arterioles, (b) by decreasing myocardial oxygen demands, and (c) by decreasing systemic arterial pressure. (pp. 640–641)

Generating Solutions: Clinical Problem Solving

CASE STUDY: Angina Pectoris

Ermelina's Situation

1. b
2. c
3. b   (pp. 638–642)
4. c

CASE STUDY: Decreased Myocardial Tissue Perfusion

Mr. Lillis' Situation

1. c
2. a
3. a
4. b   (pp. 645–649)
5. a
6. d

Chapter 29

I. Knowledge-Based Questions

Multiple-Choice

1. d (p. 678)
2. c (p. 678)
3. a (pp. 679–680)
4. a (pp. 679–680)
5. d (p. 680)

6. c (pp. 683–684)
7. c (p. 685)
8. c (p. 686)
9. a (pp. 687–688)
10. a (pp. 687–688)

11. d (pp. 688–690)
12. a (pp. 690–693)
13. a (p. 690–693)

Fill-In

1. Mitral valve prolapse syndrome is a dysfunction of the mitral valve leaflets, resulting in valve incompetency and regurgitation. Valve dysfunction progresses, and symptoms of heart failure ensue. (pp. 678)

2. Left ventricular hypertrophy develops with mitral valve insufficiency because incomplete valve closure allows a regurgitation of blood from the left ventricle to the atrium during ventricular systole. This regurgitated blood is returned to the left ventricle, increasing the volume of blood that the left ventricle must handle. Hypertrophy of the left atrium and left ventricle develops. (p. 679)

3. An inflamed endothelium causes a fibrin clot to form (vegetation), which converts to scar tissue that thickens, contracts, and causes deformities. (pp. 687–689)

4. Myocarditis is an inflammatory process that usually results from an infection. The infectious process can cause heart dilation, thrombi formation, infiltration of blood cells around the coronary vessels and between the muscle fibers, and eventual degeneration of the muscle fibers themselves. (p. 690)

5. Listen at the left sternal edge of the thorax in the fourth intercostal space where the pericardium comes in contact with the left chest wall. (pp. 691–692)

Matching

1. a
2. e
3. d   (pp. 678–680)
4. b
5. c

II. Critical Analysis Questions

Generating Solutions: Clinical Problem Solving

CASE STUDY: Infective Endocarditis

Mr. Fontana's Situation

1. toxicity of the infection, heart valve destruction, and embolization of fragments of vegetations.
2. a
3. headache, transient cerebral ischemia, focal neurologic lesions, and strokes.
4. total eradication of the invading organism.   (pp. 688–690)
5. c
6. congestive heart failure, strokes, valvular stenosis, and myocardial erosin.
7. d

Chapter 30

I. Knowledge-Based Questions

Multiple-Choice

1. c (p. 697)
2. a (p. 697)
3. c (p. 697)
4. d (p. 700)
5. b (pp. 699–701)

6. d (pp. 699–701)
7. a (pp. 701–707)
8. d (p. 702)
9. a (pp. 702–704)
10. b (pp. 702–704)

11. b (p. 706)
12. d (pp. 706–707)
13. a (p. 707)
14. d (pp. 715–716)

Fill-In

1. Cardiomyopathy, ischemic heart disease, congenital heart disease, valvular disease, and rejection of previously transplanted hearts are the most common indicators. (p. 697)

2. orthotopic transplant. (p. 697)

3. Answer should include four of these responses: dysrhythmias, hemorrhage, myocardial infarction, cerebral vascular accident, embolization, and organ failure secondary to shock, embolis, or adverse drug reactions. (pp. 701–702)

4. Symptoms of hypoxia include: restlessness, headache, confusion, dyspnea, hypotension, and cyanosis. (pp. 701–707)

5. bradycardia, tachycardia, and ectopic beats. (p. 714)

II. Critical Analysis Questions

Generating Solutions: Clinical Problem Solving

CASE STUDY: Cardiac Surgery Patient

Mrs. Effgen's Situation

1. patient's functional level, coping mechanisms, and support systems. (p. 700)

2. renal, respiratory, gastrointestinal, integumentary, hematologic, and neurologic systems. (p. 702)

3. fear of the unknown, fear of pain, fear of body image change, and fear of dying. (pp. 700–702)

4. decreased cardiac output. (pp. 703–704)

5. a (p. 715)

6. d (p. 705)

7. a (p. 707)

8. apply antiembolic stockings, avoid use of knee gatch on the bed, omit pillows under the popliteal space, discourage crossing of legs, and institute passive exercises. (p. 706)

9. 10% to 40% of patients. (p. 707)

10. hypovolemia. (p. 707)

Chapter 31

I. Knowledge-Based Questions

Multiple-Choice

1. d (p. 723)
2. b (p. 724 [Table 31–2])
3. b (pp. 724–725)
4. a (pp. 729–732)
5. b (pp. 729–732)
6. b (p. 736)
7. c (p. 736)
8. b (p. 737)

9. d (p. 737)
10. d (pp. 737–738)
11. b (pp. 739–740)
12. b (p. 740)
13. d (p. 740)
14. c (pp. 743–744)
15. a (pp. 755–757)
16. c (pp. 755–757)

17. c (pp. 757–758)
18. d (pp. 758–760)
19. b (p. 761)
20. d (p. 761)
21. a (pp. 761–762)
22. a (pp. 762–763)

Matching

1. a
2. b
3. a
4. a
⎫
⎬ (pp. 724–728)
⎭

5. b
6. b
7. a
8. a
⎫
⎬ (pp. 724–728)
⎭

II. Critical Analysis Questions

Analyzing Comparisons

1. Flow = $\Delta P/R$. The pressure difference between the two ends of the vessel (arterial and venous) provides the impetus for the forward propulsion of blood. The rate of blood flow is determined by dividing the pressure difference by the resistance. (p. 722)

2. $R = 8\,nL/\pi r^4$. Resistance to blood flow is proportional to the thickness of the blood and the length of the vessel; it is inversely proportional to the fourth power of the vessel radius. (p. 722)

3. Answer may include angiotensin, histamine, bradykinin, or prostaglandin. (p. 723)

4. systemic venous congestion (p. 723)

5. the accumulation of lipids, fibrous tissue, and such (p. 728)

Generating Solutions: Clinical Problem Solving

CASE STUDY: Peripheral Arterial Occlusive Disease

Fred's Situation

1. a
2. a
3. d
4. d
⎫
⎬ (pp. 733–736)
⎭

CASE STUDY: Essential Hypertension

Georgia's Situation

1. b
2. b
3. d
4. c
5. d
⎫
⎬ (pp. 741–750 [Table 31–5])
⎭

400

Pathophysiology of Atherosclerosis

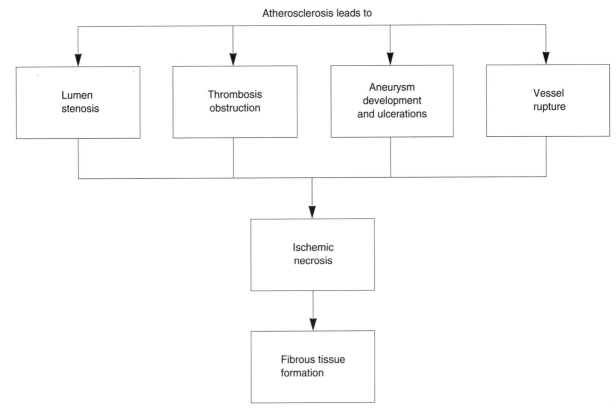

See textbook pages 728–731 [Figure 31–5] for assistance in this assignment.

Chapter 32

I. Knowledge-Based Questions

Multiple-Choice

1. a (p. 776)
2. d (p. 776)
3. b (p. 782)
4. d (pp. 788–789)
5. d (p. 779)
6. c (p. 780)
7. a (pp. 780–781)

8. b (p. 781)
9. a (pp. 781–783)
10. d (pp. 781–783)
11. d (pp. 782–783)
12. d (p. 783)
13. d (pp. 783–784)
14. d (pp. 790–791)

15. b (pp. 791–792)
16. d (pp. 791–792)
17. d (pp. 791–793)
18. b (p. 796)
19. c (pp. 796–797)
20. c (pp. 797–798)
21. d (p. 798)

22. d (pp. 800–801)
23. b (pp. 802–803)
24. c (p. 803)
25. c (pp. 802–804)

Fill-In

1. 5. (p. 768)

2. bone marrow and the lymph nodes. (p. 768)

3. ribs, vertebral column, and other flat bones. (pp. 768–769)

4. transport of oxygen between the lungs and the tissues. (p. 769)

5. 15. (p. 770)

6. 120. (p. 770)

7. protect the body from invasion by bacteria and other foreign entities. (p. 771)

8. sebumin and globulins. (p. 772)

9. the sternum and the iliac crest. (p. 774)

10. *Primary* polycythemia or polycythemia vera is a proliferative disorder in which all cells are nonresponsive to normal control mechanisms; *secondary* polycythemia is due to excessive production of erythropoietin. (pp. 790–791)

II. Critical Analysis Questions

Generating Solutions: Clinical Problem Solving

CASE STUDY: Hodgkin's Disease

Ian's Situation

1. a
2. b
3. c
4. d

(pp. 794–795)

CASE STUDY: Transfusion

Jerry's Situation

1. d
2. b
3. b
4. b

(pp. 805–807)

Chapter 33

I. Knowledge-Based Questions

Multiple-Choice

1. b (p. 816)
2. c (p. 816)
3. a (p. 817)
4. b (p. 817)
5. d (pp. 818–819)
6. b (pp. 818–819)

7. d (p. 819 [Table 32–2])
8. c (p. 819)
9. d (pp. 819–820)
10. d (p. 820)
11. a (pp. 819–821)

12. a (pp. 820–821)
13. d (p. 821)
14. b (p. 823)
15. d (pp. 823–824)
16. c (pp. 824–825)
17. d (pp. 827–828)

18. d (p. 827)
19. d (pp. 827–828)
20. b (pp. 827–828)

Matching

1. f
2. a
3. e
4. c
5. b
6. d

(p. 818 [Table 33–1])

Chapter 34

I. Knowledge-Based Questions

Multiple-Choice

1. d (p. 832)	**9.** b (pp. 832–834)	**17.** b (p. 843)
2. d (p. 832)	**10.** b (p. 835)	**18.** a (pp. 844–845)
3. d (pp. 833–834 [Table 34–1])	**11.** d (pp. 836–837)	**19.** a (p. 848)
4. b (pp. 833–834 [Table 34–1])	**12.** c (p. 837)	**20.** a (pp. 849–850)
5. a (pp. 833–834 [Table 34–1])	**13.** d (pp. 842–844)	**21.** a (pp. 851–852)
6. d (p. 832)	**14.** c (pp. 842–844)	**22.** a (pp. 852–853)
7. c (p. 832)	**15.** b (pp. 842–844)	**23.** a (pp. 852–855)
8. b (p. 832)	**16.** b (pp. 842–844)	

Matching

1. f
2. g
3. e
4. a
5. d   (pp. 833–834 [Table 34–1])
6. b
7. c
8. h

II. Critical Analysis Questions

Generating Solutions: Clinical Problem Solving

CASE STUDY: Mandibular Fracture

William's Situation

1. The latest treatment for mandibular fractures involves the placement of metal plates and screws into the bone to approximate and stabilize the bone. The lower jaw is no longer wired to the upper jaw.
2. b
3. b
4. Nasogastric suctioning is needed to remove stomach contents, thereby reducing the danger of aspiration.
5. c
6. b
7. c
8. a wire cutter

(pp. 835–836)

Chapter 35

I. Knowledge-Based Questions

Multiple-Choice

1. c (pp. 858–859 [Figure 35–1])
2. a (p. 858)
3. b (p. 858)
4. a (p. 860)
5. d (pp. 858–859)
6. d (p. 859)

7. c (pp. 860–861)
8. a (pp. 860–861)
9. c (p. 864)
10. d (p. 868)
11. d (p. 866)
12. b (pp. 866–868)

13. a (pp. 869–871)
14. b (pp. 869–871)
15. b (pp. 869–871)
16. b (pp. 874–875)
17. c (pp. 874–875)
18. d (pp. 877–879)

II. Critical Analysis Questions

Generating Solutions: Clinical Problem Solving

CASE STUDY: Cantor Tube

Martin's Situation

1. d
2. d
3. c   (pp. 858–860)
4. d
5. a

CASE STUDY: The Dumping Syndrome

Nancy's Situation

1. (a) zinc deficiency, (b) contaminated formula, (c) malnutrition, and (d) medication therapy.

2. a. Cleocin
b. digitalis
c. Inderal
d. Lincocin
e. theophylline
f. quinidine

3. a

4. d

(pp. 864–868)

Chapter 36

I. Knowledge-Based Questions

Multiple-Choice

1. b (p. 884)
2. a (pp. 885–886)
3. b (p. 886 [Table 36–1])
4. d (p. 886)
5. d (p. 887)
6. a (p. 887)
7. d (p. 887)

8. d (pp. 887–888)
9. c (pp. 888–889)
10. a (p. 893)
11. d (pp. 894–895)
12. b (pp. 894–895)
13. d (p. 893)
14. d (p. 893)

15. d (p. 895)
16. d (pp. 889–890 [Table 36–2])
17. a (p. 892 [Table 36–3])
18. d (pp. 889–890 [Table 36–2])
19. a (pp. 901–903 [NCP 36–2])
20. c (pp. 901–903 [NCP 36–2])
21. b (pp. 901–903 [NCP 36–2])

Fill-In

1. Dilute and neutralize the corrosive acid by using common antacids such as milk and aluminum hydroxide. (p. 884)

2. Patients with type A gastritis exhibit antibodies against intrinsic factor, which interferes with vitamin B_{12} absorption. (pp. 884–885)

3. Hypersecretion of acid pepsin and a weakened gastric mucosal barrier predispose to peptic ulcer development. (pp. 885–887)

4. *Helicobacter pylori* is the bacillus commonly associated with ulcer formation. (p. 884)

5. Answer may include hypersecretion of gastric juice, multiple duodenal ulcers, an increase in parietal cell mass, hypertrophied duodenal glands, and gastrinomas. (p. 887)

6. An "ulcer personality" seems to be correlated with several personality traits: the repression of strong dependency needs, the lack of opportunity to express hostility, and emotional tenseness frequently associated with occupational stress. (p. 887)

7. *Stress ulcer* refers to mucosal ulceration of the duodenal or gastric area. (p. 887)

8. The objective of the ulcer diet is to avoid oversecretion and hypermotility in the gastrointestinal tract. Extremes of temperature should be avoided, as well as overstimulation by meat extractives, coffee, alcohol, and seasonings. Current therapy recommends three normal-sized meals per day eaten at the same time each day, with no evening snack. (p. 888)

9. Hemorrhage, perforation, pyloric obstruction, and intractable ulcer. (p. 892)

10. When peptic ulcer perforation occurs, the patient experiences severe upper abdominal pain, vomiting, collapse, and an extremely tender abdomen that can be boardlike in rigidity; signs of shock will be present. (pp. 894–895)

11. Endoscopic therapy (coagulation by laser, heat probes, or drug injection such as epinephrine), intra-arterial vasopressin infusions via pump, and selective embolization. (p. 894)

12. Early symptoms of gastric cancer are a progressive loss of appetite, blood in the stools, vomiting (occasionally vomitus is coffeeground in appearance), and the appearance of or change in gastrointestinal symptoms that have been obvious for several weeks. (p. 897)

II. Critical Analysis Questions

Generating Solutions: Clinical Problem Solving

Extracting Inferences

Answer needs to include content found on pp. 885–888.

Chapter 37

I. Knowledge-Based Questions

Multiple-Choice

1. d (p. 908)
2. b (pp. 909–910)
3. c (p. 911)
4. c (p. 912)
5. a (pp. 912–913)
6. b (p. 916)
7. d (pp. 917–918)

8. d (pp. 917–918)
9. a (pp. 921–922)
10. d (pp. 921–922)
11. d (pp. 924–925)
12. d (pp. 925–926)
13. a (p. 926)
14. c (p. 928)

15. c (pp. 935–936)
16. c (p. 937)
17. d (p. 943)
18. b (pp. 946–947 [Proced 37–3])
19. c (pp. 946–947 [Proced 37–3])
20. b (pp. 946–947 [Proced 37–3])

Matching

1. a
2. b
3. c
4. b
5. d
6. b

(pp. 910, 916, 918, 920, 925–926)

II. Critical Analysis Questions

Recognizing Contradictions

1. Diarrhea refers to more than 3 bowel movements per day. (pp. 911–912)

2. Appendicitis, the most common cause of emergency abdominal surgery, occurs in about 7% of the population. (p. 915)

3. Perforation, the major complication of appendicitis occurs in 10% to 32% of cases. (p. 916)

4. The distal ileum and colon are the most common areas affected by Crohn's disease. (p. 921)

5. Change in bowel habits is the most common symptom of colon cancer. (p. 937)

Generating Solutions: Clinical Problem Solving

CASE STUDY: Appendicitis

Rory's Situation

1. c
2. c
3. d
4. d

} (pp. 915–917)

CASE STUDY: Peritonitis

Sharon's Situation

1. d
2. a
3. a
4. a

} (pp. 919–921)

Chapter 38

I. Knowledge-Based Questions

Multiple-Choice

1. b (p. 960)
2. c (p. 961)
3. d (p. 962)
4. c (p. 962)
5. b (p. 962)
6. d (pp. 964–965)
7. d (p. 970)
8. b (pp. 971–972)
9. a (pp. 976–978 [Table 38–3])

10. a (pp. 976–978 [Table 38–3])
11. b (p. 979)
12. a (pp. 979–980)
13. d (pp. 980–981)
14. d (p. 982)
15. d (pp. 982–983)
16. d (pp. 983–984)
17. d (p. 983)
18. d (pp. 985–986)

19. d (p. 986)
20. c (p. 994)
21. d (pp. 986 and 993)
22. b (pp. 992–994)
23. d (pp. 1000–1001)
24. d (pp. 1004–1005)
25. a (pp. 1004–1006)
26. c (pp. 970–971)
27. b (pp. 1008–1009)

II. Critical Analysis Questions

Generating Solutions: Clinical Problem Solving

CASE STUDY: Liver Biopsy

Veronica's Situation

1. d
2. b
3. c
4. b
5. d

} (p. 966 [Guideline 38–1 and Figure 38–4])

CASE STUDY: Laennec's Cirrhosis

Nathan's Situation

1. c (p. 983)

2. d (p. 964 [Table 38–1])

3. c (pp. 983–985; 1kg = 2.2 lb)

4. c (p. 985; normal protein intake is 0.8 to 1 g/kg)

5. c (p. 985; normal sodium intake is 3 to 6 g/24 hr without ascites; sodium restriction is minimal rather than severe)

CASE STUDY: Paracentesis

Wendy's Situation

1. c
2. d
3. a

} (pp. 973–974 [Guideline 38–2 and Figure 38–7])

CASE STUDY: Liver Transplant

Denise's Situation

1. d
2. d
3. c
4. a

} (pp. 1000–1003)

Brenda's Preoperative Situation		*Brenda's Postoperative Situation*	
1. d		**1.** a	
2. b	(pp. 1009–1011)	**2.** d	(pp. 1011–1012)
3. d		**3.** c	

Chapter 39

I. Knowledge-Based Questions

Multiple-Choice

1. c (pp. 1016–1018 [Table 39–1])
2. c (p. 1016)
3. d (pp. 1019–1020)
4. d (p. 1019)
5. a (p. 1018)
6. d (p. 1020)
7. d (p. 1018)
8. c (pp. 1017–1020 [Table 39–1])
9. d (p. 1020)
10. b (p. 1020)
11. a (pp. 1021–1022, use 15 to 20 kcal/kg of IBW for weight)

12. d (pp. 1024–1025)
13. d (pp. 1025–1026)
14. a (p. 1028 [Table 39–4])
15. c (p. 1028 [Table 39–4])
16. a (p. 1036)
17. c (pp. 1035–1036)
18. d (pp. 1037–1038)
19. d (pp. 1038–1039)
20. d (pp. 1042–1043)
21. a (p. 1043)
22. b (pp. 1043–1044)
23. d (pp. 1046–1047)

24. b (pp. 1050–1052)
25. d (p. 1051)
26. d (p. 1053)
27. c (p. 1053)
28. d (pp. 1056–1057)
29. d (p. 1056)
30. d (p. 1056)
31. d (pp. 1058–1059)
32. c (p. 1058)

Fill-In

1. II	
2. II	
3. I	
4. I	
5. I	
6.	(pp. 1016–1018 [Table 39–1])
7. I	
8. II	
9. II	
10. I	

Matching

1. c	
2. a	
3. b	(pp. 1018–1059)
4. e	
5. d	

II. Critical Analysis Questions

Generating Solutions: Clinical Problem Solving

CASE STUDY: IDDM

Albert's Situation

1. b
2. d   } (pp. 1019–1020)
3. b

CASE STUDY: Hypoglycemia

Betty's Situation

1. a
2. d
3. d   } (pp. 1043–1045)
4. d

CASE STUDY: Diabetic Ketoacidosis

Christine's Situation

1. d
2. a
3. d
4. a   } (pp. 1045–1047)
5. b
6. d

Identifying Patterns

Illustrate in diagram format the pathophysiologic sequence of changes that occur with type I diabetes. (pp. 1018–1020)

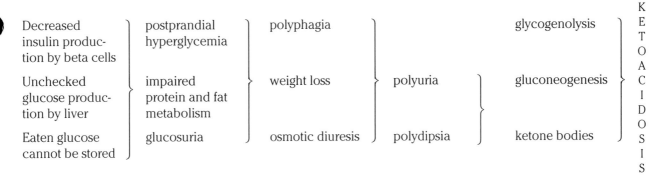

Chapter 40

I. Knowledge-Based Questions

Multiple-Choice

1. c (p. 1074)
2. d (p. 1074)
3. a (p. 1080)
4. d (p. 1080)
5. b (pp. 1083–1084)
6. b (p. 1084)
7. c (p. 1084)

8. a (pp. 1085–1086)
9. d (pp. 1085–1086)
10. d (pp. 1085–1086)
11. a (pp. 1091–1092)
12. d (pp. 1091–1092)
13. a (pp. 1093–1094)
14. d (pp. 1093–1095)

15. c (p. 1096)
16. d (pp. 1097–1098)
17. d (pp. 1098–1099)
18. a (pp. 1098–1099)
19. a (pp. 1099–1100)
20. a (pp. 1106–1107)
21. a (pp. 1106–1107)

22. d (pp. 1107–1108)
23. d (p. 1115)
24. d (pp. 1116–1117)
25. a (p. 1117)

Matching

1. h
2. g
3. i
4. d
5. a
6. c   (pp. 1069–1070 [Table 40–1])
7. f
8. e
9. j
10. b

II. Critical Analysis Questions

Generating Solutions: Clinical Problem Solving

CASE STUDY: Primary Hypothyroidism

Connie's Situation

1. d
2. d
3. b   (pp. 1076–1080 [NCP 40–1])
4. d
5. b

CASE STUDY: Subtotal Thyroidectomy

Darrell's Situation

1. d
2. d
3. d
4. a   (pp. 1090–1091)
5. b
6. a

Chapter 41

Knowledge-Based Questions

Multiple-Choice

1. b (pp. 1127–1129)
2. b (pp. 1127–1129)
3. c (pp. 1127–1129)
4. a (pp. 1130)
5. d (pp. 1129–1131)

6. b (pp. 1130–1131)
7. c (pp. 1130–1132)
8. a (p. 1132 [Chart 41–1])
9. d (p. 1133)
10. a (p. 1134)

11. a (p. 1135)
12. d (pp. 1135–1136)
13. d (p. 1136)
14. d (pp. 1137–1138)

Fill-In

1. nephron. (p. 1126)

2. 500 mOsm/L and 800 mOsm/L. (p. 1129)

3. creatine clearance. (pp. 1130–1131)

4. the antidiuretic hormone (ADH). (p. 1130)

5. the loss of the ability of the kidney to concentrate and dilute urine. (p. 1130)

II. Critical Analysis Questions

Identifying Patterns

Draw the sequence of pathophysiologic events that is triggered when the blood pressure decreases and the hormone renin is released from the cells in the kidneys.

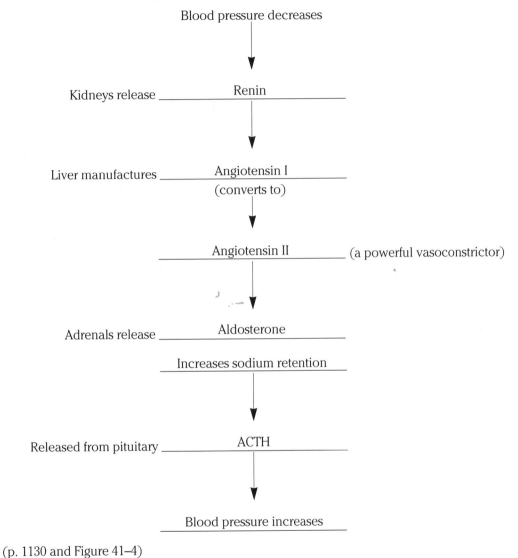

(p. 1130 and Figure 41–4)

Chapter 42

I. Knowledge-Based Questions

Multiple-Choice

1. d (p. 1146)
2. c (p. 1147)
3. c (p. 1147)
4. d (p. 1149 [Chart 42–2])
5. c (pp. 1149–1150)
6. d (p. 1153)
7. b (p. 1153)
8. b (p. 1153)

9. d (p. 1155)
10. d (p. 1157)
11. b (pp. 1161–1162)
12. d (p. 1164)
13. b (pp. 1161–1164 [1 liter = 1 kg = 2.2 lbs])
14. b (p. 1168)
15. d (1168–1169)

Matching

1. a
2. b
3. c
4. e
5. d
6. j
7. h
8. f
9. g
10. i

(p. 1146 [Chart 42–1])

Fill-In

1. a. to determine the amount of residual urine in the bladder.
   b. to bypass an obstruction that blocks urine flow.
   c. to provide postoperative drainage following bladder surgery.
   d. to monitor hourly urinary output in critically ill patients. (p. 1145)

2. *Escherichia coli, Klebsiella, Proteus, Pseudomonas, Enterobacteriaceae, Serratia,* and *Candida.* (p. 1147)

3. Signs and symptoms seen in catheter-induced urinary tract infections may include cloudy urine, hematuria, fever, chills, anorexia, and malaise. (p. 1147)

4. Sudafed. (p. 1150)

5. Arteriosclerotic cardiovascular disease is the leading cause of death. (pp. 1157–1158)

6. hypotension, air embolism, chest pain, pruritus, dialysis disequilibrium, muscle cramping, nausea, and vomiting. (pp. 1157–1158)

7. Peritonitis is the most common and most serious complication of CAPD. (p. 1165)

8. Abdominal distention and paralytic ileus are common complications of renal surgery. (pp. 1168–1169)

II. Critical Analysis Questions

Recognizing Contradictions

1. Almost <u>50%</u> of patients with a closed drainage system will experience bacteriuria within a 2-week period. (pp. 1146–1147)

2. About <u>10 million</u> adults in the United States suffer from urinary incontinence. (p. 1151)

3. <u>Greater than 50%</u> of nursing home residents suffer from urinary incontinence. (p. 1151)

4. Hemodialysis <u>does not cure or reverse</u> renal disease; it prevents death. (pp. 1155–1157)

5. CAPD is done on an <u>ongoing, 24-hour schedule</u>, usually in the patient's home. (pp. 1161–1164)

Generating Solutions: Clinical Problem Solving

CASE STUDY: CAPD

Edward's Situation

1. d
2. a
3. a } (pp. 1161–1167)
4. d
5. c

Chapter 43

I. Knowledge-Based Questions

Multiple-Choice

1. a (p. 1180)
2. d (p. 1180)
3. b (pp. 1181–1182)
4. d (pp. 1183–1184)
5. d (p. 1185)
6. d (p. 1187)
7. c (pp. 1187–1188)
8. d (pp. 1188–1189)
9. b (p. 1188)
10. b (pp. 1188–1189)

11. a (pp. 1189–1190)
12. c (pp. 1190–1191)
13. c (pp. 1192–1193)
14. d (pp. 1192–1193)
15. a (pp. 1192–1193)
16. b (pp. 1193–1195)
17. c (pp. 1196–1197)
18. d (p. 1197)
19. a (pp. 1197–1198)
20. d (p. 1204)

21. d (pp. 1204–1206)
22. d (p. 1207)
23. a (pp. 1208–1209)
24. d (pp. 1209–1210 [Chart 43–5])
25. b (p. 1215)
26. c (pp. 1216–1217)
27. a (p. 1216)
28. d (p. 1217 [Figure 43–7])

Fill-In

1. *Escherichia coli* (80% frequency). (pp. 1180–1181)

2. Cystitis is usually associated with feelings of urgency, burning, and pain on urination, frequent urination, and sometimes urination accompanied by spasms in the region of the bladder. (p. 1183)

3. *fever*, flank pain, costrovertebral angle tenderness, leukocystosis, bacteria, and white blood cells in the urine. (p. 1187)

4. The urine in the early stages of acute glomerulonephritis is characteristically *cola-colored.* (pp. 1188–1189)

5. proteinuria
hypoalbuminemia
edema
hypercholesterolemia $\left.\begin{array}{l} \\ \\ \\ \end{array}\right\}$ (pp. 1190–1191)

6. Five conditions that reduce blood flow to the kidneys and impair kidney function are hypovolemia, hypotension, reduced cardiac output and congestive heart failure, obstruction of the kidney or lower urinary tract, and bilateral obstruction of the renal arteries or veins. (pp. 1192–1193)

7. Clinical manifestations seen in chronic renal failure include fatigue and lethargy, headache, weakness, gastrointestinal symptoms, bleeding tendencies, and mental confusion. There are also decreased salivary flow, thirst, a metallic taste in the mouth, loss of smell and taste, and parotitis or stomatitis. (pp. 1196–1197)

8. Threatened graft rejection is suspected in a patient who evidences oliguria, edema, fever, apprehension, increased blood pressure, weight gain, or tenderness over the graft. (pp. 1205–1206)

9. Urinary tract stones are formed by calcium oxalate, calcium phosphate, and uric acid. (pp. 1206–1207)

10. wound infection, wound dehiscence, urinary leakage, ureteral obstruction, hyperchloremic acidosis, small-bowel obstruction, and stomal gangrene. (p. 1219)

II. Critical Analysis Questions

Generating Solutions: Clinical Problem Solving

CASE STUDY: Acute Renal Failure

Fran's Situation

1. c
2. d
3. b
4. b
5. c
6. b $\left.\begin{array}{l} \\ \\ \\ \\ \\ \end{array}\right\}$ (pp. 1192–1196)

Chapter 44

I. Knowledge-Based Questions

Multiple-Choice

1. a (p. 1236)
2. a (pp. 1240–1242 [Table 44–1])
3. c (p. 1240)
4. a (p. 1240)
5. c (pp. 1244–1245)

6. b (pp. 1245–1246)
7. a (pp. 1246–1247)
8. c (pp. 1248–1249)
9. c (pp. 1251–1252)
10. a (pp. 1251–1252 [Chart 44–2])

11. b (pp. 1255–1256)
12. c (p. 1257)
13. d (pp. 1260–1261)
14. b (pp. 1262–1264)
15. c (pp. 1262–1264)

Fill-In

1. irregular or excessive vaginal bleeding, abnormal discharge, bleeding after menopause, painful intercourse (dyspareninia), bleeding after intercourse, urinary disturbances, and painful menstruation. (p. 1236)

2. endometrial biopsy. (p. 1241)

3. Answer may include headache, fatigue, low back pain, engorged or painful breasts, abdominal fullness, mood swings, general irritability, fear of loss of control, binge eating, crying spells. (p. 1246)

4. 49 to 52, with a median age of 51.3 years. (p. 1251)

5. The pill blocks the stimulation of the ovary by preventing the release of follicle-stimulating hormone (FSH) from the anterior pituitary. (pp. 1253–1254)

6. Risk factors would include a history of thromboembolic disorders, uterine fibroids, neuro-ocular disturbances, liver or gallbladder disease, smoking over age 35, and scanty or irregular menses. (pp. 1253–1255)

7. Depo-Provera, a long-acting progestin that is injected IM, effectively inhibits ovulation for 3 months. (p. 1256)

8. Vaginal rings; RU-486 (mifepristone)   (pp. 1256–1258)

9. A highly hygroscopic seaweed tent is placed into the cervix; it swells to four to five times its original size and dilates the cervix. (pp. 1259–1260)

10. ovarian, tubal, cervical, or uterine. (pp. 1260–1262)

11. For *in vitro fertilization,* at an appropriate time, the egg is recovered by transvaginal ultrasound retrieval. Sperm and egg are coincubated for up to 36 hours so that fertilization can occur. Forty-eight to 80 hours after retrieval the embryo is transferred to the uterine cavity by means of a trancervical catheter. Implantation should occur in 2 to 3 days. (p. 1262)

II. Critical Analysis Questions

Recognizing Contradictions

1. Nurses conducting a health assessment need to know that more than 20% of women are incest survivors. (pp. 1236–1237)

2. Women born to mothers who took DES during their pregnancy have a higher than average chance of developing cancer of the cervix. (p. 1239)

3. A biopsy excision of an inverted cone of tissue is done when a Pap smear is "suspicious." The patient must be anesthetized for this procedure. (p. 1240)

4. Magnetic resonance imaging uses a magnetized field to produce an image. Radiation is not necessary. (p. 1244)

5. Progesterone is the most important hormone for preparing the endometrium for the fertilized ovum. (p. 1245)

6. Painful cramps result from an excessive production of prostaglandins. (p. 1246)

7. More than 3 million yearly pregnancies in the United States are unintended and one-third of these occur in teenagers. (p. 1252)

8. An aborted fetus usually weighs less than 1000 g and is considered viable after 6 months. (pp. 1258–1260)

9. Potency is not altered after a bilateral vasectomy. (p. 1254 [Chart 44–3])

10. The pregnancy rate after treatment for an ectopic pregnancy is enhanced. (pp. 1260–1261)

Chapter 45

I. Knowledge-Based Questions

Multiple-Choice

1. d (p. 1270 [Table 45–1])
2. d (pp. 1270–1272 [Table 45–1])
3. d (pp. 1273–1274)
4. c (pp. 1275–1277)
5. a (pp. 1277–1278)
6. a (pp. 1281–1283)
7. b (pp. 1286–1287)
8. c (pp. 1286–1287)

9. d (pp. 1285–1286)
10. d (pp. 1286–1287)
11. c (pp. 1286–1287)
12. d (pp. 1286–1287)
13. b (p. 1287 [Table 45–2])
14. b (p. 1288)
15. d (pp. 1288–1289)
16. c (pp. 1288–1289)

17. d (p. 1291)
18. d (p. 1291)
19. d (pp. 1292–1293)
20. c (p. 1294)
21. c (p. 1294 [Table 45–4])
22. b (pp. 1295–1296)
23. d (pp. 1295–1297)

Scramblegram

1. vulvodynia (p. 1270)
2. Micostatin (pp. 1271–1272)
3. Flagyl (p. 1272)
4. acyclovir (p. 1275)
5. septic shock (pp. 1275–1277)
6. cystocele (p. 1281)

7. Pap smear (p. 1287)
8. Hysterectomy (p. 1289)
9. menorrhagia (p. 1270)
10. fibroids (p. 1284)
11. DES (p. 1286)
12. HRT (p. 1289)

13. Kegal (pp. 1282–1283)
14. fistula (p. 1280)
15. prolapse (pp. 1281–1283)
16. dermoid (pp. 1294–1295)

	E			^{16}D	^{4}A	C	Y	C	L	O	V^1	I	R
	L			E		M^2				U			
	E			R		Y		L			^{15}P		
	C	^{7}P	A	M			C	V	Y		^{9}M	R	
	O	A	L	O			O		G		E	O	
	T	P	U	I		D	S		A		N	L	
Y	S	S	T	D	Y	L	T		L		O	A	
M	Y	M	S	N			A		F^3		R	P	
O	^{6}C	E	I				T	G			R	S	
T		A	^{14}F			^{10}F	I		E		H	E	
C		R				I	N			K^{13}	A		
E						B					G		
R						R			^{11}D		I		
E						O			E		A		
T		^{5}S	E	P	T	I	C	S	^{12}H	O	C	K	
S						D			R				
Y						S			T				
^{8}H													

II. Critical Analysis Questions

Generating Solutions: Clinical Problem Solving

CASE STUDY: Vaginal Discharge

Maryanne's Situation

1. a
2. b
3. c   (pp. 1270–1272 [Table 45–1])
4. a
5. a

CASE STUDY: Toxic Shock Syndrome

Irene's Situation

1. c
2. a
3. b   (pp. 1275–1277)
4. d
5. c

CASE STUDY: Intracavitary Irradiation

Jill's Situation

1. c
2. a   (pp. 1296–1297)
3. d

Chapter 46

I. Knowledge-Based Questions

Multiple-Choice

1. b (pp. 1303–1305)
2. b (pp. 1303–1305)
3. b (pp. 1305–1307)
4. a (pp. 1305–1307)
5. c (pp. 1305–1307)
6. b (p. 1310)
7. d (pp. 1309–1310)

8. a (p. 1310)
9. d (p. 1310)
10. c (p. 1310)
11. d (p. 1310)
12. c (p. 1311)
13. d (p. 1311)
14. b (p. 1311)

15. b (p. 1313)
16. b (p. 1313)
17. b (p. 1313)
18. b (p. 1315)
19. d (pp. 1314–1315)
20. d (pp. 1318–1319)
21. c (pp. 1321–1325)

22. a (pp. 1321–1325)
23. d (p. 1324)
24. a (p. 1325)
25. c (pp. 1329–1331)

II. Critical Analysis Questions

Generating Solutions: Clinical Problem Solving

CASE STUDY: Simple Mastectomy

Louise's Preoperative Situation

1. c
2. d   (pp. 1320–1321)
3. b
4. c

Louise's Postoperative Situation

1. b
2. c   (pp. 1321–1325)
3. a

Identifying Patterns

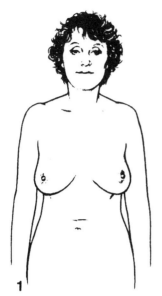

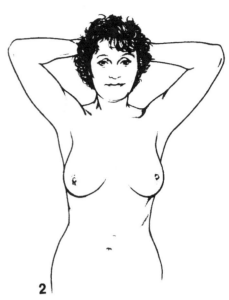

Figure 1: Stand before a mirror. Check both breasts for anything unusual. Look for a discharge from the nipples, puckering, dimpling, or scaling of the skin.

Figure 2: Watching closely in the mirror, clasp your hands behind your head and press your hands forward.

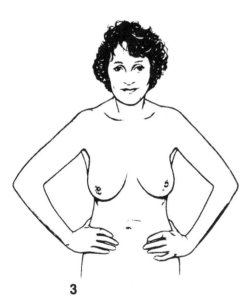

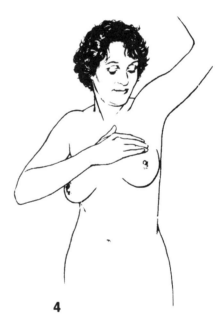

Figure 3: Press your hands firmly on your hips and bow slightly toward the mirror as you pull your shoulders and elbows forward.

Figure 4: Raise your left arm. Use three or four fingers of your right hand to feel your left breast firmly, carefully, and thoroughly. Beginning at the outer edge, press the flat part of your fingers in small circles moving the circles slowly around the breast. Gradually work toward the nipple. Be sure to cover the whole breast. Pay special attention to the area between the breast and the underarm, including the underarm area itself. Feel for any unusual lump or mass under the skin.

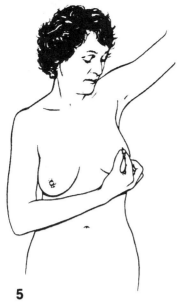

5

Figure 5: Gently squeeze the nipple and look for a discharge. (If you have any discharge during the month—whether or not it is BSE—see your doctor.) Repeat the examination on your right breast.

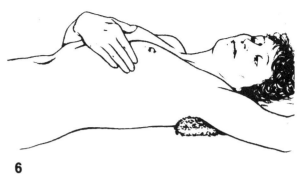

6

Figure 6: Steps 4 and 5 should be repeated lying down. Lie flat on your back, with your left arm over your head and a pillow or folded towel under your left shoulder. This position flattens the breast and makes it easier to check it. Use the same circular motion described above. Repeat on your right breast. (pp. 1306–1307; [Chart 46–2])

Chapter 47

I. Knowledge-Based Questions

Multiple-Choice

1. d (p. 1341)
2. b (pp. 1340–1341)
3. d (pp. 1341–1342)
4. a (p. 1342)
5. c (p. 1346)
6. b (pp. 1344–1345)

7. a (pp. 1346–1347)
8. d (pp. 1345–1347)
9. b (p. 1347)
10. a (p. 1347)
11. d (p. 1347)
12. c (pp. 1347–1348)

13. a (pp. 1354–1356)
14. c (pp. 1354–1356)
15. b (p. 1356)
16. a (p. 1356)
17. c (p. 1357)

Fill-In

1. PSA and DRE. (p. 1337)

2. burning, urgency, perineal discomfort, frequency, and pain with or after ejaculation. (pp. 1340–1341)

3. frequency of urination, nocturia, urgency and a sensation that the bladder has not emptied completely, abdominal straining, and a decrease in the volume and force of the urinary stream. (p. 1341)

4. Heparin is given prophylactically because there is a high incidence of deep vein thrombosis and pulmonary embolism postprostatectomy. (pp. 1345–1346)

5. diethylstilbestrol. (p. 1348)

6. Epididymitis is an infection of the epididymis that usually descends from an infected prostate or urinary tract. It passes upward through the urethra and ejaculatory duct and along the vans deferens to the epididymis. (p. 1349)

7. Priapism is an uncontrolled, persistent erection of the penis that causes the penis to become large, hard, and often painful. (p. 1357)

Chapter 48

I. Knowledge-Based Questions

Multiple-Choice

1. d (p. 1366)   **5.** b (p. 1369)   **9.** b (pp. 1372–1373)
2. d (p. 1367)   **6.** d (p. 1369)   **10.** d (p. 1374 [Table 48–2])
3. c (p. 1368)   **7.** a (p. 1369 [Chart 48–1])   **11.** c (p. 1374)
4. b (p. 1369)   **8.** c (pp. 1371–1372)   **12.** d (pp. 1373–1374)

Fill-In

1. Disorders arise from excesses or deficiencies of immunocompetent cells, alterations in cellular functioning, immunologic attack on self-antigens, and inappropriate or exaggerated responses to specific antigens. (p. 1366)

2. *Natural immunity,* which is nonspecific, is present at birth. *Acquired immunity* is more specific and develops throughout life. *Passive acquired immunity* is a temporary immunity transmitted from another source that has developed immunity through previous disease or immunization. (pp. 1366–1368)

3. Complement is a term used to describe circulating plasma proteins that are made in the liver and activated when an antibody couples with an antigen. (pp. 1373–1374)

4. Biologic response modifiers (BMRs) suppress antibody production and cellular immunity. (p. 1374)

5. Trace elements include: copper, iron, manganese, selenium, and zinc. (pp. 1376–1378)

Matching

1. c
2. e
3. c
4. d   (pp. 1371–1372)
5. a
6. b
7. a

Chapter 49

I. Knowledge-Based Questions

Multiple-Choice

1. d (pp. 1382–1384)   **5.** d (p. 1384)   **9.** b (pp. 1386–1387)
2. d (p. 1382)   **6.** c (p. 1384)   **10.** d (pp. 1386–1387)
3. d (pp. 1382–1385)   **7.** a (p. 1385)
4. b (p. 1382)   **8.** b (p. 1386)

II. Critical Analysis Questions

Identifying Patterns

1. phagocytic dysfunction. (p. 1382)
2. B-cell deficiency, probably CVID. (pp. 1382–1385)
3. T-cell deficiency. (pp. 1384–1385)
4. ataxia-telangiectasia. (p. 1384)
5. a secondary immunodeficiency. (p. 1385)

Chapter 50

I. Knowledge-Based Questions

Multiple-Choice

1. b (p. 1390)
2. c (pp. 1390–1391)
3. b (pp. 1390–1391)
4. d (pp. 1390–1391)
5. d (p. 1391)
6. d (pp. 1392–1393)
7. c (pp. 1393–1394)
8. b (p. 1394)
9. a (p. 1395)
10. d (pp. 1396–1397)
11. a (pp. 1396–1397)
12. c (p. 1400)
13. b (pp. 1400–1401)

Recognizing Contradictions

1. The HIV virus carries its genetic material in RNA. (p. 1390)

2. There is a substantial increase in AIDS in the heterosexual population on the East Coast. (pp. 1390–1391)

3. Greater than 10% of those with AIDS are age 50 or older. (p. 1395)

4. Trimethoprim–sulfamethoxazole (TMP/SMZ) is the drug of choice for *Pneumocystis carinii* pneumonia. (pp. 1398–1399)

5. The most effective chemotherapy regimen is a combination of doxorubicin (Adriamycin), bleomycin, and vincristine. (p. 1401)

Generating Solutions: Clinical Problem Solving

CASE STUDY: AIDS

Brenden's Situation

1. risky sexual practices and intravenous drug use.
2. c
3. c
4. answer may include opportunistic infections, impaired breathing or respiratory failure, wasting syndrome, fluid and electrolyte imbalance, and untoward reaction to medications.
5. d
6. d

(pp. 1403–1409)

Chapter 51

I. Knowledge-Based Questions

Multiple-Choice

1. d (p. 1422)
2. d (p. 1423)
3. a (p. 1424)
4. b (p. 1427)
5. d (pp. 1430–1431)

6. d (p. 1427)
7. d (p. 1431)
8. a (pp. 1432–1433)
9. b (p. 1433)
10. d (pp. 1433–1435)

11. d (p. 1431)
12. b (p. 1431)
13. c (p. 1440)
14. c (p. 1431; a minimum of 0.1 mg/kg is recommended)

II. Critical Analysis Questions

Generating Solutions: Clinical Problem Solving

CASE STUDY: Allergic Rhinitis

Chris' Situation

1. Potential ineffective breathing patterns, related to an allergic reaction; knowledge deficit about allergy and recommended modifications in lifestyle; and impaired adjustment, related to chronicity of condition and need for environmental modifications.

2. Restorations of a normal breathing pattern, knowledge about the causes and control of allergic symptoms, adjustment to alternations and modifications, and absence of complications.

3. d
4. d
5. d   (pp. 1432–1438)
6. c

Chapter 52

I. Knowledge-Based Questions

Multiple-Choice

1. d (p. 1446)
2. d (pp. 1445–1448 [Chart 52–2])
3. b (p. 1445)
4. d (pp. 1450–1451 [Table 52–1])
5. c (pp. 1452–1453 [Table 52–3])
6. b (pp. 1452–1453 [Table 52–3])
7. d (p. 1445 [Figure 52–1])

8. a (pp. 1445–1446)
9. d (pp. 1445–1446)
10. c (pp. 1460–1461)
11. a (pp. 1461–1462)
12. a (p. 1461)
13. d (pp. 1461–1462 [Figure 52–3])

14. d (p. 1463)
15. b (p. 1462)
16. b (pp. 1464–1465)
17. d (pp. 1464–1466)
18. b (p. 1466)
19. b (pp. 1466–1467)
20. a (p. 1467)

II. Critical Analysis Questions

Generating Solutions: Clinical Problem Solving

CASE STUDY: Rheumatoid Arthritis

Jane's Situation

1. b
2. b
3. fever, anemia, fatigue, and Raynaud's phenomenon
4. HLA-DR4
5. d
6. c
7. d

(pp. 1460–1461 [Tables 52–1 and 52–3])

Chapter 53

I. Knowledge-Based Questions

Multiple-Choice

1. b (pp. 1481–1482)
2. a (pp. 1481–1482)
3. b (p. 1482)

4. a (pp. 1483–1485 [Table 53–2])
5. b (pp. 1483–1485 [Table 53–2])
6. c (pp. 1486–1488 [Chart 53–2])

II. Critical Analysis Questions

Analyzing Comparisons

1. skin coloring (pp. 1478–1479)
2. jaundice (p. 1479)
3. scurvy (p. 1482)

4. inspection (pp. 1483–1484)
5. scales (p. 1486 [Chart 53–2])

Identifying Patterns

1. telangiectasis
2. syphilis
3. ecchymosis or petechia
4. urticaria
5. Kaposi's sarcoma

(p. 1480 [Table 53–1])

Chapter 54

I. Knowledge-Based Questions

Multiple-Choice

1. c (pp. 1494–1495)
2. c (pp. 1494–1495)
3. d (p. 1495)
4. d (p. 1495)
5. b (pp. 1494–1495 [Table 54–1])
6. c (p. 1496 [Table 54–2])
7. b (p. 1503)
8. d (pp. 1507–1508)
9. b (p. 1510)
10. d (p. 1511)
11. a (pp. 1511–1512)
12. d (p. 1513)
13. d (p. 1513)
14. c (pp. 1513–1514)
15. c (p. 1516)
16. a (pp. 1516–1517)
17. d (pp. 1520–1521)
18. d (pp. 1524–1526)
19. b (p. 1527)
20. a (pp. 1527–1528)
21. c (pp. 1529–1530)
22. d (pp. 1529–1530)
23. d (p. 1534)
24. c (pp. 1534–1535)
25. d (pp. 1535–1537)

II. Critical Analysis Questions

Generating Solutions: Clinical Problem Solving

CASE STUDY: Malignant Melanoma

Steve's Situation

1. b
2. d
3. c   (pp. 1529–1534 [Table 54–4])
4. c
5. a

Chapter 55

I. Knowledge-Based Questions

Multiple-Choice

1. d (p. 1546)
2. c (p. 1548)
3. c (p. 1548)
4. b (p. 1549)
5. b (pp. 1548–1549)
6. b (pp. 1549–1550 [Table 55–1])
7. a (p. 1549)
8. c (pp. 1550–1551)
9. a (pp. 1550–1551)
10. a (p. 1552)
11. a (p. 1551)
12. a (pp. 1553–1555 [Table 55–3])
13. a (pp. 1553–1555 [Table 55–3])
14. d (p. 1555 [Chart 55–2])
15. b (pp. 1554–1555 [Chart 55–2])
16. b (p. 1555)
17. c (pp. 1556–1557)
18. b (pp. 1558 and 1563 [Table 55–4])
19. d (pp. 1558 and 1563)
20. b (pp. 1549–1550 [Table 55–1])
21. c (pp. 1564–1565)
22. c (pp. 1564–1565)
23. b (pp. 1565–1566)
24. c (pp. 1567–1568)
25. b (p. 1569)
26. d (protein requirement should be 3 g/kg; p. 1569)
27. b (p. 1572)

II. Critical Analysis Questions

Recognizing Contradictions

1. Survival chances are greatest for children <u>over age 5</u> and young adults <u>age 40 and younger</u>. (p. 1546)

2. Localized responses <u>do not exceed 20%</u> of their body surface area. (p. 1546)

3. About <u>33%</u> of all burn injuries greater than 25% of body surface area are associated with a pulmonary injury. (pp. 1548–1549)

4. During the acute phase of burn care, <u>diuresis occurs</u>, fluid resuscitation has been completed, and the wound nears closure. (pp. 1551–1552 [Table 55–2])

5. Fluid replacement with colloids and crystalloids usually takes <u>48 hours</u> to restore normal plasma levels. (pp. 1553–1555 [Chart 55–2])

Generating Solutions: Clinical Problem Solving

Nursing Care Plans

See Chapter 55 and Nursing Care Plans 55–1 and 55–2 in the textbook for assistance with the completion of the assignment. **Sample:**

Aimee's Situation

Nursing diagnosis:	Altered comfort, related to pain resulting from a burn injury
Immediate goal:	Pain relief
Intermediate goal:	Continue developmental growth patterns while providing for skin healing and grafting
Long-term goal:	Maintain socialization patterns consistent with Aimee's peer group
Nursing interventions:	Assess Aimee's respiratory status
Expected outcomes:	Aimee has a patent airway and does not exhibit any respiratory distress

Chapter 56

I. Knowledge-Based Questions

Multiple-Choice

1. d (p. 1596)
2. c (pp. 1635–1636 [Table 56–2])
3. d (pp. 1635–1636 [Table 56–2])
4. b (pp. 1605–1606 [Table 56–1])
5. c (pp. 1602–1603)
6. a (p. 1607)
7. c (p. 1608)
8. c (p. 1615 [Chart 56–3])
9. d (p. 1603)
10. d (pp. 1619–1620)
11. c (pp. 1619–1620)
12. b (pp. 1622–1623)
13. d (p. 1625)
14. c (p. 1627)
15. d (pp. 1624–1627)
16. d (p. 1629)
17. c (pp. 1629–1630)
18. d (pp. 1632–1634)
19. d (pp. 1638–1639)

Matching

1. b
2. c
3. f
4. j
5. a
6. e
7. g
8. d
9. h
10. i

} (pp. 1588–1590 and Chart 56–1)

Crossword Puzzle (reference pages throughout chapter)

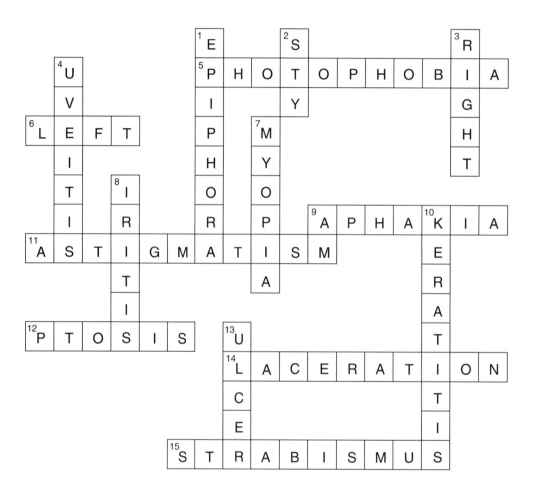

II. Critical Analysis Questions

Identifying Patterns

1. blepharitis (pp. 1605–1606)
2. sty (external hordeolum). (pp. 1606–1607)
3. conjunctivitis. (p. 1608)
4. keratitis. (pp. 1609–1610)
5. cataract. (pp. 1612–1613)

Generating Solutions: Clinical Problem Solving

Nursing Care Plan: Cataract Surgery

Elise would have several immediate, intermediate, and long-term goals. Following is an example of one with a nursing diagnosis. Page references for assistance with the completion of this care plan are Chapter 2 and Chapter 56, pages 1616–1619 (Nursing Care Plan 56–1). **Sample:**

Nursing diagnosis:	Altered visual sensory perception related to cataract formation.
Immediate goal:	Make Elise familiar with her new environment.
Intermediate goal:	Prepare the affected eye for surgery.
Long-term goal:	Encourage Elise to walk with her cane as independently as possible.
Nursing intervention:	Assess Elise's level of knowledge about her surgery.
Expected outcomes:	Elise understands the purpose, process, and expected outcomes of her surgery.

Chapter 57

I. Knowledge-Based Questions

Multiple-Choice

1. a (p. 1644)
2. a (p. 1644)
3. a (p. 1647)
4. b (p. 1647)
5. d (p. 1648)
6. d (p. 1649)
7. d (pp. 1647–1648)
8. b (p. 1651)
9. c (p. 1656)
10. d (p. 1655)
11. b (pp. 1655–1657)
12. a (p. 1657 [Table 57–2])
13. c (p. 1656 [Table 57–2])
14. d (p. 1656)
15. d (pp. 1655–1656)
16. c (pp. 1658–1660)
17. b (p. 1663)

II. Critical Analysis Questions

Generating Solutions: Clinical Problem Solving

CASE STUDY: Mastoid Surgery

Amber's Situation

1. Answer may include infection, otalgia, otorrhea, hearing loss, vertigo, erythema, edema, and odor of discharge.

2. Answer may include reduction of anxiety, freedom from discomfort, prevention of infection, stabilization/improvement of learning, absence of injury or vertigo, absence of or adjustment to altered sensory perception, return of skin integrity, and knowledge about the disease process and surgical intervention.

3. a sense of aural fullness or pressure.

4. b

5. an elevated temperature and purulent drainage.

6. d

7. c

8. bending at the waist and moving or lifting heavy objects. (pp. 1658–1660 and Table 57–3)

Chapter 58

I. Knowledge-Based Questions

Multiple-Choice

1. a (p. 1676)	**7.** c (p. 1679)	**13.** c (pp. 1686–1687)
2. a (p. 1676)	**8.** b (pp. 1681–1682)	**14.** d (p. 1698)
3. c (p. 1676)	**9.** a (p. 1685)	**15.** b (pp. 1699–1700)
4. a (p. 1676)	**10.** d (p. 1686)	**16.** c (pp. 1700–1702 [G 58–1])
5. a (pp. 1677–1678)	**11.** b (pp. 1686–1687)	
6. d (p. 1678)	**12.** a (p. 1687)	

II. Critical Analysis Questions

Generating Solutions: Clinical Problem Solving

Nervous System Effects

Column I	*Parasympathetic Effect*	*Sympathetic Effect*
a. bronchi	constriction	dilation
b. cerebral vessels	dilation	constriction
c. coronary vessels	constriction	dilation
d. heart	inhibition	acceleration
e. iris	constriction	dilation
f. salivary glands	secretion	secretion
g. smooth muscle of		
(1) bladder wall	constriction	inhibition
(2) large intestine	increased motility	inhibition
(3) small intestine	increased motility	inhibition

See textbook pages 1687–1688 for assistance in completing this chart.

Cranial Nerves

Nerve no.	Column I	Column II
1	olfactory	smell
2	optic	vision
3	oculomotor	eye movement
4	trochlear	eye movement
5	trigeminal	facial sensation
6	abducens	eye movement
7	facial	taste and expression
8	acoustic	vestibuolcochlear
10	vagus	swallowing, gastric motility, and secretion
11	spinal accessory	trapezius and sternomastoid muscles
12	hypoglossal	tongue movement

Use textbook page 1692, Table 58–2 as a reference.

Chapter 59

I. Knowledge-Based Questions

Multiple-Choice

1. d (pp. 1706–1709)
2. d (pp. 1709–1710)
3. c (pp. 1709–1711)
4. b (pp. 1709–1712)
5. d (p. 1711)
6. a (p. 1713)

7. a (pp. 1714–1715)
8. c (p. 1715)
9. d (pp. 1718–1719)
10. c (p. 1725)
11. d (pp. 1725–1726)
12. d (pp. 1725–1726 [Chart 59–2])

13. c (pp. 1735–1736)
14. b (pp. 1735–1736)
15. c (pp. 1737–1739)
16. d (pp. 1745–1747)

Matching

1. a and f
2. c and e
3. b
4. a
5. c

(pp. 1706–1709)

II. Critical Analysis Questions

Generating Solutions: Clinical Problem Solving

Nursing Care Plan: Unconscious Patient

Use Chart 59–1 and pages 1718–1724 as a guide for a plan of care for Miss Potter.

Nursing Care Plan: CVA

See textbook pages 1725–1735 for development of Mrs. Coe's care plan.

Chapter 60

I. Knowledge-Based Questions

Multiple-Choice

1. b (p. 1754)
2. c (p. 1755)
3. d (pp. 1755–1757)
4. a (p. 1758)
5. a (pp. 1761–1762)
6. d (pp. 1761–1762)
7. d (p. 1763)
8. b (pp. 1771–1772)

9. a (pp. 1772–1773)
10. d (pp. 1775–1776)
11. c (pp. 1778–1779)
12. a (p. 1781)
13. b (pp. 1782–1783 [G 60–1])
14. b (p. 1784 [Chart 60–4])
15. d (p. 1788)
16. d (p. 1791)

17. a (p. 1796)
18. b (p. 1796)
19. b (p. 1799 [Chart 60–8])
20. b (pp. 1800–1801)
21. c (pp. 1813–1815)
22. b (pp. 1815–1816)
23. c (pp. 1818–1819)

II. Critical Analysis Questions

Generating Solutions: Clinical Problem Solving

CASE STUDY: Multiple Sclerosis

Toni's Situation

1. d
2. d
3. a
4. d

(pp. 1767–1771)

CASE STUDY: Parkinson's Disease

Charles' Situation

1. d
2. c
3. d
4. b

(pp. 1771–1775)

Nursing Care Plan: Huntington's Disease

See Chapter 60, pages 1775–1777 [Chart 60–3] in the textbook for assistance with the development of a nursing care plan for Mike.

Nursing Care Plan: Cervical Spine Injury

See Chapter 60, pages 1776–1805 in the textbook for assistance with the development of a nursing care plan for Katie.

Nursing Care Plan: Paraplegia

See Chapter 60, pages 1805–1809 in the textbook for assistance with the development of a nursing care plan for Matthew.

Chapter 61

I. Knowledge-Based Questions

Multiple-Choice

1. b (p. 1832)
2. a (p. 1832)
3. a (p. 1833)
4. c (p. 1834)
5. a (p. 1836)

6. a (p. 1837)
7. d (p. 1837)
8. b (pp. 1837–1838)
9. b (p. 1838)
10. b (p. 1841)

Matching

1. h
2. i
3. b
4. j
5. g
6. e
7. d
8. c
9. a
10. f

} (pp. 1837–1838)

Fill-In

1. General functions of the musculoskeletal system include protection, support, locomotion, mineral storage, hematopoiesis, and heat production. (p. 1832)

2. 99. (p. 1832)

3. 206. (p. 1832)

4. sternum
   ileum
   vertebrae
   ribs

} (pp. 1833–1834)

5. Vitamin D increases calcium in the blood by promoting calcium absorption from the gastrointestinal tract and by accelerating the mobilization of calcium from the bone. (p. 1834)

6. parathyroid hormone and calcitonin. (p. 1834)

Scramblegram

1. periosteum. (p. 1833)
2. ligaments. (p. 1836)
3. sarcomere. (p. 1837)
4. tendons. (pp. 1836–1837)
5. osteoporosis. (p. 1838)
6. scoliosis. (p. 1839)

Chapter 62

I. Knowledge-Based Questions

Multiple-Choice

1. b (p. 1846)
2. d (p. 1847)
3. b (p. 1849 [Figure 62–2])
4. c (p. 1849 [Table 62–2])
5. d (p. 1849 [G 62–2])
6. b (p. 1854)
7. d (p. 1855)
8. b (p. 1855)
9. c (pp. 1855–1856 [G 62–3])

10. d (pp. 1858–1859)
11. b (pp. 1860–1861)
12. b (p. 1860)
13. b (p. 1862)
14. c (pp. 1861–1863)
15. c (p. 1863)
16. d (pp. 1864–1865)
17. d (pp. 1865–1866)
18. c (p. 1866)

19. a (p. 1866)
20. b (p. 1868)
21. d (p. 1869)
22. a (pp. 1869–1870)
23. a (p. 1869)
24. a (p. 1870)
25. a (p. 1870)

Fill-In

1. • reduce a fracture
   • correct a deformity
   • apply uniform pressure to underlying soft tissue
   • provide support and stability for weakness joints (p. 1848)

2. anhydrous calcium sulfate gypsum crystals. (p. 1848)

3. Circulatory impairment can be noted by assessing toes or fingers, which should be pink, warm, and easily moved (wiggled). The blanch test may be carried out to determine capillary refill. (p. 1852)

4. Danger signs of possible circulatory constriction include unrelieved pain, swelling, discoloration, tingling, numbness, inability to move fingers or toes, or any temperature changes. (p. 1852)

5. to minimize muscle spasms, to reduce, align, and immobilize fractures; to lessen deformities; and to increase space between opposing surfaces within a joint. (p. 1857)

6. • Buck's extension traction
   • pelvic traction   (p. 1857)

7. pulmonary embolism (p. 1866)

8. leg shortening, abnormal rotation, malalignment, inability to move the leg, and increased localized discomfort. (pp. 1869–1870)

II. Critical Analysis Questions

Generating Solutions: Clinical Problem Solving

CASE STUDY: Buck's Traction

1. a

2. the patient's body weight and the bed position adjustments.

3. Inspect the skin for abrasions and circulatory disturbances and make certain the skin is clean and dry before any tape or foam boot is applied.   (pp. 1860–1861)

4. 3 kg.

5. skin color, skin temperature, capillary refill, edema, pulses, sensations, and ability to move.

6. a positive Homans' sign indicates deep vein thrombosis.

(pp. 1860–1861)

Chapter 63

I. Knowledge-Based Questions

Multiple-Choice

1. c (p. 1880)
2. b (p. 1880)
3. b (p. 1881)
4. a (pp. 1881–1882 [Figure 63–1])
5. c (pp. 1882–1883 [Figures 63–2 and 63–3])
6. a (pp. 1882–1884)
7. d (p. 1894)

8. b (pp. 1896–1897)
9. d (pp. 1896–1897)
10. b (pp. 1897–1898)
11. d (pp. 1897–1899)
12. c (pp. 1899–1900)
13. b (p. 1900)
14. a (pp. 1900–1901)

II. Critical Analysis Questions

Generating Solutions: Clinical Problem Solving

CASE STUDY: Osteoporosis

Emily's Situation

1. The rate of bone resorption is greater than the rate of bone formation.

2. Women have a lower peak bone mass than men, and estrogen loss affects the development of the disorder.

3. c
4. a
5. c
6. d

(pp. 1891–1894)

Chapter 64

I. Knowledge-Based Questions

Multiple-Choice

1. d (p. 1908)
2. b (p. 1908)
3. a (p. 1909)
4. b (pp. 1909–1910)
5. d (p. 1912)
6. d (p. 1914 [Table 64–1])
7. a (p. 1916)

8. b (p. 1917)
9. d (p. 1917)
10. b (pp. 1919–1920)
11. a (pp. 1920–1921)
12. d (pp. 1923–1925)
13. b (pp. 1923–1925)
14. a (p. 1925)

15. b (p. 1925)
16. d (pp. 1925–1928)
17. a (pp. 1928–1935)
18. c (pp. 1936–1937)
19. d (pp. 1936–1937)
20. d (pp. 1939–1941)

Matching

II. Critical Analysis Questions

Generating Solutions: Clinical Problem Solving

CASE STUDY: Above-the-Knee Amputation

William's Situation

1. d
2. d
3. d
4. d
5. a
6. d
7. b
8. d

(pp. 1936–1944)

Chapter 65

I. Knowledge-Based Questions

Multiple-Choice

II. Critical Analysis Questions

Recognizing Contradictions

1. The purpose of OSHA, by law, is the <u>protection of health care workers</u> from hazards recognized in particular industries. (p. 1960)

2. The underlying premise of Universal Precautions is that barrier precautions are to be used <u>routinely for all patients</u>. (pp. 1960–1961)

3. Used needles should <u>never be recapped</u>. (p. 1960)

4. Gohorrhea and syphilis <u>are different diseases caused by different microorganisms</u>. They attack the body in different ways but are spread in the same manner. A person may have gonorrhea, syphilis, and other sexually transmitted diseases at the same time. (pp. 1968–1970 [Table 65–3])

5. <u>Hepatitis A</u> is the virus almost always transmitted by the fecal–oral route. (pp. 1976–1977)

6. Eighty percent of the cases of Rocky Mountain spotted fever occur in the <u>south Atlantic and south central United States</u>. (p. 1983)

7. There are currently <u>28 vaccines</u> licensed in the United States, the most recent being the vaccine for chickenpox in 1995. (pp. 1983–1984)

8. Rubeola is another name for <u>measles</u>. (pp. 1984–1985)

Chapter 66

I. Knowledge-Based Questions

Multiple-Choice

1. c (p. 2000)
2. b (pp. 2001–2002 [G 66–1])
3. b (pp. 2003–2005 [G 66–3])
4. d (p. 2005)
5. c (p. 2009)

6. b (pp. 2010–2012)
7. a (pp. 2012–2013)
8. c (pp. 2012–2013)
9. d (pp. 2015–2016)
10. d (pp. 2014–2016)

11. c (pp. 2016–2018)
12. d (p. 2018)
13. d (pp. 2019–2020)
14. a (pp. 2037–2038)

II. Critical Analysis Questions

Generating Solutions: Clinical Problem Solving

1. See textbook pages 2003–2005 for assistance with nursing actions to clear an obstructed airway.

2. See textbook pages 2014–2015 for assistance with nursing care for a patient who has experienced blunt, abdominal trauma.

3. See textbook pages 2020–2021 for assistance with emergency measures to manage an anaphylactic reaction.

4. See textbook pages 2021–2025 (Figure 66–5 and G 66–7) to develop nursing measures to assist with gastric lavage.

5. See textbook pages 2027–2031 (Table 66–1) for assistance with nursing actions necessary for drug abuse reactions.

6. See textbook pages 2036–2037 for assistance with nursing actions necessary for the management of psychiatric patients.

blood dM .
colon   (+15)

20